The World of Worm: Physician, Professor, Antiquarian, and Collector, 1588–1654

This monograph offers the first comprehensive treatment of the multi-faceted scholarly interests of Ole Worm, professor of medicine at the University of Copenhagen. Scholarship about Worm has focused mainly on Worm's collecting and the creation of his cabinet of curiosity, the Museum Wormianum, resulting in Worm's rationale for his research being largely overlooked. Worm shared his many interests with a number of other physicians of the age, but in terms of breadth, few matched the variety of his concerns. For a man who considered himself first and foremost a physician and anatomist, his interests in Paracelsianism and collecting can at times be baffling, while his interests in antiquarianism, runes, and chronology strike the modern reader as at odds with his medical and natural philosophical interests. It is important to comprehend that Worm's multi-faceted interests in the created world were underpinned by his Lutheran, Melanchthonian natural philosophy, and this served to unify all Worm's scholarly undertakings, inquiries, and experiments in the single aim of reaching a better understanding of God's creation, the Book of Nature.

Ole Peter Grell is Emeritus Professor of Early Modern History at the Open University, UK.

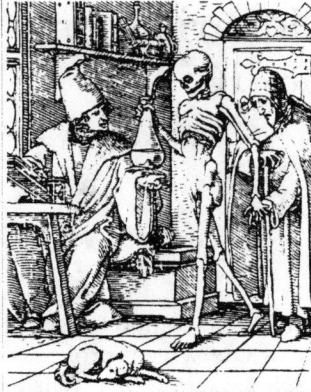

The History of Medicine in Context

Series Editors: Andrew Cunningham (Department of History and Philosophy of Science, University of Cambridge) and Ole Peter Grell (Department of History, Open University)

Titles in the series include

Authority, Gender, and Midwifery in Early Modern Italy
Contested Deliveries
Jennifer F. Kosmin

Forty Days
Quarantine and the Traveller, c. 1700 – c. 1900
John Booker

The World of Worm: Physician, Professor, Antiquarian, and Collector, 1588–1654
Ole Peter Grell

'I Follow Aristotle': How William Harvey Discovered the Circulation of the Blood
Andrew Cunningham

For more information about this series, please visit: https://www.routledge.com/The-History-of-Medicine-in-Context/book-series/HMC

The World of Worm:
Physician, Professor, Antiquarian, and Collector, 1588–1654

Ole Peter Grell

Routledge
Taylor & Francis Group

LONDON AND NEW YORK

Cover credit: The Worm family painting 1648; photo by Lennart Larsen, courtesy of the Danish National Museum.

First published 2022
by Routledge
4 Park Square, Milton Park, Abingdon, Oxon OX14 4RN

and by Routledge
605 Third Avenue, New York, NY 10158

Routledge is an imprint of the Taylor & Francis Group, an informa business

British Library Cataloguing-in-Publication Data
A catalogue record for this book is available from the British Library

Library of Congress Cataloging-in-Publication Data
Names: Grell, Ole Peter, author.
Title: The world of worm: physician, professor, antiquarian, and collector, 1588-1654 / Ole Peter Grell.
Description: Milton Park, Abingdon, Oxon ; New York, NY : Routledge, 2022. |
Series: The history of medicine in context | Includes bibliographical references and index. |
Identifiers: LCCN 2022002651 (print) | LCCN 2022002652 (ebook) | ISBN 9781032270104 (hardback) | ISBN 9781032270111 (paperback) | ISBN 9781003290940 (ebook)
Subjects: LCSH: Worm, Ole, 1588-1654. | Worm, Ole, 1588–1654—Influence. | Physicians—Denmark—Biography. | Anatomists—Denmark—Biography.
Classification: LCC R542.W67 G74 2022 (print) | LCC R542.W67 (ebook) | DDC 610.92 [B]—dc23/eng/20220209
LC record available at https://lccn.loc.gov/2022002651
LC ebook record available at https://lccn.loc.gov/2022002652

ISBN: 978-1-032-27010-4 (hbk)
ISBN: 978-1-032-27011-1 (pbk)
ISBN: 978-1-003-29094-0 (ebk)

DOI: 10.4324/9781003290940

Typeset in Sabon
by codeMantra

For Maximilian and Oliver

Contents

Figures

Acknowledgements

My interest in Ole Worm and the world of learning he inhabited goes back a fair number of years and has resulted in several articles. Nearly thirty years ago a Danish friend, Erland U. Jessen, arrived in Cambridge with H. D. Schepelern's three-volume edition of Ole Worm's correspondence, which served to get me started on this line of research while forming the foundation for this book. Ole Worm's productivity and the survival of so much of his correspondence, manuscripts, and publications offer an extraordinary insight into the republic of letters in the first half of the seventeenth century and of how knowledge was acquired and certified. However, the richness of the sources and Worm's many intellectual contacts which have proved so interesting and valuable for this book also served to delay it while new avenues of investigation had to be pursued. Over the years many hours have been spent in the manuscript and rare book departments of the Royal Library in Copenhagen, which were made pleasant by its ever helpful staff. In 2019 I was able to spend considerable time in Copenhagen as a visiting professor at the Department of Church History at the University of Copenhagen. This also provided me with a further opportunity to discuss my interest in Ole Worm and his circle with a number of Scandinavian colleagues, expanding the contacts which had been made at a workshop in 2013 on medicine, natural philosophy, and religion in post-reformation Scandinavia which I co-organised with Dr Carsten Selch Jensen at the University of Copenhagen with support from the Wellcome Trust. In 2015 I benefited from spending the autumn in New York as a visiting professor at the Centre for Society and Science, at Columbia University, where I had the opportunity to discuss my interests with its Director, Professor Pamela H. Smith, and several of her colleagues at the Centre.

While the Covid-19 pandemic and lockdowns restricted further visits to archives and libraries, forcing me to rely on electronic resources, it also served to enhance my productivity, resulting in far fewer interruptions and competing demands while writing. However, my offer to my offspring and their girlfriends, sheltering here during lockdowns, to read them extracts of my work after dinner was gently rebuffed, even if the odd snippet was appreciated. Secondary works which were not available online were, in many cases, forwarded to me in either electronic or printed form by colleagues, and I am particularly grateful to Dr Karen Skovgaard Petersen for sending me her book *Historiography at the Court of Christian IV* and to Dr Håkan Håkansson at the University of Lund for sending me his book on Johannes Bureus.

As always I have benefitted from the interest and encouragement of my colleagues in the History Department of The Open University. A number of friends and fellow historians have read and commented on individual sections of the book, but in particular I should like to thank my friend and collaborator Dr Andrew Cunningham, for reading yet another of my manuscripts and providing helpful suggestions for improvement of the text. Likewise, I should like to thank Dr Morten Fink-Jensen at the University of Copenhagen for reading the whole manuscript and offering many valuable comments. The responsibility of the final product remains, of course, mine.

Introduction

Few scholars in Northern Europe equalled Ole Worm in the gathering and dissemination of knowledge during the first half of the seventeenth century. Like many, if not most of them, Worm had been trained as a physician, but his interests were diverse, stretching from natural philosophy, medicine, botany, natural history, iatrochemistry, astrology, to antiquarianism, and collecting. His pursuits were encyclopaedic, even if his main focus was on the natural world, something the Lutheran Worm shared with a number of other scholars of this period, as religiously diverse as the Calvinist Johann Henrich Alsted and the Jesuit Athanasius Kircher. Even so, Ole Worm's research interests and engagement with the natural world – the Book of Nature – can only be understood if his roots in a Melanchthonian natural philosophy and Lutheran theology are fully taken into account. Worm's modes of acquiring knowledge were typical for the age: he depended on books, correspondence, travel, face-to-face discussions, collecting unusual objects, and finally empiricism, observation, experiment, and description, all of them closely interrelated and interdependent.

Ole Worm's grandparents had fled the Netherlands for religious reasons after the Dutch Revolt in 1567 and subsequently settled in the town of Aarhus in Denmark. Born in 1588 as the grandchild to these immigrants Ole Worm belonged to what had become a wealthy merchant family towards the end of the sixteenth century.[1] Having attended the Cathedral School in Aarhus Ole Worm was barely thirteen years old when he set out on what in effect became a twelve-year peregrinatio academica. Even in an age characterised by the Grand Tour and growing academic travel Worm's peregrinatio proved of exceptional duration, offering him the chance to spend extended periods at some of the most significant urban and academic centres. Thus, Worm set out on the first of his educational journeys in 1601. He spent the next four years at 'gymnasia' (grammar schools) – the first year in Lüneburg and the following three years in Emmerich where he lodged with members of his Dutch family. In 1605 he briefly returned to the family

---

1 E. Hovesen, *Lægen Ole Worm*, Aarhus 1987, 30–44, and *Dansk Biografisk Leksikon*, 3rd ed., 16 vols., Copenhagen 1979–84, henceforth *DBL*.

DOI: 10.4324/9781003290940-1

home in Aarhus before setting out for the then Lutheran University of Marburg where he intended to study theology. However, shortly after Worm's arrival, the university turned Reformed, having come under the authority of the Calvinist Duke Moritz of Hesse-Kassel. Worm joined his Lutheran teachers and moved to Giessen where he continued his theological studies.

In 1607 Worm left Giessen for Strasbourg in order to continue his studies at the Lutheran Academy there. Here he abandoned theology for medicine and took up residence with one of his teachers, Dr Johann Rudolf Salzmann, a keen anatomist and botanist. In August 1608 on his way to Basle to further his medical studies, Worm received a letter from Salzmann informing him that the 'medical exercises had temporarily been halted' in Strasbourg, but that Salzmann intended to dissect a calf in order to keep his skills honed, and that he hoped to obtain a corpse for dissection the following winter. If we can trust Worm's autobiography, it was Salzmann's experimental and practical approach to medicine that encouraged him to further his anatomical and botanical studies at the University of Basle under the tutelage of the famous professors Felix Platter, Caspar Bauhin, and Jacob Zwinger. When in Basle, Worm did not limit his medical studies to the university curriculum, but actively participated in Bauhin's private botanical classes and anatomical dissections, as well as Zwinger's practical bedside teaching.

After a little over a year in Basle, Worm continued his training in Padua, where he matriculated in October 1608.

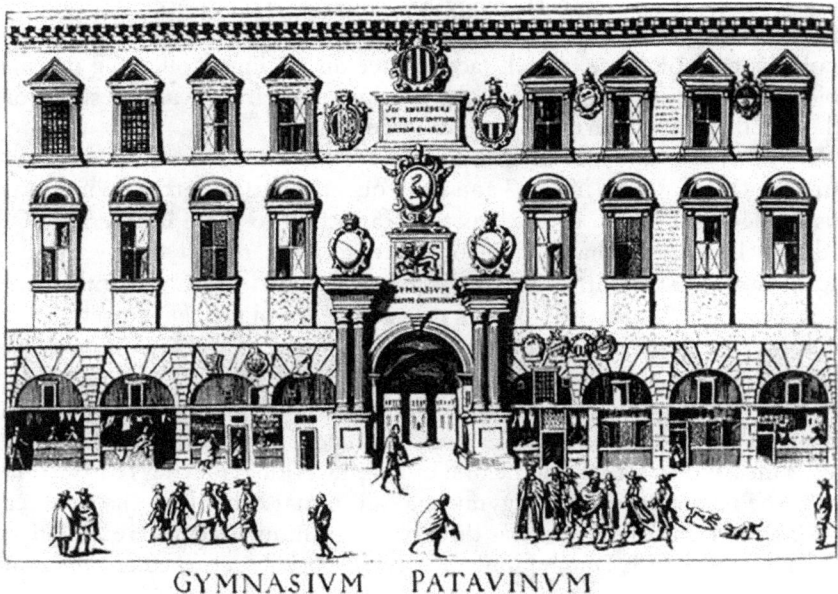

GYMNASIVM   PATAVINVM

Figure 0.1 Palazzo Bo, University of Padua ca. 1600; courtesy of Andrew Cunningham.

During his eighteen-month stay, Worm studied anatomy under Fabricius Aquapendente, and he claimed that his knowledge of surgery was much improved by the teaching of Julius Casserius Placentinus. He also found time to regularly treat and visit patients during the last six months of his stay in Padua. In recognition of his qualities Worm was elected Consiliarius for the German nation at the University of Padua. Considering Worm's interests in botany, it is noteworthy that he did not refer to the botanical garden in Padua created in 1545.

Before leaving for France, Worm spent the summer of 1609 touring Italy as far as Naples in the company of, among others, Heinrich Petraeus, later professor of medicine at the University of Marburg, who, like Worm, was interested in iatrochemistry and sought to find a way of uniting Galenism with Paracelsianism. Ole Worm wished to go to France in order to study iatrochemistry, which by the spring of 1609 had become a primary interest for him, as he informed his Basle teacher Jacob Zwinger, who would have approved. Worm specifically asked for letters of introduction to the famous Parisian Paracelsians Joseph du Chesne and Theodore de Mayerne. Travelling by boat from Genoa to Marseilles Worm quickly reached Montpellier. Here he spent the next six months delighted with the excellence of the local professors of medicine and the way medicine was taught at the university, befriending the two professors of medicine Jean Varandal and Jacques d'Esterre Signeur de Pradilles, and the well-known botanist Pierre Richter de Belleval. In fact his stay in Montpellier left such a positive impression on Worm that he repeatedly recommended his students to go there twenty years later. However, when Worm finally arrived in Paris in early March 1610, Joseph du Chesne had died and the Huguenot Theodore de Mayerne had left France for England. Instead, Worm managed to befriend the anatomist Jean Riolan (the Younger) and the philologist Issac Casaubon while also practising medicine in the French capital. Worm's stay in Paris came to a sudden end when King Henry IV was assassinated on 14 May 1610 and many foreigners left France concerned about their safety. Worm left Paris for the United Provinces, spending the next few weeks at the University of Leiden.

By June 1610 Ole Worm was back in Denmark, visiting the nobleman Holger Rosenkrantz, the Learned, who became a close friend and patron. In September that year Worm matriculated at the University of Copenhagen, and he also found time to practise medicine, so successfully, according to his autobiography, that people begged him to stay. This, however, proved a brief stay of not much more than four months. Worm's interests in Paracelsianism and iatrochemistry remained fervent, and by early 1611 he was already on his way back to the University of Marburg. This time it was the Paracelsian physician, Johannes Hartmann, who occupied the first European professorship in chemistry, who drew Worm to Marburg. On his way there Worm stopped in Hamburg to visit the famous iatrochemist Konrad Khunrath. According to his autobiography Worm spent his time in Marburg on iatrochemical studies and experiments under Hartmann's supervision. However, Worm found Hartmann's teaching expensive, not least because the Marburg professor was reluctant to part with any important alchemical information unless he had been well paid.

Worm probably long intended to obtain his MD from the University of Basle, as he wrote to his mentor Caspar Bauhin in October 1611. This was the university where Worm had studied longest and the contacts between the medical faculties of Basle and Copenhagen remained close. Furthermore, for years most of the professors of medicine at the University of Copenhagen had obtained their MDs from Basle. Although Worm stated in his autobiography that he had contemplated obtaining his MD from the University of Marburg, this was probably more a statement of appreciation rather than intent. Despite the plague that caused the University of Marburg to close over the summer of 1611, Worm might easily have returned from nearby Kassel in the autumn if he had wanted to obtain his MD there. In Kassel Worm was staying with his old friend, the alchemist physician, Arnold Gillenius, who had become court physician to Duke Moritz of Hesse-Kassel. Gillenius was heavily involved in the duke's alchemical laboratory and Worm's stay offered him an opportunity to become personally involved in alchemical experiments, getting his hands dirty, something he constantly encouraged his students to do after having become professor at the University of Copenhagen. Meanwhile, Worm made sure that his promoters within the medical faculty in Basle occupied the positions where they might best further his interests before he defended his doctoral dissertation, *Selecta Controversiarum Medicarum Centuria*, in December 1611.

The hundred medical controversies were briefly covered by Worm in ten pages. Significantly Worm accepted Paracelcus's division of illnesses in four groups in the first controversy he discussed in his dissertation. He was clearly inspired by Paracelsus without being fully converted to Paracelsianism. More importantly in his preface Worm referred to Julius Cæsar Scaliger, 'the most shrewd philosopher and physician', who claimed,

> That nothing is more disgraceful than to enslave our intellect, the dictator and ruler of all things, to the pleasure of others. Who can therefore, I ask, blame me that I have not sworn allegiance to one teacher in this my investigation of selected controversies about the most substantial sufferings of the human body? On the contrary I have attached myself to everyone to the same extent as I have found they have attached themselves to truth. Because truth alone is the unstained virgin whom everyone with sound judgement properly has to woo as opposed to all others. Since it is the manifold practical knowledge that is needed by the physician, rather than plentiful words, I have in this dissertation

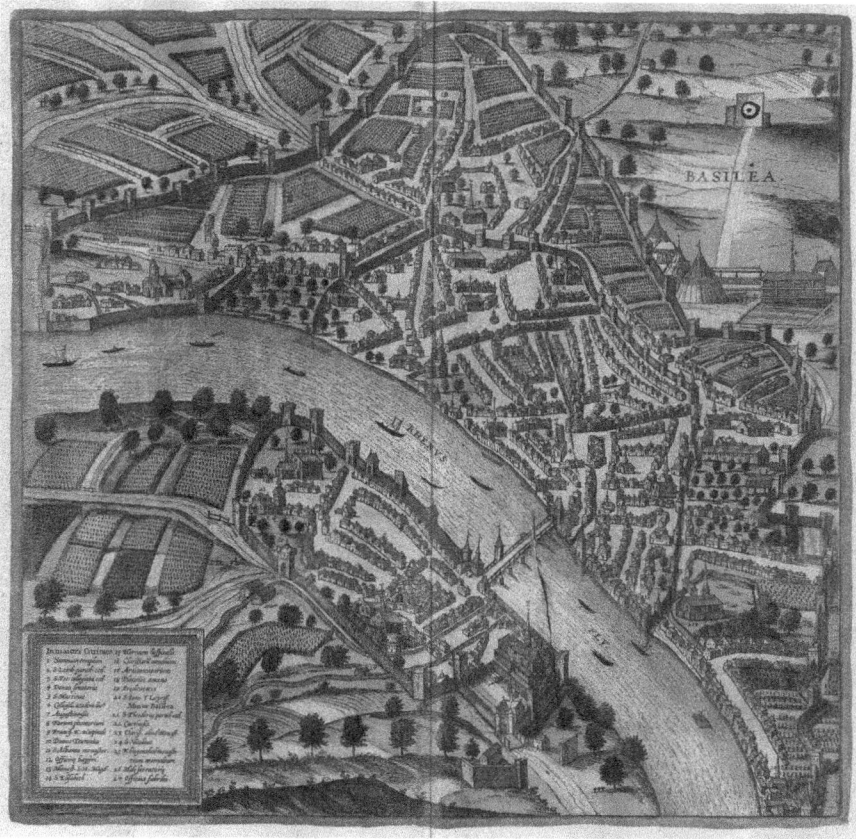

Figure 0.2 Map of Basle ca. 1600, Braun/Hogenberg; courtesy of the Royal Danish Library.

in particular attached importance to making it richer in facts rather than words, all chosen and different and especially aimed at practice. I therefore present it to those who are initiated into Asklepios's secrets for honest assessment on the scales of rational considerations.[2]

Ole Worm, in other words, was neither a Galenist nor a Paracelsian. Instead he was open to any school of thought which could be tested, observed, and

2 H. D. Schepelern, *Museum Wormianum. Dets Forudsætninger og Tilblivelse*, Copenhagen 1971, 80. For Ole Worm's *Selecta Controversiarum Medicarum Centuria*, see Hovesen, *Worm*, 64–116.

validated through medical practice. This was a position he reiterated again and again over the years and never deviated from.

Having obtained his MD, Worm travelled down the Rhine from Basle to Amsterdam with the intent of crossing over to London, where he arrived in February 1612. Within three months he had become personal physician to Robert Rich, the later Earl of Warwick. This evidently provided Ole Worm with an opportunity to befriend the Huguenot Paracelsian, Theodore de Mayerne, then physician to James I of England, whom he had been unable to meet when in Paris. While in London Worm was asked by his friend, the physician Christen Lauritsen Bording, whether another Huguenot, Paracelsian physician Felix Rotmund, still practised medicine and remained in London with Theodore de Mayerne. If so Bording wanted Worm to greet them both.[3] After a year and a half in London Ole Worm returned to Denmark for good in July 1613 on the encouragement of family and friends.[4]

At the time of his appointment to his first professorship in pedagogy at the University of Copenhagen in September 1613, Ole Worm had sampled the best medical education available at the leading universities in Europe. He had been educated by some of the most prominent medical figures of the age, often having participated in their private colloquia and classes. Through his varied experiences Worm had developed a hands-on, observationally based experimental approach to natural philosophy and medicine, happily mixing a Galenic/Hippocratic approach with aspects of Paracelsianism, a sound scepticism with an open-minded inquisitiveness. Worm had also practised medicine in several of the larger European cities, mastering several languages, while simultaneously finding time to benefit from the company of some of the leading intellectual figures of the age. By the time he returned to Copenhagen, he had established a comprehensive network of friends and contacts across Europe that would prove particularly important for a man who was to spend the rest of his life practicing medicine and serving as a professor at the University of Copenhagen. Without it, Worm's entry into the international republic of letters would have been virtually impossible, as would his attempts to keep abreast of the discoveries and challenges to established knowledge in the early seventeenth century. However, from the outset, the driving force behind Worm's thirst for knowledge

---

3 H. D. Schepelern (ed.), *Breve fra og til Ole Worm*, 3 vols., Copenhagen 1965–68, nos. 13 and 1040; for Felix Rotmund, see H. Trevor-Roper, *Europe's Physician. The Various Life of Sir Theodore de Mayerne*, New Haven 2006, 61–62.

4 Ole Worm's autobiography was printed in an abbreviated form in Thomas Bartholin, *Cista Medica Hafniensis*, Copenhagen 1662, 579–82; cited and supplemented with information from Worm's two *album amicorum*, in Schepelern, Museum, 42–97. See also O. P. Grell, 'In Search of True Knowledge: Ole Worm (1588–1654) and the New Philosophy', 215–17 in P. H. Smith and B. Schmidt (eds.), *Making Knowledge in Early Modern Europe. Practices, Objects, and Texts, 1400–1800*, Chicago 2007.

was rooted in his hope of obtaining true and comprehensive knowledge and understanding of the natural world as created by God.

The view that Nature had been created by God as a source for his plan for Man and the world was forcefully expressed by the professor of theology Cort Aslaksen, whom Ole Worm considered the leading light at the University of Copenhagen. Aslaksen was a Melanchthonian if not a cryto-Calvinist in his theology and had served as an assistant to Tycho Brahe on the island of Hven. In his *De Mundo Disputatio Prima*, 1605, he stated that God had created the Natural world as a mirror through which Man could see the wisdom and power of God. Nature had been created in order that Man could reach a better understanding of God by studying it carefully.[5]

For a relative outsider to the university establishment in Copenhagen such as Ole Worm a good marriage which linked him with influential families was of paramount importance. Worm demonstrated his awareness of this when in November 1615 he married Dorothea Fincke, third daughter of the leading professor of medicine Thomas Fincke, who was one of the most powerful men within the University of Copenhagen. Not only did this make him Thomas Fincke's son-in-law, but it also made him brother-in-law of the other professor of medicine Caspar Bartholin, the prominent Copenhagen physician Jørgen Fuiren, and the later professor of theology Hans Rasmussen Brochmand. Dorothea died thirteen years later from the plague. Worm only remained a widower for two years; if nothing else, he needed a mother for his four young girls. This time he married Susanne, the daughter of the Bishop of Lund, Mads Jensen Medelfar. Worm is likely to have made the acquaintance of Mads Jensen Medelfar while the latter served as court preacher to Christian IV before he was promoted to the bishopric of Lund in 1620. Like his first marriage an alliance with a leading ecclesiastical family made good sense. Unfortunately Worm's marriage to Susanne lasted only seven years. She died in 1637 during the next plague epidemic. Once again Ole Worm found himself a widower with young children and once again he quickly married. A year and a half later he married his third and last wife in February 1639. This time he allied himself with one of the wealthier merchant families in Copenhagen when he married Magdalene Motzfeldt, daughter of Peter Motzfeldt.[6]

However, this book is not a biography of Ole Worm and his personal life is only of secondary importance. It will only be referred to in so far as it had an effect on his scholarly interests. Worm was a dedicated and conscientious scholar whose life centred on four main concerns, all of which were rooted in his natural philosophical outlook. First among them came his role as a physician. Worm always thought of himself as first and foremost

---

5 See M. Fink-Jensen, *Fornuften under troens lydighed. Naturfilosofi, medicin og teologi i Damark 1536–1636*, Copenhagen 2004, 203 and J. R. Christianson, *On Tycho's Island. Tycho Brahe and His Assistants, 1570–1601*, Cambridge, 252–53.

6 See Hovesen, *Ole Worm*, 266–71.

a physician and, on all his publications he added his academic title of MD to his name. Throughout his life he never stopped working as a physician caring for his patients.

Accordingly Chapter 1 of this book is concerned with his work as a physician. Like a number of medical men Ole Worm began practising medicine before he was awarded his MD. Before his return to Denmark and appointment to his first professorship in the Faculty of Philosophy at the University of Copenhagen Worm had practised medicine in several European cities. Only a few years after his appointment to the professorship at the university he had developed a flourishing medical practice in Copenhagen where his services were much in demand, especially among his academic colleagues and the leading burghers of the city. Gradually, however, Worm also became the physician of choice to a number of influential noble families. Thus, his medical practice continued to grow and become more lucrative.

By 1630 his reputation was such that he was increasingly consulted in medical matters by the royal household. Initially his assistance was sought by more peripheral members of the royal family, but gradually his advice and treatment was needed by the Elected-Prince Christian and eventually by the king himself.

Worm, who became professor of medicine in 1624, was a strong advocate of learned medicine and a promoter of medical regulation under the auspices of the country's leading physicians. Within the community of physicians Worm was highly valued and his advice was often sought. Worm treated his medical colleagues with respect and when in a position of authority tried to look after their interests as best as he could.

An important and somewhat unusual aspect of Ole Worm's medical practice was the number of consultations by letter he undertook. This was brought about by his many contacts and friends from Iceland and the Faroe Isles. These islands situated far from Denmark were without both physicians and apothecaries. Most of Worm's patients had also been his students at the university prior to their return. Worm provided diagnoses and medical remedies for these patients; aware of the problems posed by the lengthy sea-journey needed, and the harsh weather conditions, his remedies had to be able to withstand to remain useful at arrival.

As a physician Ole Worm adhered in the main to the Galenic humoral system. Patients' lifestyles and diets were significant for Worm as were bloodletting and other evacuations of bodily fluids. However, Worm also relied on other sources of inspiration and believed in Hippocratic ideas about the sources of disease to be found within as well as without the human body. He drew on Paracelsian alchemical ideas and developed his own chemical remedies. Similarly he held a strong belief in astrological medicine and paid great attention to when a medical intervention could best be made. It is in that context his concern for his own health and the belief in the grand climacterium should be seen.

In terms of importance Ole Worm's position as professor at the University of Copenhagen came a close second to his role as a physician. This is the subject of Chapter 2. For more than forty-one years Worm served the university in this capacity. The first eleven years were spent in a variety of professorships in the Faculty of Philosophy before he was awarded a chair in medicine in 1624. He was a dedicated member of both faculties, hard-working, and trusted by his colleagues. He was repeatedly elected as dean and vice chancellor. Initially his career progressed well until May 1616 when he was prevented from becoming dean to the Faculty of Philosophy, formally because he had never obtained an MA. Whatever the reason the issue was resolved a couple of years later and Worm was awarded the deanship. In this connection the backing of his in-laws from the Faculty of Medicine, Thomas Fincke and Caspar Bartholin, proved important.

Ole Worm took the opportunity in 1619 in his inaugural address as dean to warn that year's graduates against Rosicrucianism. Bearing in mind that Worm had been fascinated by this movement since 1611, even if, at times, expressing his doubts about it, his warning was surprising. That he should have decided to publicly label the movement a dangerous sect and distance himself from it by spring 1619 tells us that Worm was alert to the changing religious climate in Denmark where a less tolerant and uniform Lutheranism was being promoted by the country's leading theologian Hans Poulsen Resen. This may also explain why Worm had been invited to give a memorial lecture on 31 October 1618 as part of the centenary celebrations for the Reformation by his brother-in-law, Caspar Bartholin, who served as the university's vice chancellor in 1618–19. Evidently Ole Worm's friends and relations wanted him to enhance his orthodox Lutheran credentials to make him less of a potential target for Hans Poulsen Resen and his associates.

Even if Worm felt the need to clear himself of any suspicions of religious heterodoxy in 1619 he maintained an interest in Rosicrucianism. His doubts about the Rosicrucians did not affect his considerable interest in Paracelsianism and iatrochemistry. These interests were very much in evidence in his inaugural address when he was promoted to the professorship in natural philosophy in April 1621 and reflected in his natural philosophical interests. Even so Worm retained a guarded and critical attitude to Paracelsianism while remaining rooted in a Melanchthonian natural philosophical tradition.

Worm tirelessly promoted the value and importance of anatomy for medicine. Bearing that in mind it is surprising that he never undertook dissections of humans in Copenhagen during his tenure as professor of medicine. That he restricted himself to animals may well have had something to do with the fact that no anatomical theatre was available in Copenhagen before 1644. Worm's extensive interests in anatomy found expression in his fascination with Aselli's discovery of the lacteals and Harvey's circulation of the blood, which he repeatedly tried to observe, demonstrate, and describe during the 1630s and 1640s. For Worm this hands-on, experimental approach was essential and characterised his interests in iatrochemistry and Paracelsianism.

Ole Worm was a conscientious teacher delivering his lectures and disputations regularly. He continued his role as a teacher for those of his students who undertook their peregrinatio academica, supporting and advising them by letter and introducing them to his contacts abroad. He persistently reminded them of the importance of anatomy and iatrochemistry for the physician to be, and he never missed an opportunity to remind them of the importance of practical experience and observation. They were told of the great benefit from lodging with local practitioners, be they surgeons, physician, or apothecaries, in order to get as much hands-on experience as possible. While his students served as his eyes and ears abroad, notifying him of new undertakings in medicine, Ole Worm was available with support, both abroad and at home.

As opposed to his role as a physician and a professor, which both helped finance and underpin his existence, Worm's antiquarian research was primarily driven by interest. More than anything else it was Worm's antiquarian publications which established his international reputation, and it is this antiquarianism which is the focus of Chapter 3. Worm started to take a serious interest in antiquarian matters around 1622. His research into the runes and ancient Danish monuments was clearly inspired by the then Chancellor Christen Friis, who was also the driving force behind the production of several histories about the kingdom of Denmark launched around the same time. That he should have encouraged Worm, who, of course, considered philology a necessary tool for physicians as well as other scholars, to take this on can hardly surprise considering how close Worm was to the Chancellor. That Worm could find the time for this research, bearing in mind his other time-consuming occupations as a physician and a professor, is more surprising. Two factors caused Ole Worm to take on the role as the country's leading antiquarian. First, he realised that the man he had initially chosen to lead the research into the runes and ancient Danish monuments was not up to the task. Second, Worm came to appreciate how significant this antiquarian enterprise might turn out to be not only to the chancellor but also to Christian IV, both keen on promoting a patriotic, cultural history of the kingdom. While Worm's personal fascination with the runes and the Danish ancient monuments grew, so did his awareness of the potential advantage of his involvement in this project, drawing him to the attention of the king and the chancellor and making him an obvious recipient of royal favours.

Ole Worm was to spend much of his time over the next thirty years researching and writing on the runes and the ancient monuments. It proved a difficult task not least because this was a new and relatively unexplored field of research. Worm was fortunate to have a host of Icelandic students and friends who were able to assist him, but he was disappointed by the lack of government support for his efforts. Initially it proved difficult for him to find publishers. His first work, *Fasti Danici*, was published by the university printer Salomon Santor and would appear to have presented few problems in publication terms, but Worm struggled to find a publisher for his second work on the runes. Eventually he was forced to pay for its publication himself and he came close to giving up his research and writing on the runes and the ancient monuments. Worm felt unappreciated, especially at home, even if he gained recognition for his work from leading international antiquarians such as Sir Henry Spelman.

This all changed with the discovery of the ancient gold horn in Southern Jutland and Worm's quickly produced tract about it, *De Aureo Cornu*, which was published in 1641. It proved this work more than anything else which came to underpin Ole Worm's fame at home and abroad. Undoubtedly Worm benefitted from the fact that the gold horn was an extremely rare and valuable object, decorated with weird and wonderful images and letters. Worm's tract about the ancient gold horn sold out within months and undeniably facilitated the publication of his work on the ancient Danish monuments, which was published in 1643 including an expanded and amended version of *De Aureo Cornu*. The gold horn fascinated scholars across Europe, many of whom wrote tracts about it. Apart from Sir Henry Spelman in London it drew Ole Worm to the attention of leading antiquarian scholars, such as Johannes de Laet in Leiden, Herman Conring in Helmstedt, Gabriel Naudé in Paris, Cassiano dal Pozzo and Athanasius Kircher in Rome, and Fortunio Liceti in Bologna. Simultaneously Ole Worm's growing reputations abroad served to enhance his standing at home at both the court and university.

Posthumously Ole Worm's fame came to rest more than anything else on his cabinet of curiosity. Throughout most of his life Worm was an avid collector of rare natural objects in particular. It is his role as a collector which is the subject of Chapter 4. Initially it was his interests in botany which drove Ole Worm's interests in collecting. This was closely linked to his interest in creating and improving his garden in the decade after his appointment to his first professorship at the University of Copenhagen. Later Worm renewed his interest in gardening and botany at intervals until 1644.

Like most of his contemporaries Worm had started to collect the odd object during his extended, educational journey in Europe. Gradually, after he had settled in Copenhagen he intensified his collection of rare natural objects until he began to apply a more systematic approach to his collecting by the early 1620s. By the end of that decade he had also started to include unusual man-made objects in his collection, the so-called artificia. Thus a cabinet of curiosity came into existence and by the end of the 1620s visitors had begun to arrive.

It was, however, not until the 1640s that Worm's cabinet of curiosity really grew and acquired an international reputation. Several factors proved crucial to this development. First among them was Worm's friendship with Johannes de Laet in Leiden, the wealthy natural historian and director of the Dutch West India Company. Through de Laet Ole Worm obtained an array of objects, plants, and animals which he would not otherwise have been able to collect, not to mention a wealth of information. Between 1642 and 1648 Worm and de Laet corresponded regularly, exchanged objects, and discussed issues of natural historical importance. Second was the importance and input by his nephews of the Bartholin and Fuiren families, who obtained a continuous stream of items for his museum while generating important contacts to leading figures within the republic of letters during their peregrinatio academica. Third was the donations coming from Ole Worm's former students and friends on Iceland as well as the Faroe Isles. Many of these gifts such as parts of the narwhale and its tooth proved important for the growing international reputation of Worm as a collector and his cabinet of curiosity. Fourth was the growing number of gifts of artificia in particular from princes and nobles in the decade leading up to Worm's death in 1654.

The fact that Worm had two catalogues printed during these years, the first in 1642 and the second in 1645, listing all the objects exhibited in his cabinet of curiosity, tells us not only how quickly his collection had expanded but also how significant his museum had become. The catalogues were widely distributed among friends and colleagues across Europe not only with the intent of demonstrating the importance of his collection but also serving as a guide and aid to provide Worm with objects missing from his museum. In August 1642 Worm received a long letter from his Icelandic friend and correspondent Arngrim Jonsson, who reserved special praise for his 1642 catalogue, which Arngrim had recently received. Worm would undoubtedly have been pleased by what Arngrim wrote about him and his catalogue:

> Its distance from the prison of his own brain (Arngrim's) is as far and distant as heaven is said to be from the earth. Heavenly is the comprehension and talents, which have been granted one individual while God must be praised for all his creations. Through the power of such divine gifts He makes us admire what we do not understand, while teaching us not to show them contempt like beasts. Because it is the intention of God when he lets one person stand way above others that we examine and recognise how much the greatest eclipse the lesser, and unite in a hymn of thanksgiving to the Creator. Stars with a weaker light do not envy those with greater radiance, but in unison they tell us about God's and Heaven's Glory.[7]

---

7 Breve fra og til Ole Worm, no. 1065.

Towards the end of his life, in 1647, Ole Worm had a large picture of himself and his extended family painted. Bearing in mind its size, 2 × 4 meters, this epitaph or painting was unlikely to have been intended for Worm's own home, but rather for the University of Copenhagen. The painting portrays Worm's three wives, their many children, and his two son-in-laws, but the two main figures are Ole Worm himself and Jesus Christ, standing next to him while looking towards him and his family. Behind them are four men, of whom one, his father-in-law, Thomas Fincke, can be clearly identified (third from left), while the figure on Fincke's left bears a resemblance to Worm's brother-in-law Caspar Bartholin. The other two figures might be those of Worm's other 'Fincke' brothers-in-law, Jørgen Fuiren and Hans Rasmussen Brochmand. A verse by Thomas Bartholin praising Worm's fertility and learning can be seen in the left corner of the painting plus a reference to Matthew 19. V. 14.[8] The painting provides a clear illustration of Ole Worm's view of himself and his activities as being firmly situated within his Lutheran faith and guided by Christ.

At the same time Worm dedicated more and more time to writing his museum history, *Museum Wormianum*, until the first draft was ready in 1648. He then spent the next six years, until his death, editing and expanding it. He spent considerable time finding a publisher, convinced that only a leading European press would do, before he settled on the Elzevirs in Amsterdam. His previous disappointments with printers caused him to take a keen interest in the publishing process, making sure that only the best paper, types, and illustrations were used. He constantly intervened to prevent unnecessary delays and mistakes, while forwarding a never-ending stream of amendments and corrections until his death.

Museum Wormianum became the crowning glory of a life-time of pre-occupation with natural philosophy and history undertaken by a Lutheran scholar who sought to understand God's creation – the Natural world – through study, observation, experiment, and description.

---

8 The painting is now in Nationalmuseet in Copenhagen. Names and identifications have been added later to the painting, see H. D. Schepelern, *Breve fra of til Ole Worm*, vol. 3, Copenhagen 1968, noter til illustationerne. Camilla Mordhorst identifies the four figures as Thomas Fincke, Mads Jensen Medelfar, Worm's two fathers-in-law, plus Hans Hansen Resen, and Jesper Brockmand, see C. Mordhorst, *Genstandsfortællinger. Fra Museum Wormianum til de modern museer*, Copenhagen 2009, 38.

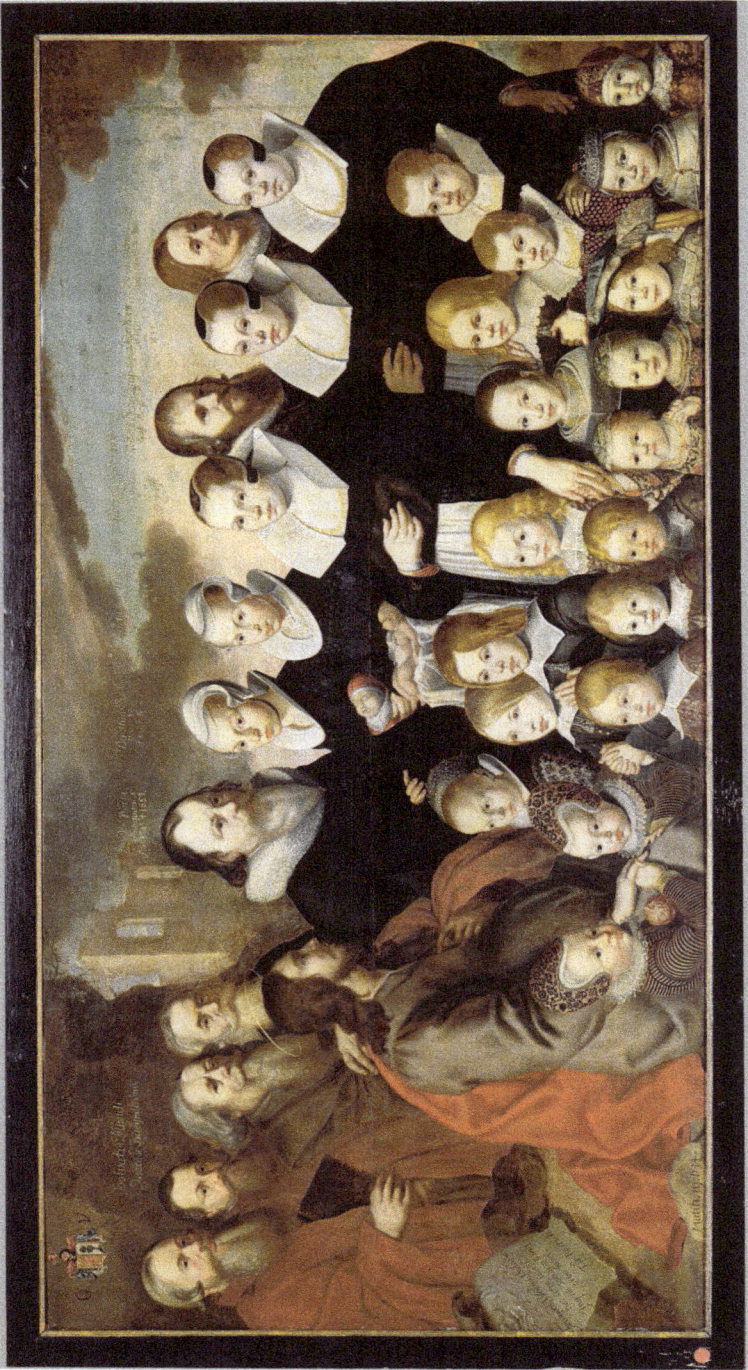

In colour: The Worm family painting 1648; photo by Lennart Larsen, courtesy of the Danish National Museum.

1 The Physician

Worm's interests and research constantly changed throughout his life. For a period he appeared to have prioritised natural philosophy, later his focus was on antiquarianism and history, and finally he became increasingly absorbed in collecting, creating his cabinet of curiosity and in particular in writing the book about his museum. Only one interest or role remained constant in his career: namely that of the physician. Worm practised medicine throughout most of his life. He never stopped looking after his patients be it through direct physical consultations or via letters, and with only two exceptions he remained in Copenhagen to look after them during major outbreaks of epidemic disease and plague. However, it is important to remember that most of Worm's activities as a practising physician have left little or no evidence behind, consisting as they did of face to face encounters between physician and patient.

Even before he had obtained his medical degree Worm had started practising medicine. He had begun his medical studies in 1607 and already three years later, at the tender age of twenty-one and yet to obtain his MD, he started practising medicine during his two month stay in Paris, as his obituary put it 'he regularly and with success practised medicine'. Later in the summer of 1610 Worm returned to Denmark most likely to his home in Aarhus. He visited the influential nobleman Holger Rosenkrantz, the Learned, on the latter's estate Rosenholm in late June. In the beginning of September Worm arrived in Copenhagen where he matriculated at the university. He would appear to have spent the next eight to ten months in Copenhagen not only studying and building up relationships with 'the leading professors at the Academy', but also adding to his reputation by providing medical assistance to a wide clientele who encouraged him to settle in the capital.[1]

Worm, however, decided to continue his academic travels, undoubtedly realising his need for an MD. First he headed for Marburg and then to Basle where he obtained his MD in December 1611. He then travelled via the Netherlands to England where he arrived in late February or beginning of March 1612. The choice of England, at this time a fairly unusual

1 See Schepelern, *Museum*, 45–46.

DOI: 10.4324/9781003290940-2

destination on the peregrinatio academica, was most likely linked to the close royal connections between England and Denmark, with the English King James I married to the Danish King Christian IV's sister, Anne of Denmark. Six years earlier Christian IV had undertaken a four week state visit to England which had seen contacts being established between English and Danish courtiers. One of them Jonas Charisius, who had married a daughter of the famous Paracelsian physician, Peter Severinus, the Dane, met Worm in London on 6th March 1612 and most likely facilitated the contact to the nobleman Robert Rich, Baron Rich who later in 1618 became Earl of Warwick. By the end of March Worm had become personal physician to Robert Rich whom he also assisted in the latter's chemical and medical research. As always Worm sought the acquaintance of many of the leading local physicians, especially the two royal physicians Theodore de Mayerne and John Craig. Worm remained as personal physician to Robert Rich for nearly eighteen months eventually returning to Copenhagen in July 1613 to take up a professorship in pedagogy.[2]

Worm began establishing his medical practice in Copenhagen at the same time he took up his professorship.

In a letter from August 1616 to his friend Anders Skytte, physician to Queen Sophie, Worm complained that his university teaching and his many patients prevented him from finding enough time for his own research.[3] Despite the demands on his time Worm was satisfied with the success of his medical practice as he informed his old teacher Caspar Bauhin in Basle a few months later.[4] Not surprisingly a number of his patients came from within the academic community, such as the professor of theology, Jesper Rasmussen Brochmand, who in 1617 had taken on the role of tutor to Christian, the elected-prince.

In this new role Brochmand had to spend much of his time away from his home in Copenhagen attending the prince at royal castles, such as at Kronborg and Frederiksborg. Over the three years Brochmand served as tutor to the prince Worm regularly supplied him with prescriptions and medical remedies.[5] Jesper Brochmand's absence from home, however, caused his wife considerable anxiety which Worm had to deal with as the family physician. Brochmand's own health also concerned Worm and writing to Brochmand in May 1617 he offered detailed advice:

> Your wife is seriously troubled about your health; thus I would appreciate if you wrote to her that you were feeling better after the bloodletting (which I hear you have agreed to) and at the same time informed

2 *Ibid.*, 46 and 83–85.
3 *Breve fra og til Ole Worm*, no. 21
4 *Ibid.*, no. 24.
5 *Ibid.*, nos. 40 and 52. In February 1618 Brochmand received a recipe for a drug against hypochondriac pain, while in November that year he asked Worm to supply him with some of his best theriac.

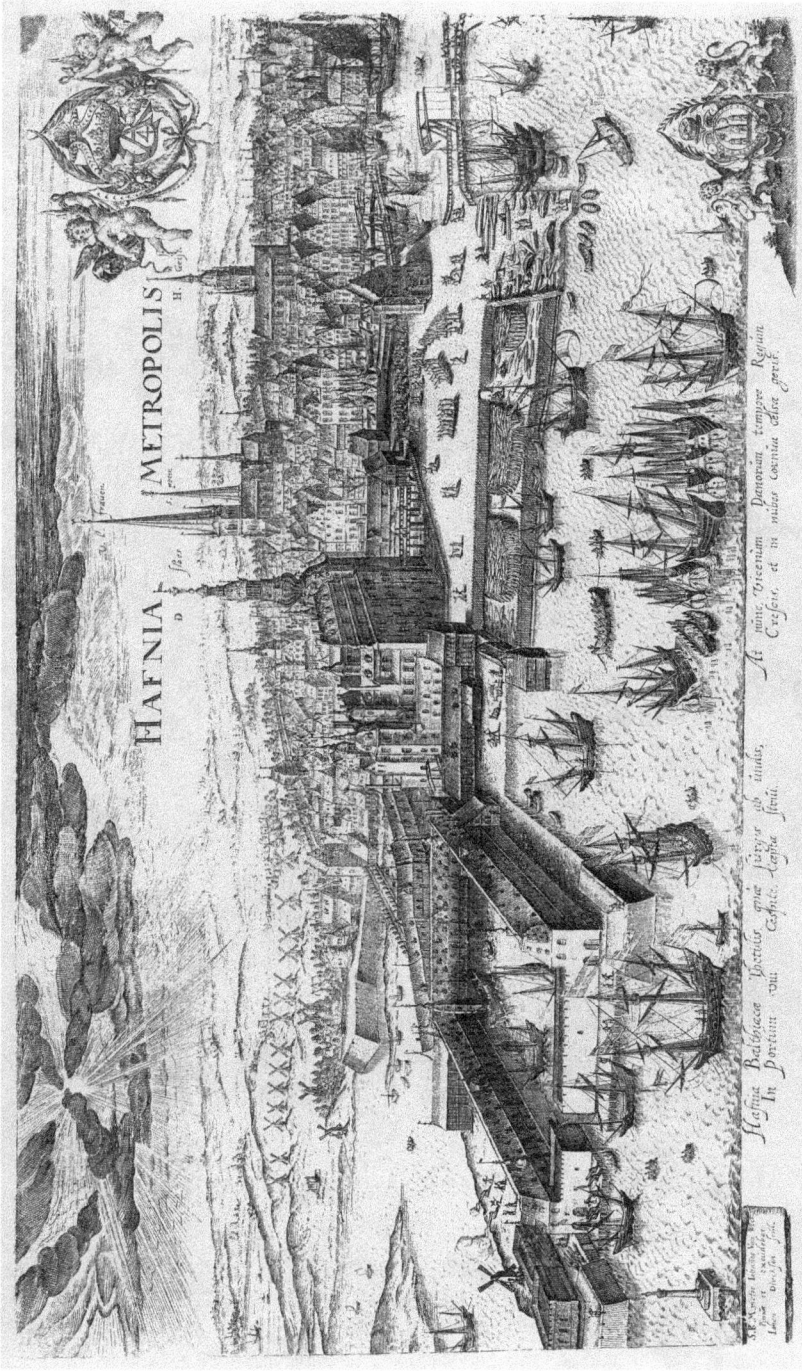

Figure 1.1 Prospect of Copenhagen 1611; courtesy of the Royal Danish Library.

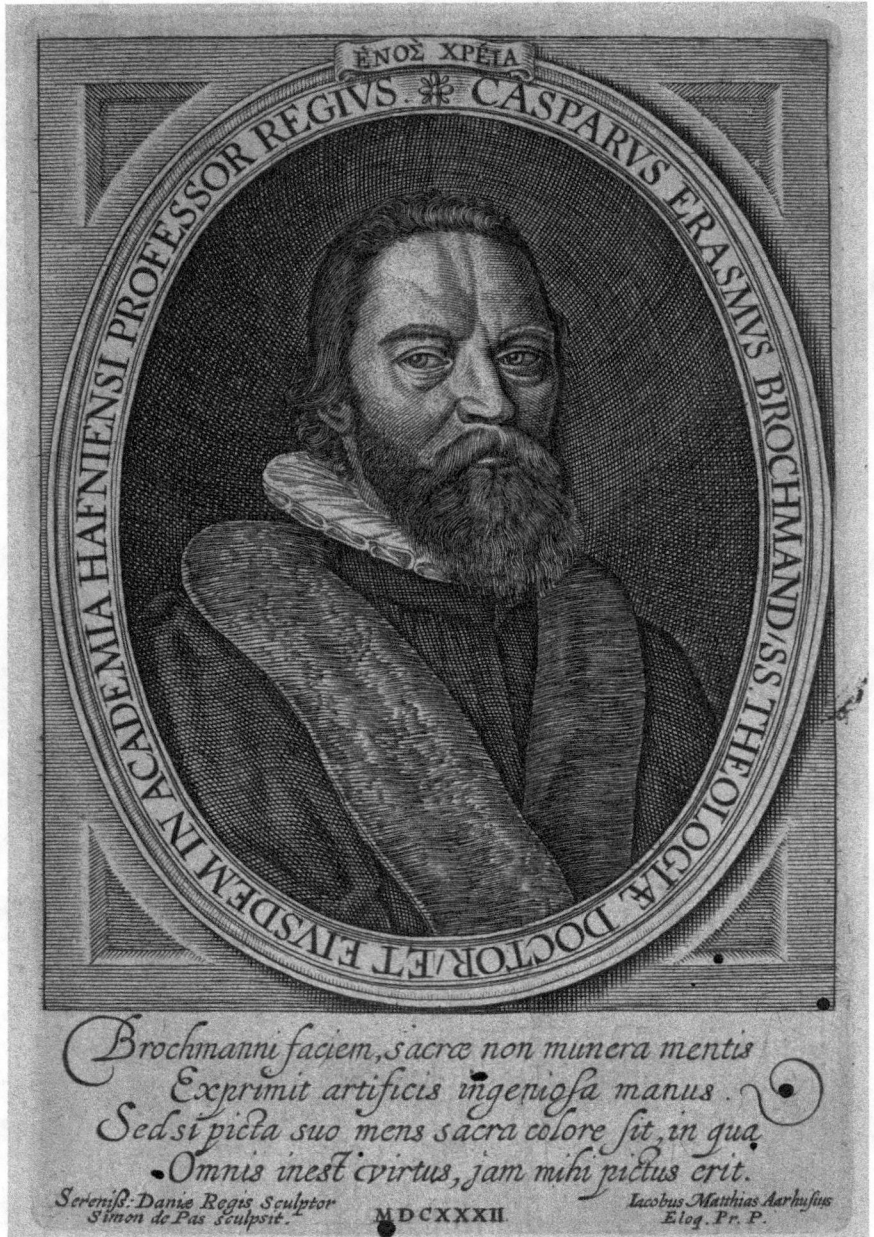

Figure 1.2 Jesper Rasmussen Brochmand (1585–1652) age 47, by Simon de Pas;
courtesy of the Royal Danish Library.

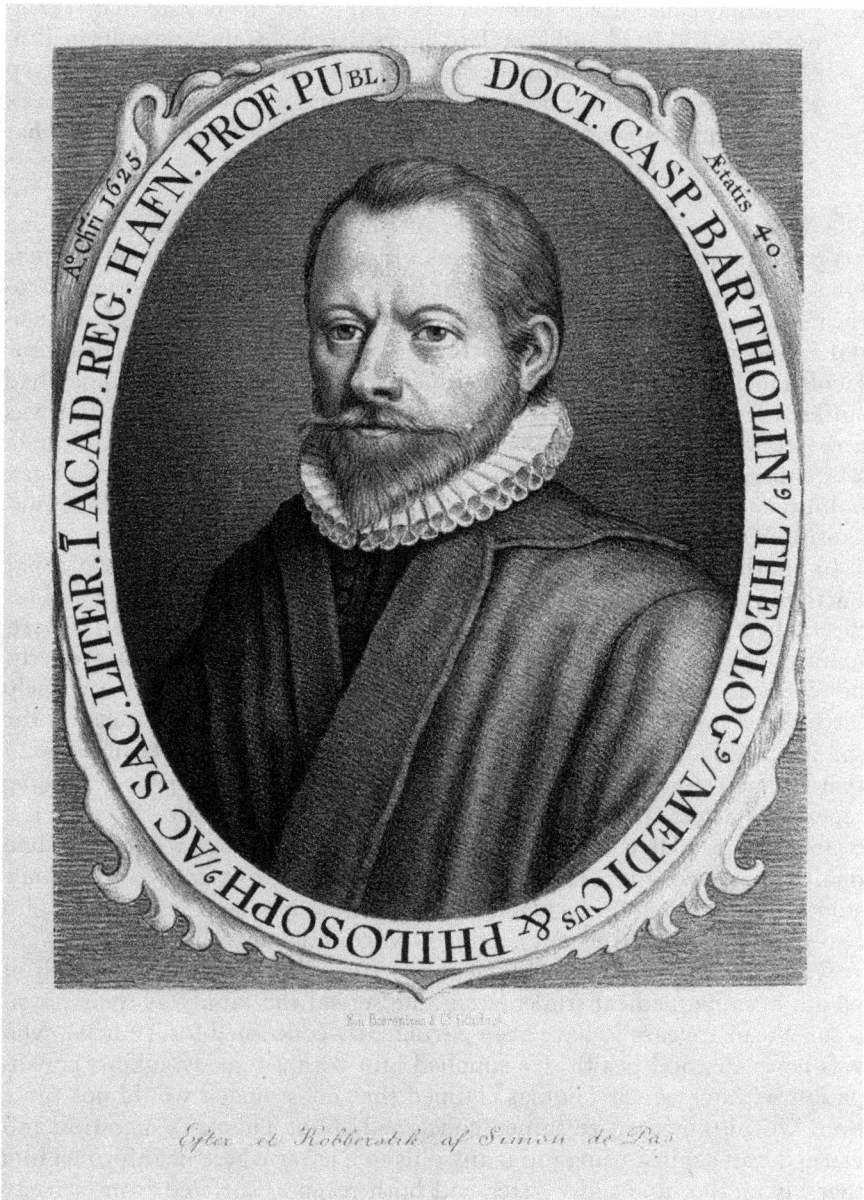

Figure 1.3 Caspar Bartholin (1585–1629) age 40; courtesy of the Royal Danish Library.

her that you feel that your body is stronger than before. This would in particular cause her to feel relieved. And please make sure that you do not work too hard and keep late hours thereby neglecting your health. Much is achieved with moderation. Make sure that your stools keep step with your intake; do not let worries and misplaced late hours tax your mental capacity thereby leaving you with a disabled body. That way I think everything will turn out well.[6]

Ole Worm counted many members of the academic community among his patients, including family, such as his father-in-law professor Thomas Fincke, and his brother-in-law Caspar Bartholin. Worm had married Dorothea Fincke in November 1615 and thereby allied himself with the influential Fincke dynasty. In December 1617 Worm informed his brother-in-law Jacob Fincke, who was studying in Giessen, that his father Thomas had suffered from an 'endemic fever' over the last couple of months, but was now recovering well.[7] In November 1623 Worm wrote to his student in Wittenberg, Hans Andersen Skovgaard informing him that Caspar Bartholin had recently been confined to bed with shooting pains in his limbs causing Worm considerable concern.

In another letter written later that month Worm indicated that Caspar Bartholin was slowly recovering while his rheumatism was abating and his 'hectic heat' had become less intense. Worm pointed out that even if Bartholin's appetite had improved his stomach did not yet function properly, nor for that matter, did his limbs, adding, that he hoped God would help his brother-in-law to a full recovery. Caspar Bartholin sought relief at the spa in Carlsbad, but to little or no avail. Worm reported in February 1625 that he had returned from the spa having failed to recover properly, being repeatedly affected by 'kidney pains' which taxed his health. However, a couple of years later Worm was able to report that Caspar Bartholin had finally recovered and did no longer suffer from pains caused by kidney stones. The fact that it was plague which eventually killed Caspar Bartholin two years later would seem to confirm Worm's diagnosis in 1627.[8]

Worm remained close to his nephews from the Fuiren family, both of whom became medical students, and he served the family as their physician. Worm appears to have been particularly concerned for Thomas, who was never in good health. He supplied him with a remedy against constipation without which Thomas claimed that his stomach would not function. Worm, however, remained concerned about Thomas's digestion and warned him against using too many pills in a letter where he informed him that his mother and older sister had both recently suffered from a nasty fever, but were recovering.[9]

6 *Ibid.*, no. 27.
7 *Ibid.*, no. 37.
8 *Ibid.*, nos. 139, 146, 173, 215, 280 and 282.
9 *Ibid.*, nos. 605 and 615.

Later when studying in Padua the Fuiren brethren regularly sought medical advice from their uncle in Copenhagen. Henrik asked Worm's advice about his brother in June 1641. He was concerned that his coughs regularly produced foaming blood which he thought might result in consumption. Despite having taken the medical remedies on the advice of the Paduan professor of medicine, Benedictus Sylvaticus during the spring which were not only intended for his chest, but which should also have served to ease his constipation and improve his urination, none of it had helped. Consequently, Worm advised his mother to ask him to return home as soon as possible, thinking that the thicker, cooler air and the Rostock beer might help him.[10]

Worm showed similar concern for his nephew Thomas Bartholin for whom he stood in loco parentis. He paid close attention to Thomas's health, which he considered delicate, while the latter studied in Leiden. Writing to Thomas in June 1638 Worm advised Thomas not to take too many medical remedies which might break down his natural heat and possibly his strength too. Thomas Bartholin was suffering from constipation and Worm advised him to eat a handful of large beans together with soup first thing in the morning; if that did not work he told his nephew to buy some pills he was familiar with which would serve to assist Nature in producing faeces. Worm recommended Thomas to try to develop a daily routine, making sure that he went to the toilet morning and evening. Such a regime would in Worm's opinion help Nature to cure him.[11] In May 1640 Worm expressed serious concern for Thomas's frailty. He warned Thomas not to weaken his already feeble body further through misplaced wakeful nights and research thereby wasting his health and 'depriving his fatherland of his glorious talents'. He impressed on Thomas to recollect the example of his late father, who in his youth exhausted himself with such strenuous studies, that when the time came, when he might best have been of use to his fatherland, he was overwhelmed with a host of emerging illnesses, achieving only the lesser part of all that he wanted to do.[12]

Worm also appears to have had the former Tycho Brahe pupil and professor of theology Cort Aslaksen among his patients. He certainly attended Aslaksen in the latter's last illness. Reporting to his friend, the physician Niels Christensen Foss in Lund, Worm described how, as he put it,

> the convulsion which had caused a paralysis in his [Aslaksen] right leg developed into gangrene and caries towards the end which the surgeons were unable to prevent or neutralise despite all their efforts. His waning strength and other things, which I shall tell you on another occasion, did not make an amputation advisable.[13]

10 *Ibid.*, nos. 950 and 957.
11 *Ibid.*, no. 722.
12 *Ibid.*, no. 844.
13 *Ibid.*, nos. 150 and 151.

Another university professor who relied on Worm for medical advice was the professor of metaphysics Jens Dinesen Jersin. In 1624, while Dinesen served as tutor to King Christian IV's illegitimate sons Christian Ulrik and Hans Ulrik Gyldenløve at the Academy in Sorø, Worm prescribed Dinesen pills which were particularly beneficial for the head and pills for his wife's complaints about her uterus which Worm had personally manufactured chemically.[14]

Thomas Wegner, who was made Bishop of Stavanger in Norway in 1627, might well have been a patient of Ole Worm from 1618 when he became vicar at St. Nicolai Church in Copenhagen. It is evident from Worm's letter of May 1628 that they had been friends for some time and that Worm had previously supplied Wegner with drugs. Offering Wegner some advice on how to deal with pills which had become stuck together Worm promised to deal with any concern Wegner might have about his health or drugs he needed. Worm also took the opportunity to inform Wegner that Copenhagen had recently been struck by a storm or tornado which had damaged many of the buildings in the capital and shattered St. Nicolai Church where Wegner had been the vicar for nearly a decade. This was according to Worm all grim proofs of the anger of the Almighty.[15]

Worm regularly supplied Wegner with medical remedies and Wegner reciprocated by sending fish and oysters to Worm after his promotion to the bishopric in Norway. In 1635 Worm had been told by his nephew, Henrik Fuiren, that Wegner suffered from colic. Worm forwarded some purging electuarium aperiens and recommended an enema, but warned that this required materials which might not be available locally to Wegner; so he suggested oil and a hot compress with laurel leaves as an alternative.[16] When Wegner's son Cort returned to Copenhagen in June 1638 to resume his studies after the plague epidemic of 1637 Worm took the opportunity to forward medical remedies and medical advice to his father. It is interesting that Wegner continued to rely on Worm as his physician after his promotion to the see of Stavanger. Obviously physicians were thin on the ground in Norway while Thomas Wegner retained great confidence in the advice and treatment by Worm even if it had to be done from a distance and via correspondence.

In February 1648 Worm filled a box he was returning to his friend the royal historiographer and professor of history at the Academy in Sorø, Steffen Hansen Stephanius, with cough lozenges against the cough Stephanius normally suffered from that time of the year. Worm was evidently both his considerate friend and physician.[17]

14 *Ibid.*, no. 166.
15 *Ibid.*, no. 241.
16 *Ibid.*, nos. 277, 467, and 576.
17 *Ibid.*, no. 1565.

Worm was appreciated by many of his patients who often thanked him for his assistance. In some cases, as in that of the young Margrethe Hansdatter, he received thank you letters and presents. Worm was happy to hear about Margrethe's improved health and showed himself a firm believer in astrological medicine:

> the plaster placed on her head had proved very useful, having extracted much of the itchy material from the eyes. But it would be wise to avoid using it together with other medical remedies during the heat of the dog days. Long ago it was pointed out by our Hippocrates that all medical remedies have less effect during and before the dog days. Take care that the rays of the sun don't hit your eyes during the dog days, or that your body becomes overheated by light or other movement. You know from experience that smoke and wind is damaging for the eyes and I should wish that you don't harm them through intensive sowing or similar fine, female activities. In the autumn I will God willing attend to the other sick. I also approve of your mother's plan, because she is a very clever lady, when she does not tire your little sister with medical remedies at this time of year which is not well suited to treatment.[18]

Ole Worm also treated many other patients most of whom have left little or no trace in his papers. Only when letters were written can their treatment be traced. Such as that of the wife of Thomas Lund in Elsinore who suffered from constipation, pains in her back and legs, and headache for whom Worm supplied both drugs and medical guidance. Occasionally Worm appears to have acted on the instigation of others such as his father-in-law Thomas Fincke, who asked him to forward a specific medical remedy to a certain gentleman of his acquaintance, whom Worm, always a firm adherent of astrological medicine, sent some pills to be taken at the waning moon, adding that the man in question should let himself be bled on the advice of a surgeon.[19] Similarly Worm forwarded a remedy against scurvy to Hans Borchardsen in Ribe, not on the patient's, but on his brother-in-law's request, recommending that the remedy be supplemented by plenty of exercise such as chopping firewood.[20] In March 1646 Worm wrote to one of his patients in Greve, Erik Mogensen, expressing his satisfaction that the medical remedies he had prescribed him had worked well, but warning him not to put the outcome in danger by not finishing the prescribed treatment.[21] An unusual case was that of Bishop Jacob Madsen in Aarhus whom Worm had been asked to contact by his mother-in-law who was concerned about the Bishop's health and the 'rigidity of his joints'. This appears to have been

18 *Ibid.*, no. 728.
19 *Ibid.*, nos. 333 and 397.
20 *Ibid.*, no. 757.
21 *Ibid.*, no. 1395.

the sole basis for Worm advising the Bishop to be bled twice a year in the side which was not in pain; to take plenty of walks outside, avoid heat and cold and to use the traditional remedies against scurvy, especially the remedy prepared by his colleague Dr Jacob Madsen in Elsinore.[22]

Worm's medical advice was sought by a variety of patients across Sealand. In July 1650 he examined a child of an Elsinore resident, Magnus Durell. He had found a swelling on the right side of the boy's abdomen. He was concerned that this might turn into a hernia as a result of strenuous exercise. He therefore informed the father that he had ordered a bandage to be applied plus the rubbing of oil. Worm recommended that the boy abstain from vigorous exercise for the time being, if so he predicted that he would recover from this complaint.[23]

Over the years Ole Worm also provided many of his students with medical advice on their study trips abroad. Writing to Willum Lange in Rome Worm expressed his sympathy for Lange's bad health, but found it surprising that the famous Roman physicians were unable deal with it, especially since some of their colleagues in the North knew how to tackle it. He suggested softening and painkilling enemas plus rosewater of Althea juice, onions, and parsley water, questioning whether he should 'bring owls to Athens', indicating that all that was well known in Rome.

1 Physician to the nobility

Ole Worm also served as physician to a number of the most prominent noble families in Denmark, especially the Rosenkrantz family. In May 1623 he looked after Holger Rosenkrantz's wife Sophie Brahe. The following year he attended Holger Rosenkrantz himself during the latter's prolonged illness in Copenhagen.[24]

A year later Worm forwarded a number of remedies including theriac against the plague for Holger Rosenkrantz's sons who were at the Academy in Sorø.[25] After King Christian IV's defeat in the Thirty Years War at Lutter am Barenberg and the subsequent occupation of Jutland in the autumn of 1627 the Rosenkrantz family was forced to flee their Jutland estates. For Holger Rosenkrantz the loss of his beloved library on Rosenholm proved particularly painful. Towards the end of 1627 when he posted medical remedies for the strengthening of the head and the spirit to Holger Rosenkrantz, now resident in Scania, Worm was busy trying to see if he could facilitate negotiations for the library's return to Rosenkrantz.[26] That

---

22 *Ibid.*, no. 1531: this is one of very few instances where Worm recommended remedies made by colleagues
23 *Ibid.*, no, 1697.
24 *Ibid.*, nos. 129, 164, and 171
25 *Ibid.*, no. 178.
26 *Ibid.*, nos. 139–40.

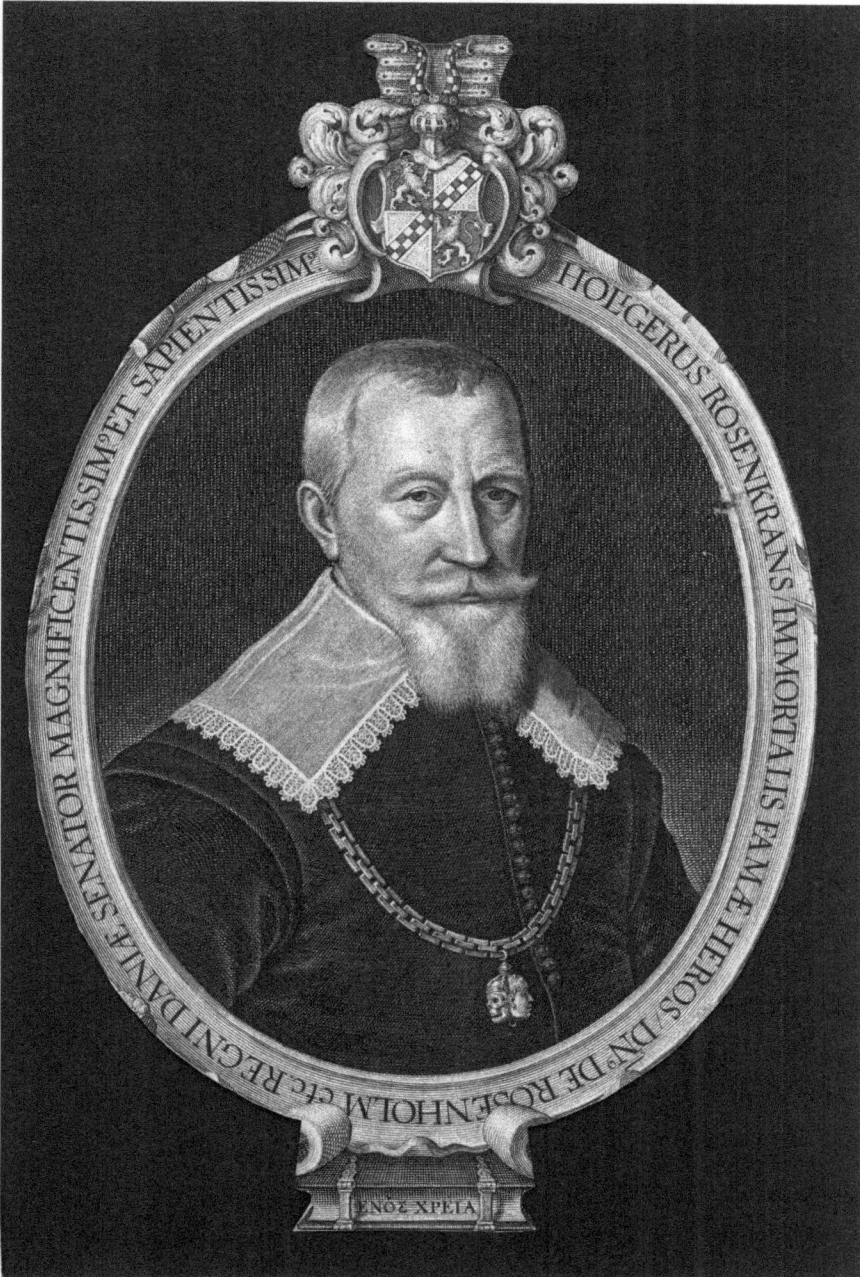

Figure 1.4 Holger Rosenkrantz, The Learned (1574–1642); courtesy of the Royal Danish Library.

year Worm was paid twenty-four Reichsthaler – a very considerable sum – for curing Holger of scurvy. And only eight days before Christmas that year he attended and cured Holger of a non-specified disease at his estate of Løberød in Scania for which he was paid eighteen Reichsthaler.[27] These two sums from the Rosenkrantz family would have amounted to more than 20% of Worm's annual salary for his university professorship.[28]

In 1629 Worm was paid twenty-four Reichsthaler for treating Holger's son Gunde Rosenkrantz for typhoid or spotted fever. This is undoubtedly the treatment referred to in Worm's letter to Holger Rosenkrantz written on Boxing Day 1628. Here Worm informed Rosenkrantz that his son was likely to have caught this disease on his journey to Copenhagen. Despite what Worm described as the use of a mild purgation the patient's headaches continued. Worm had also ordered some preventive drugs against what he described as an epidemic fever. However, due to, as Worm put it, someone else's negligence the treatment had been delayed for three days which had resulted in Gunde developing skin rashes, which Worm was now treating with salt of hartshorn and bezoar stone. Worm concluded optimistically that the crisis had been dealt with. That year Worm also received a payment of twelve Reichsthaler for curing Holger Rosenkrantz's daughters of an infectious blood disease.[29]

Rosenkrantz's wife Sofie Brahe apart from managing the family estate also operated a small bank taking deposits from a number of individuals such as Ole Worm and his father-in-law Thomas Fincke. The fact that both of them placed 1,000 Reichsthaler on deposit with Sofie Brahe in March 1629 tells us that they were comfortably off. When Worm withdrew his capital at the end of 1630 he received 120 Reichsthaler in interest.[30]

When forwarding medical remedies to Holger Rosenkrantz in Helsingborg in July 1629, containing among other things a description of Emplastrum uterinum for Rosenkrantz and Aqua vitæ antherita for Mette Gøye, Worm referred to the fact that there was much fever and dysentery in Copenhagen. This had clearly spread to Helsingborg across the Sound by August when Holger Rosenkrantz's son-in-law requested Worm to attend his son Axel who suffered from diarrhoea and to bring his own drugs. Three weeks later Worm received a similar request from Holger himself asking him to attend his daughter Beate in Helsingborg who was suffering from diarrhoea, vomiting, back pains and nightly shivering fits followed

27 See H. Paulsen (ed.), *Sophie Brahes Regnskabsbog 1627–1640*, Jysk Selskab for Historie, Sprog og Litteratur, Aarhus 1955, 8 under 'Vdgifft til doctorer'.
28 For university salaries in this period see H. Matzen (ed.), *Kjøbenhavns Universitets Retshistorie 1478–1879*, II, Copenhagen 1879, 33ff.; W. Norvin, *Københavns Universitet i Reformationens og Orthodoxiens Tidsalder*, I, Copenhagen 1937, 170–73; and S. Ellehøj et al. (eds.), *Københavns Universitet 1479–1979*, IV, Copenhagen 1980, 9ff.
29 *Ibid.*, 35 and *Letters to and from Ole Worm*, no. 265
30 Paulsen (ed.), *Sophie Brahes Regnskabsbog*, 26 and 42.

by a hot fever. Worm responded a couple of days later informing Holger Rosenkrantz that he was unable to attend her, because he himself suffered badly from diarrhoea. However, he forwarded drugs with directions for their use, pointing out that the fever would subside if and when the body had been purged. He recommended bezoar stone, terra sigillata, and rice pudding with nutmeg.[31] Apart from some drugs which Worm supplied to Holger Rosenkrantz during the Parliament of 1633 this proved Worm's last service to the Rosenkrantz family as their physician.[32] This is explained by the fact that the Rosenkrantz family's exodus from their main estates in Jutland and Funen came to an end by the beginning of October 1629 when they left Helsingborg as a result of the peace treaty with the Holy Roman Emperor which Christian IV had signed in Lübeck the previous May.[33] The services of Worm, however, remained in high demand among the nobility in Sealand. This was obviously financially important to Worm. Such people could afford his services, but they also demanded his full attention. In the middle of writing a letter to his nephew in Leiden, Thomas Bartholin, to be brought by his brother Caspar who was just about to leave Copenhagen for Leiden Worm was called away to attend a noble lady out of town who had suffered a stroke. While Worm was caring for her Caspar left Copenhagen without his letter to Thomas causing Worm considerable irritation.[34]

When medical intervention failed or was perceived to have gone wrong resulting in damage or death to the patient physicians like Worm might find themselves in serious trouble, especially if the patient belonged to the nobility and a complaint was made to the king and the university. Thus, by June 1639 rumours began to circulate that Tycho (Axelsøn) Brahe, a namesake and relative of the famous astronomer and husband of Jytte (Birgitte) Brock, had raised a complaint against the treatment of his wife by the Copenhagen physician Tancred Leyel. Worm became heavily involved in this case. Together with some of his colleagues, following the complaint by Brahe, he had advised Leyel to try and get everything settled amicably through intermediaries. After pressure from Leyel Worm had agreed to take on this role. Subsequently he claimed to have managed to convince Tycho to let matters rest for a month; Leyel, however, wanted to get the case fully settled and sought the advice of others.[35]

In late September 1639 Ole Worm felt obliged to provide his friend, the physician Ægidius Gjøde Jensen in Randers with a detailed description of the case undoubtedly because Gjøde was the family physician to the influential Brok family.

---

31 *Breve fra og til Ole Worm*, nos. 283, 286, 292, and 294.
32 Paulsen (ed.), *Sophie Brahes Regnskabsbog*, 85.
33 *Ibid.*, XI.
34 *Breve fra og til Ole Worm*, no. 793.
35 *Ibid.*, nos. 782 and 790.

Jytte Brok had arrived in Copenhagen in late January 1639 suffering from a slight eye infection, but otherwise strong and healthy. She had consulted Tancred Leyel whom she had often used while in Copenhagen and asked him for a remedy. He insisted that her impure body needed to be purified. She pointed out that her physical condition was unsuitable for purifying remedies, revealing that she was three months pregnant. He doubted that this could be the case since she had already been barren for many years, and claimed that her body could still be purified by the proper remedies even if she was pregnant. Jytte Brok continued to reject his advice, pointing out that she knew of several cases where purifying remedies had caused an abortion. Eventually she was convinced by Leyel and took some grains of skammonia-resin together with crème of tartar on his advice. This had an immediate effect, and she had a violent evacuation combined with severe pain in the abdomen. This repeated itself over the next couple of days until on the third day what she ate went straight through her undigested. Leyel was called back and made futile efforts to alleviate the pain through the use of external remedies. On the fourth day Jytte Brok produced a slimy stool mixed with blood during the night, and shortly afterwards she expelled pure blood accompanied by terrible pain, feebleness, and wakefulness. Worm was told all this by Jytte Brok herself after her husband, Tycho Brahe, had fetched him in the middle of the night to attend his wife. He had found her exhausted by pain and unable to sleep with all her strength gone. He was then shown three bedpans totally filled with blood evacuated with her stools. At this point Jytte Brok wanted nothing else than a blissful death. Worm had then briefly discussed her illness, its start and development, with Leyel, on which he declared that the discharge had to be stopped immediately and the pains soothed or death could be expected sooner rather than later. Leyel initially disagreed with Worm insisting that his cure should be continued. Eventually Worm convinced the 'trembling and irresolute' Leyel and ordered a small pill from the apothecary. On taking it Jytte Brok calmed down, the pains passed, and the unrestricted discharges diminished with the result that she slept the whole night without any discharge. The following day Worm followed up with strengthening remedies even if the pain had not totally disappeared. Whereupon Jytte Brok insisted that Worm alone should continue her treatment and Leyel be dismissed. Worm accepted this with some hesitation because he was unsure what symptoms would result from a pregnant woman suffering such extreme exhaustion. Eventually he consented overcome by both the patient's and her husband's entreaties, and he spent the following month seeking to strengthen the mother and foetus while making the symptoms of scurvy disappear.

By the beginning of March Jytte Brok had recovered enough to return home from Copenhagen, even if not fully healed and still complaining about considerable weakness. All this Worm knew at first hand. As expected Jytte Brok gave birth in August to a healthy baby as Worm was informed by her husband a couple of days later. However, the mother died unexpectedly a few days after having given birth. Worm had been informed by the noble ladies who prepared her for the funeral that her body had suddenly become distended and disfigured by a considerable sallowness which they attributed to the damaging effects of Leyel's medical remedies. Worm, however, told them that these surprising impacts were more likely to have been caused by the scurvy from which Jytte Brok had suffered since childhood. Shortly after Jytte Brok's recovery from her initial treatment, however, her husband had begun proceedings at the university against Tancred Leyel for medical malpractice to be adjudged by the medical faculty. Until then Worm still believed that the case had been successfully hushed up through his and others' interventions.[36]

For Leyel the treatment of Jytte Brok came close to destroying his career and reputation. It also underlined the risks physicians were exposed to when the treatment of influential, noble patients went awry. The fact that Worm became involved may well have saved Leyel, even if Worm clearly took care to distance himself from Leyel's approach and treatment. Worm may have been able to calm things in the short term, but not for long, since Tycho Brahe submitted his complaint to the king and the University Council on 2 May. In his complaint of malpractice against Leyel Brahe, helpfully for Worm, had pointed out that it was Worm's involvement which had saved his wife's life. The medical faculty presided over by Thomas Fincke found that Leyel had acted properly and could not be held responsible for Jytte Brok's ailment. Thomas Bartholin found the documents from the case, Tycho Brahe's complaint, Tancred Leyel's statement, and the judgement by the dean of the medical faculty, Thomas Fincke, significant enough to include them in his *Cista Medica Hafniensis* published in 1662.[37]

2 Forensic medicine

It is an open question whether Ole Worm was directly involved in the case against Tancred Leyel which was brought before the medical faculty. As one of the two professors in the medical faculty he would normally have been involved in adjudging such a case. However, the fact that he had been involved in her case as a physician might well have disqualified him from joining Thomas Fincke in making a decision in the case. Something which would appear to be confirmed by the fact that only Thomas Fincke signed the faculty's votum.

Forensic medicine had become a growing area for the medical faculty of Copenhagen to exercise its expertise within during the early seventeenth

---

36 *Ibid.*, no. 808.
37 See Thomas Bartholin, *Cista Medica Hafniensis*, ed. Niels W. Bruun and H-O. Loldrup, Copenhagen 1982, 159–63; for Tancred Leyel, see V, Ingerslev, *Danmarks Læger og Lægevæsen fra de ældste Tider indtil Aar 1800*, vol. 1, Copenhagen 1873, 338–39; see also E. Hovesen, *Lægen Ole Worm*, Aarhus 1987, 212–13.

century. The two professors of medicine at the university were generally joined by a couple of specially appointed physicians for each case, mainly recruited from among the royal physicians or the Copenhagen based physicians. This group would then either discuss the case based on written evidence or supplement it by an examination of the people involved in the case, but at this point in time they had yet to undertake forensic dissections.[38]

After he had been appointed professor of medicine in 1624, Worm was involved in a number of forensic medical cases which were referred to the medical faculty by the chancellor and the king.

In April 1630 the king asked the medical faculty to provide a statement about a presumed murder of an unborn baby in Scania, killed by an attack on the mother. They were ordered to examine witnesses before reaching a verdict and summoned the accuser, Gertrud Mortens, the accused, Jens Nielsen, and all the witnesses. Worm and Thomas Fincke were joined by the royal physician Henning Arnisæus, and another two Copenhagen physicians. Each of the physicians provided a statement before a joint verdict was given. Arnisæus, who held an MD from the University of Helmstedt and had been professor of moral philosophy at that university before becoming physician to Christian IV in 1619, appears to have had a particular interest in forensic medicine.

First the physicians concluded that it was possible for a foetus to die inside the mother and putrefy there. It could remain unborn not only for a couple of weeks, but for several months until it was expelled through the normal or 'even abnormal' routes. A pregnant woman would be able to conduct her regular housework during this period. They concluded that Gertrud Mortens was a good example of that. The physicians determined this not only from the evidence given by the women who were present when Gertrud gave birth to the dead baby's bones, but also from having inspected the small bones which she had continued to expel. That the foetus, as claimed by the mother, was more than twenty weeks old they accepted from the size and strength of the bones.

From all the evidence they had heard they were, however, unsure about the reason and time of the death of the foetus. Even if Gertrud had produced a witness who declared that he had seen Gertrud brutally attacked by Jens Nielsen, he had been forced to admit that he was too far away to be able to determine whether Jens Nielsen had hit her with his stick or his hands. They believed that she had been flogged with bare hands, but did not find proof that the strokes were of such a nature or so violent that they could have killed the foetus. Daily experience informed the physicians that even if pregnant women often were mistreated with too forceful medical remedies, or strokes and violence, it did not affect their health, and they were able shortly afterwards to give birth to healthy children.

---

38 *Cista Medica Hafniensis*, 127

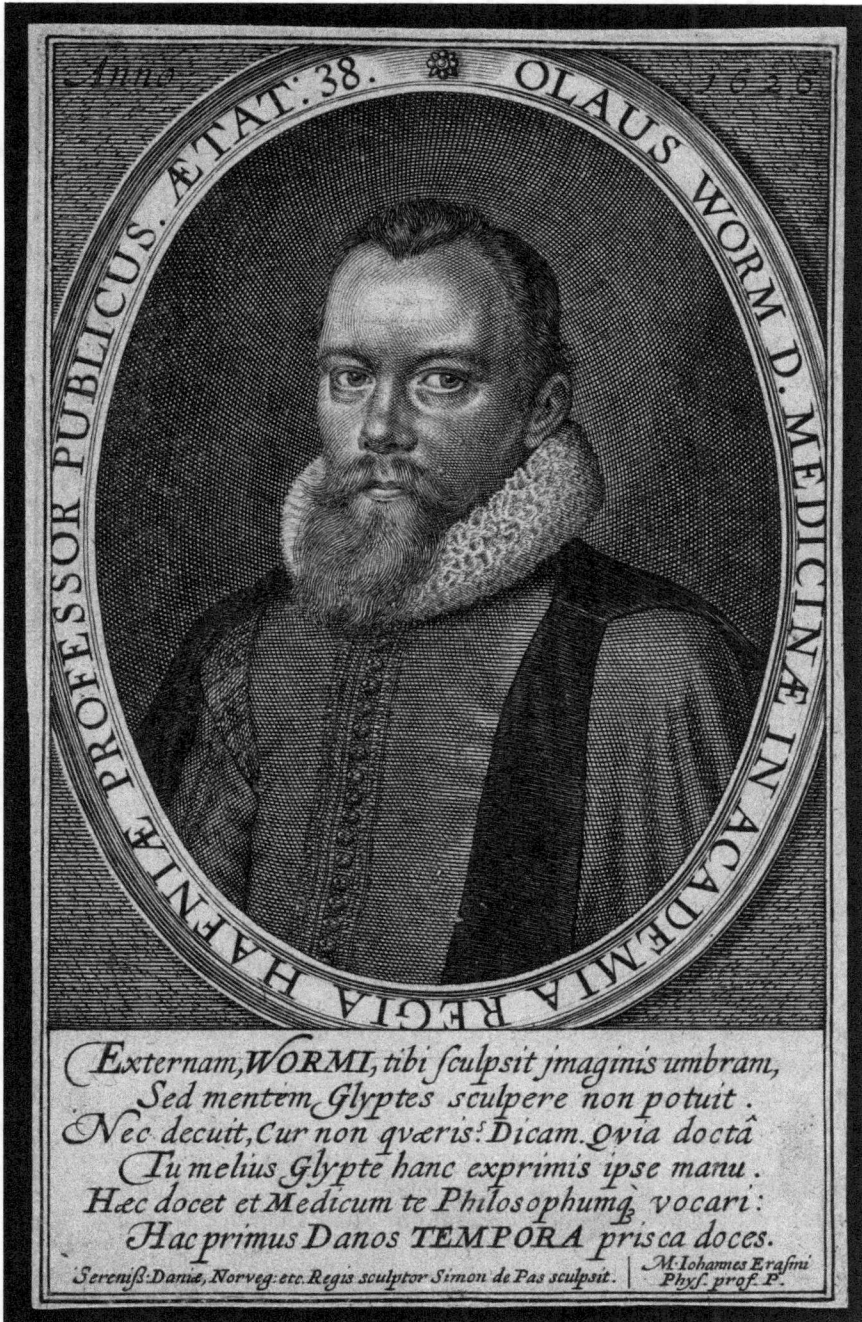

Figure 1.5 Ole Worm (1588–1654) age 38, by Simon de Pas; courtesy of the Royal Danish Library.

Furthermore, it was commonly accepted that foetuses did not exclusively die from strokes, beatings and other physical violence, but to a considerable degree also from other internal causes, such as a disadvantageous position of the foetus, or if the mother was exposed to extreme mental and bodily movements. Likewise many other conditions could cause the vessels in the tiny body of the foetus to burst, especially in women who were already disposed to abort. Gertrud had freely admitted that her first child had been stillborn, only an hour after she had last noticed the foetus had moved. She had neither been hit nor beaten up on that occasion.

Concerning the blue spot or pustule on her right hypochondrium about a hand's breath from her naval which had been drawn to their immediate attention by the judge, and which they had inspected carefully, the physicians felt unable to reach any decision, except that it was too high up for the foetus to have been affected. Furthermore, the physicians noted that Gertrud eight days after the incident had walked to church – a trip of a quarter of a mile – before she fell unconscious and had a discharge. They therefore concluded that these symptoms had proved of greater danger to the foetus after the long and exhausting walk rather than the earlier attack.[39]

Not all cases put before the medical faculty had necessarily reached the courts first. In 1632 the chancellor asked them to summon a surgeon from Malmø, Hans Kröger, and his patient, Peder Rasmussen, in order to determine whether the patient had suffered injury through the surgeon's treatment. The two of them appeared before Ole Worm and Thomas Fincke on 25 October. First the petition of Peder Rasmussen was read out, accusing the surgeon of having caused him disagreeable suffering which prevented him from opening his mouth; the injury was supposed to have been caused by the remedies containing mercury used by the surgeon after he had made an incision in the patient's throat. Johannes Kröger claimed that he had used no mercury remedies in his treatment. The surgeon provided a detailed list of the remedies he had deployed. He also explained how he had gently applied the necessary ointments which was confirmed by the patient. The surgeon also denied that he had made an incision in Peder Rasmussen's throat. He had only loosened the flesh around a tooth he intended to pull. After careful consideration of the evidence Worm and Fincke decided that they had found no evidence that the surgeon had used mercury based remedies, or that he had made an incision in the patient's throat. They therefore decided that the surgeon was not responsible for Peder Rasmussen's suffering.[40]

The case of a woman from Elsinore who stood accused of having murdered her foetus in September the following year caused Ole Worm to seek the advice of his friend the royal physician Henning Arnisæus. Worm

39 *Cista Medica Hafniensis*, 138–39; see also 140–48.
40 *Ibid.*, 148–49.

evidently felt exposed having been ordered by the chancellor to take charge of this case which had been referred to the medical faculty for its opinion, while the dean, Thomas Fincke, was absent on other business. In this instance Arnisæus was not officially appointed to join Worm and his colleagues in assessing the case, but only asked for his advice. Bearing in mind Henning Arnisæus's particular interest in this area of medicine his opinion would have been highly valued.[41]

An affidavit given by some local women in early April 1633 stated that the accused, Margrethe Johannesen, had been found to have milk in her breasts and traces of skin lesions on her stomach and abdomen as if she had given birth. Three weeks later Margrethe had admitted that she had had sex with a young man three weeks before Easter the previous year and fallen pregnant. She had then lost the foetus around Midsummer Day. It had not been bigger than a goose egg and not knowing what it was she had thrown it on the dunghill. Henning Arnisæus provided Worm and his colleagues with a detailed report on the case. Interestingly Arnisæus suggested a much harder approach to the case finding Margrethe's explanation far from convincing. Evidently the moral philosopher Arnisæus found there was a case to answer.

The verdict by Worm and Fincke proved less incisive. They had no doubt that Margrethe Johannesen had been pregnant, but felt unable to conclude that it had been her fault that the foetus had died or had been expelled, because of her taking remedies to bring this about, based on the documentation they had been provided with. Furthermore, they felt unable to decide whether or not the foetus had been further developed than the accused claimed.[42]

The medical faculty was asked to examine a similar case in 1635 about a woman from Halland who had been found to have milk in her breasts and was suspected of having killed her foetus. This time round, however, the professors of medicine felt the evidence provided made it impossible for them to provide a judgement and returned the case to the court for clarification.[43]

To judge from this small sample dealing with medical malpractice and foetus or child murder which were referred to the medical faculty for evaluation, the two professors Ole Worm and Thomas Fincke proved careful and guarded in their responses and considered any medical doubt to benefit the accused. They proved reluctant to condemn the women who had been accused of having murdered their recently born or unborn children on the

---

41 See Henning Arnisæus, *Disquisitiones de Partvs Hvmani legitimis terminis. Ejusdemque Observationes & Controversiæ Anatomicæ*, Frankfurt 1641
42 *Cista Medica Hafniensis*, 151–56 and *Breve fra og til Ole Worm*, nos. 494, 496 and 497.
43 *Cista Medica Hafniensis*, 165–57.

basis of the evidence presented to them.[44] Similarly they sided with their medical colleagues in the two cases of malpractice they adjudged. This was not particularly surprising in the case of the Malmø surgeon, but certainly in the case of their Copenhagen colleague, Tancred Leyel, who clearly had a case to answer and having found himself accused by the influential nobleman, Tycho Axelsen Brahe. Here evidently shared professional interest and collegiality won the day.

3 Patients from Iceland and the Faroe Islands

Among Ole Worm's many patients were a number of Icelanders, many of whom had made Worm's acquaintance while studying at the University of Copenhagen. Some had resided with him, while others he had become acquainted with through his interest in history and antiquarianism. These Icelanders consulted him by letter and Worm offered his diagnosis as best he could and sent them medical remedies which were capable of tolerating the long voyage between Copenhagen and Iceland. Worm's interests in the runes and ancient monuments also brought him into contact with Icelanders he had not encountered before such as the learned headmaster of the Latin school at Holar, Arngrim Jonsson, whom he made contact with in the summer of 1628.[45] Until he approached Ole Worm for medical advice the following year Jonsson appears to have been a patient of Worm's father-in-law Thomas Fincke. However, he wanted Worm's advice on how 'to face the difficulties of old age'. Jonsson explained that this evil was well known to many of those who were inclined towards the phlegmatic. He appears to have suffered from two complaints. The first being slime which gathered in his lungs and was difficult to dislodge by coughing; the second being a complaint about itching skin. Arngrim had received plenty of advice from learned friends none of whom appears to have been medically trained. Some had recommended syrup and juice to cleanse his chest; others advised him to have 'a general purgation' which would benefit both brain and blood; he had also been told to have sweating treatment. On top of that, he had been

---

44 Ole Worm clearly retained a considerable interest in illegitimate pregnancies and births as can be seen from the disputation he held with his student Jacob Hasebard in May 1621 where the question, whether the presence of milk in women's breasts proved they were pregnant, was debated, *Cista Medica Hafniensis* 128–37; see also the disputation with Caspar Ringelman from November 1632 where it was discussed whether a foetus born in the eighth month of pregnancy could survive, Hovesen, *Ole Worm*, 170. In February 1638 Ole Worm asked Henrik Ernst in Paris about a sentence he had heard had been pronounced by the Parliament of Grenoble, acquitting a woman as honest and innocent, who had fallen pregnant and given birth without having had intercourse with her husband. Worm was inclined to consider it a tall story, but if it was true, he was keen to see what medical rationale the judges had relied on, *Breve fra og til Ole Worm*, no. 701.

45 *Ibid.*, no. 202.

advised to use the acidic springs available in Iceland, but this did not appeal to him, nor did he believe that he would gain any benefit from bathing in them. His preference was the use of some of the sweeter syrups which did not generate vomiting, or remedies which would bring about sweating without any danger to him, but he was open to whatever treatment Worm might suggest. Finally, Arngrim also wanted Worm to discuss an 'old complaint' of his with Thomas Fincke. For some time he had suffered from a headache in one side of his head accompanied by deafness in his left ear. Furthermore, symptoms in his lungs and diaphragm had made him short of breath and his voice less sonorous. When walking 'his tired chest' quickly affected him. His head could tolerate neither cold nor heat, and the slightest coolness affected the back of his head. This was evidently a major concern for Arngrim, because that was where he thought the memory was situated. If that was weakened he considered it an omen of his approaching death.[46] Worm provided a supportive response:

> I would be delighted to offer you advice on your health if I could be with you; however you shall find me a faithful Achates [Aeneas's loyal companion on his journey to Sicily], because I shall not remain totally idle. As far as I can determine the cause of your headache and difficulties in hearing, and even your difficulty in breathing and the itching (which appears in a particular smarting and sharp form) is a, for your age, particularly threatening catarrh, which partly runs into the head and chest and partly affects the whole condition of your body; from what you yourself so sensibly explain I have no doubt that you have drawn your own conclusions. And even if a number of remedies are needed to root this out which cannot easily be forwarded over such long distances without the risk of being spoilt I shall not be seen as someone who totally deserts his friend, but forward some pills; I have no doubt that if you take thirteen at a time when need demands it, that they will drive away most of the cause for so many signs of illness. But I forward three doses in order that you can keep them for when need arises.[47]

Later that year the Bishop of Holar, Thorlak Skulason, a former student of Worm's, sought his advice on an intestinal disease he had suffered from for three years. From the symptoms he was convinced it was an illness of the spleen, because the food he had eaten appeared undigested in his stools. He admitted that even if this might also happen as a consequence of an illness of the diaphragm, or in the liver, or as a result of a stomach chill, he was convinced that it was due to the spleen being clogged up. In

46 *Ibid.*, no. 288.
47 *Ibid.*, no. 354.

his response Worm stated that he was sorry to hear that the illness had become so severe that it was wasting Skulason and confirmed the Icelander's diagnosis. Worm explained that it would have been better if the disease had been treated much earlier; before it had set such deep roots, as he put it. However, he forwarded some remedies which he hoped would help. They consisted of some cut herbs which he advised Skulason to infuse in either wine or beer for a minimum of twenty-four hours. The infusion should then be drunk at six in the morning and the same medicine should be taken six hours later, while fasting. If needed, this should be repeated. Worm also added a single dose of pills which were to be taken if the infused wine/beer did not deliver the expected result. In order to strengthen the stomach and the intestines Worm included a powder, half a spoon of which should be dissolved in either soup or wine and taken at lunch and dinner. He also recommended that an electuary be taken at bedtime. If all these remedies proved too much for Skulason Worm advised him to stop taking the infusion for a couple of days. But first and foremost Worm advised him to watch his lifestyle and to enjoy good, juicy, and easy to digest food, such as meat from young animals and poultry and only to take drinks without sediment and have the occasional sip of bitters.[48]

The following year the headmaster Arngrim Jonsson wanted to know about the medical application of tobacco. He had encountered it through some of the sailors arriving in Iceland who had emphasised its medical value. Worm responded by first referring him to the work of Carolus Clusius and then a recent book by Johannes Neander, *Tabacologia*[49], published in Bremen in 1622. Then he went on to explain that it was a plant that was particularly beneficial to cold and moist constitutions, when used in moderation as with other medical remedies. When it was smoked in a pipe, as done by sailors, Worm claimed it removed slime from the brain and the sensory organs and made the brain dry by removing inflammation. Worm emphasised that the drug had absolutely no damaging effects on moist constitutions. He claimed that an amount similar to the size of a nutmeg dissolved in a glass of wine at night time worked as an emetic, but pointed out that he did not know whether it could be consumed in its pure form.[50]

Bishop Thorlak Skulason continued to rely on Worm's medical advice for decades. He was complaining to Worm about his failing health in the mid-1640s. Worm concluded from his letter that the Bishop suffered from scurvy which he claimed affected Skulason in a variety of ways. Worm argued that this was a well-known illness among people living in coastal

48 *Ibid.*, nos. 368 and 404.
49 Johannes Neander, *Tabacologia: Hoc est, Tabaci, Seu Nicotianæ descriptio Medico-Cheirurgico-Pharmaceutica: Vel Eius præparatio & usus in omnibus corporis humani incommodes*, Bremen 1622.
50 *Ibid.*, nos. 416 and 440.

areas. The best way to cure it was through constant exercise and a diet aiming at dryness. He recommended the use of mustard and horseradish mixed into the food, and the plant cochlearia, known as scurvy-grass, which normally grew plentifully at the seaside, as a particularly efficient remedy. Worm advocated the use of its juice or simply eating its leaves three to four times a day. He emphasised that he recommended these remedies because he expected them to be readily available in Iceland. Worm also forwarded some of his own remedies which he was convinced would improve Skulason's health if they were taken at the right time. For an astrological physician such as Worm timing remained essential. Worm also included an ointment which Skulason should brush onto his loose teeth several times a day in order to restore and fix them.

When Bishop Skulason thanked Worm nearly a year later he sent him a copy of the first Icelandic Bible he had had printed at Holar, plus two pairs of winter stockings his wife had knitted. However, only the letter reached Worm because the Icelandic merchant who was supposed to take the goods and the Bible to Copenhagen had been shipwrecked.[51] The following summer Worm received another copy of the Icelandic Bible, and stockings for his whole family from Skulason. His medical remedies, however, had proved a disappointment. Worm pointed out that the lengthy transport in summer temperatures was likely to have destroyed much of their power. Once more he told Skulason to make use of the local plants he had recommended and to change his diet. He took the opportunity to include a small treatise in Danish about the treatment of scurvy he had written for the medical faculty on the order of King Christian IV.[52]

Bishop Skulason continued to suffer from ill health and to struggle with his loose teeth. A year later he requested Worm to supply him with a remedy which could fix his teeth. He had already lost two molars while the rest of his teeth were close to falling out. As always Worm offered his support and despaired of the distance separating them which made it impossible for him to properly examine Skulason, while the medical remedies he could supply were in danger of being spoiled by the long journey. Worm remained convinced that Skulason suffered from scurvy and recommended the use of a variety of local plants such as scurvy grass. He forwarded a powder for Skulason's loose teeth which he instructed him to apply to his gums repeatedly. Worm was convinced that it would work especially if Skulason made an effort to cleanse his body of damaging fluids at the same time.[53] However, the plants Worm recommended were not available in Iceland, so Skulason asked him to send extracts of them and instructions for their use. Consultation by letter between Iceland and Copenhagen was never

51 *Ibid.*, nos. 1221 and 1238.
52 *Ibid.*, nos. 1336 and 1425.
53 *Ibid.*, nos. 1445 and 1506.

a speedy process often taking a year before medical remedies and advice could be provided.

By the autumn of 1647 Bishop Skulason also wanted Worm to prescribe medical remedies for his wife to cleanse her brain and chest. She had been badly affected by an illness which Skulason was unable to identify. Accordingly he had failed to find an 'antidote'. He emphasised that his wife was increasingly affected by palpitations and absent-mindedness.[54] When Worm responded in June 1648 he forwarded medical remedies which were less likely to lose their efficacy over time. They included pills which would cleanse the body of evil liquids, but had to be taken in large quantities. Herbs in paper which were useful against scurvy, when marinated for twenty-four hours in whey, resulting in a juice to be regularly drunk at six in the morning. To fortify themselves Skulason and his wife should drink a spoonful or two of the water Worm had forwarded. As a remedy against his wife's complaint Worm sent her a fine purging powder which should be dissolved in thin soup or wine and drunk. He added that it was difficult to prescribe remedies at such a great distance without having been able to see the patient. Furthermore, he underlined that what he had sent would have to do until he received further information about its effect and other conditions.[55]

Worm also provided the other Icelandic Bishop, Brynjulf Sveinsson on Skalholt, another former student of his, with occasional medical advice such as in July 1648 when Brynjulf wanted him to supply him with a recipe for a remedy for the evacuation and cleansing of all fluids, and the driving out of superfluous liquids 'to be used by healthy people'. Ten months later Worm dispatched two doses of pills for general use advising Brynjulf to take no less than fifteen at a time by a waning moon at six in the morning, staying inside all day, avoiding sleep and not taking lunch until noon. As always Worm demonstrated his dedication to astrological medicine.[56]

Ole Worm also continued to provide the headmaster of the Latin school in Holar, Arngrim Jonsson, with medical advice. He informed him that the ointment he used was ineffective against scurvy. Instead, he advised him to use extracts from the same plants he had pointed Skulason towards. He told Jonsson to put his legs in a decoction of those plants, forcing the sweat out which would prove particularly beneficial for his tibias. Worm also forwarded ginger, liquorice juice, and two rings of walrus tooth to prevent convulsions. Furthermore, for a woman who had an illness of the spleen Worm sent a 'lump of ointment', part of which should be rubbed into a cloth on a daily basis and used to cover the 'diseased spot'. Born in 1568 Arngrim Jonsson was close to eighty in 1647 when he asked Worm for more liquorice juice and some medical remedies which had previously been

---

54 *Ibid.*, no. 1533.
55 *Ibid.*, no. 1591.
56 *Ibid.*, nos. 1596 and 1632.

prescribed by either Worm or his father-in-law Thomas Fincke. Added to that Jonsson had also lost his spectacles and wanted Worm to find replacements, preferably two pairs.[57]

Worm also provided Jonsson's son Thorkel, a student at the University of Copenhagen, with medical care and reported back to his father about his health. The pills Arngrim Jonsson wanted proved impossible for Worm to supply because he had not previously prescribed him any, and he had no idea what diseases they were meant to treat; had he known, he would have forwarded some. However, instead he supplied some 'common' pills which he expected would prove useful. They had to be taken in large quantities, between nine and thirteen at a time. Worm also included herbs and plants which were useful against scurvy and intestinal diseases, and would have a mild purifying effect on the body. Detailed instructions for their preparation and use were included. Similarly, for obvious reasons, Worm had reservations about finding Jonsson replacement spectacles. Worm knew nothing about Jonsson's sight, but after having taken the advice of his son, he forwarded a couple of pairs, which he hoped might serve him. Bearing in mind the time it took for letters and goods to be transported between Iceland and Copenhagen it is unlikely that they reached Arngrim Jonsson before his death that year.[58]

Worm was also approached directly by some of the Icelandic students at the University of Copenhagen for medical advice as can be seen from the letter of Torfi Jonsson. Jonsson was approaching Worm on behalf of his uncle, the surgeon Magnus Gissurarson. He was seeking Worm's advice on how to heal his wife who often lost consciousness. Gissurarson was of the opinion that this was caused by her womb or uterus moving upwards, causing her heart to tremble with fear, while her lungs seeking to cool the heat were pulling back towards the collarbone and the chest like bellows, causing a compression of the windpipe, thereby impeding her breathing. He referred to Marsilio Ficino, Albertus Magnus, and others who prescribed beverages against the rising of the lungs as evidence for this view. However, whether this was so, or whether her loss of consciousness had another cause, he left for Worm to decide. Torfi Jonsson asked Worm to prescribe a remedy which he would then obtain from the apothecaries in Copenhagen and send to his uncle in Iceland.[59]

Even Icelanders such as the wealthy grandee, Gisli Magnussen, occasionally sought medical advice from Worm. In 1648 he wanted him to recommend medical remedies for a number of people in his locality who suffered from a variety of diseases such as leprosy, the French pox, and paralysis of the feet.[60]

57 *Ibid.*, nos. 1503 and 1529.
58 *Ibid.*, no. 1590.
59 *Ibid.*, no. 1328.
60 *Ibid.*, no. 1609.

Worm also provided medical advice to a few Faroe Islanders. Thus, he provided the minister Hans Rasmussen from Thorshavn with cleansing and sweating remedies for his wife in the summer of 1646.[61] In May the following year Rasmussen sent his wife to Copenhagen for treatment of a catarrh which affected her eyes, knees, and ankles. Hans Rasmussen considered the moist climate in the Faroe Isles to be the cause of many diseases while there were no barbers to bleed people on the islands.[62] A year later his wife was back in Thorshavn and Rasmussen thanked Worm for his service. However, she was now menstruating two to three times a month and he asked Worm for medical remedies.[63] They were duly dispatched and Hans Rasmussen expressed his gratitude in September 1650 pointing out how he had observed his wife's illness peak every month around the time of the new moon, the full moon, when the sun turned towards Equator, and during storms and when the wind blew from the south.[64]

In April 1652 Worm supplied drugs for the widow of the predecessor of the new minister in Thorshavn, Lucas Jacobsen Debes. Pills and theriac was sent with Debes son and Worm advised that there were two doses of pills, in case the first did not solve the problem. She could then take the second or keep it for later use if the symptoms returned. Since the widow had seen an improvement in one side of her body after an opening had been placed in her arm to drain off impure matter Worm recommended that the same procedure be applied to the other arm.[65]

Evidently medical expertise was difficult to find on both Iceland and the Faroe Iles and the fact that Ole Worm was closely engaged with students from these remote parts of the kingdom made him an obvious person to seek medical advice from. Worm was known to them and proved a loyal friend. Furthermore, Worm's interests in Nordic history and antiquarianism served to reinforce these contacts. Many of his former students who also became his patients proved absolutely essential for his antiquarian interests and enquiries. He was indirectly remunerated by important historical and antiquarian information and with objects for his cabinet of curiosity, while also being directly paid in woollen stockings, barrels of butter, and stock fish.

4 The interactions of Worm with other physicians

When sending Danish plants and seeds to his former tutor Caspar Bauhin, in Basle in 1618, Worm pointed out that many of them remained unknown to most learned botanists. This was according to Worm due to the fact that they had for the most part been named by peasants and common

---

61 *Ibid.*, nos. 1444 and 1493.
62 *Ibid.*, no. 1497.
63 *Ibid.*, no. 1604.
64 *Ibid.*, nos. 1653 and 1700.
65 *Ibid.*, no. 1720.

people, something he linked to the fact that medicine in Denmark to a large extent remained dominated by barbers, women, and charlatans.[66] Understandably Worm was a forceful advocate of learned medicine. Not surprisingly he favoured medical regulation and control by him and his fellow physicians. A year later he approvingly informed his friend Niels Christensen Foss, then in France, that a royal order had been issued stopping all empirics and quacks from plying their trade without the permission of the medical faculty, adding that further regulations had been introduced for apothecaries and surgeons which he hoped would have a positive effect.[67]

Six years later Worm was involved in the treatment of a patient together with his friend Niels Christensen Foss, now a physician in Lund. Evidently things had not gone to plan for the two of them. Foss had clearly prescribed too forceful a laxative for the patient. Worm, however, argued that was not the reason the patient's life had been in danger, but rather the patient's own carelessness. He had not only neglected to take the prescribed drugs at the recommended time, but he had also neglected the medical advice given. Worm had repeatedly informed those present to that effect, but had left immediately when an 'empirical herbalist', as he described him, had been summoned with whom Worm refused to be associated. That the patient had been cured had according to Worm been due to good fortune rather than the treatment given.[68]

By the late 1620s Worm's medical practice kept him busy and he claimed that he simply did not have the necessary time available to take on the role of historian and antiquarian too. That this was not just an excuse can be seen from the evidence of others. Thus, his student Hans Andersen Skovgaard, when briefly back in Copenhagen from Padua at the end of 1625, had found it impossible to see Worm because of the daily demands from Worm's extended medical practice. Some years later when writing to his friend Johannes Cabeljau in Germany Worm complained that the daily demands of his medical practice prevented him from serious studies and research.[69] In the autumn of 1638 he referred to the burden of his medical practice which lately had forced him away from home to attend patients in the most remote areas of Sealand.[70] In 1640 when writing to his friend the physician Ambrosius Rhode in Norway Worm even claimed that his considerable medical practice prevented him from fulfilling his duties at the university. A view which may well have been influenced by the fact that he suffered from a dangerous fever at the time.[71]

---

66 *Ibid.*, no. 42.
67 *Ibid.*, no. 55.
68 *Ibid.*, no. 150.
69 *Ibid.*, nos. 220, 193, and 489.
70 *Ibid.*, no. 735.
71 *Ibid.*, nos. 848 and 852.

Throughout his life Worm discussed medical cases with colleagues and provided them with advice and second opinions. Thus in September 1629 the physician Otto Sperling informed him that he had been called to Sorø, presumably to the Academy, to treat the young Henrik Fuiren, Worm's nephew, who had suffered from diarrhoea with blood in his stools for some days, without serious stomach pains, but accompanied by vomiting. Sperling was of the opinion that this might have been caused by Fuiren having eaten nuts and raw fruit. He asked Worm to send him medical remedies since there was no pharmacy in Sorø. A few days later Sperling informed Worm that Henrik Fuiren still suffered from vomiting which he in vain had tried to treat through the use of enema and theriac, the universal panacea. Worm approved of Sperling's use of rhubarb and tormentilla root. The latter an obvious choice for a botanist like Sperling and supposed to be particularly effective against chronic diarrhoea. Worm, however, took the opportunity to provide Sperling with the recipes for his own theriac and laxative when forwarding the requested remedies and rhubarb.[72]

Worm also corresponded about medical matters with his former student, the German, Ambrosius Rhode who had become town physician and professor in natural philosophy at the local gymnasium in Kristiania in Norway in the late 1630s. He agreed with Rhode that *nobilis hepatica* – liverleaf – was useful against scurvy. Worm pointed out that liverleaf also worked well against dropsy, neutralised constipation, encouraged the production of blood and strengthened Nature so that much evil matter is excreted and replaced by good. In his opinion it could also heal wounds. Finally he concluded that 'Nature was still hiding many treasures in its womb, but since one day must inform the next, we are forced to leave much to our successors'.[73] This was a statement which corresponded closely with ideas and thoughts Worm had put forward decades earlier when he took up his chair in natural philosophy.

In October 1647 Worm was consulted by his colleague in Aarhus, the German physician Johan Christoph Creuzauer, about the treatment of his brother-in-law Bishop Jacob Madsen. Creuzauer explained that the Bishop suffered from anxiety during the night and dizziness, pressure in the hypochondrium and numbness in right hand and foot. Creuzauer had applied cleansing remedies and remedies against scurvy without any result. Worm informed Creuzauer that he agreed with his treatment and in his opinion his brother-in-law stood a good chance of recovery if he followed his medical advice properly.[74] Not exactly a vote of confidence in his brother-in-law by Worm.

72 *Ibid.*, nos. 296–98.
73 *Ibid.*, no. 835. For Ambrosius Rhode, see J. Shackelford, *A Philosophical Path for Paracelsian Medicine. The Ideas, Intellectual Context, and Influence of Petrus Severinus: 1540–1602*, Copenhagen 2004, 377–81.
74 *Ibid.*, nos. 1546 and 1548.

Likewise his former student and friend, the physician Poul Moth, who was practising medicine in Funen, sought his advice in April 1648 about the treatment of two noblemen. The first, Axel Brahe (son of Tycho Axelsøn Brahe, who had died eight years earlier), had suffered from constipation since his youth most likely, in Moth's opinion, as a consequence of an unhealthy lifestyle typical of the Nordic region; even so Axel Brahe had travelled abroad with his tutor. In Barcelona he contracted smallpox, but having been healed, he did not have the necessary patience to cleanse the evil fluids, preferring instead the Spanish wine. Consequently he started to suffer from piles and sank into melancholy on the way home. After he came back his relations left his recovery to God and Nature. Now eighteen months after his return Moth had been sent for by his aunt [Birgitte Brahe]. Having provided Worm with his case history Moth wanted to know whether or not Worm agreed with his proposed treatment: cleansing through bleeding and the placement of a 'fontenelle' in Brahe's leg, followed by strengthening remedies. The second, Eiler Bille to Nakkebølle, forty-four years old, suffered badly from hypochondriac aches, and pains in arm and shoulder. A journey to the spas had given him some relief, but three weeks later the pains had returned. Nature had now found an opening through the leg which had resulted in the evacuation of water and matter, but he was at risk of developing gangrene. Moth had sent for his colleague Joachim Timmermann from Odense and several surgeons. Worm agreed with Moth's proposed treatment, adding that it was difficult to deal with patients – a reference to Axel Brahe – who refrained from following medical advice.[75]

A couple of years later Poul Moth once more sought Worm's opinion in a case where the patient had repeatedly refused to take both his and the professor of medicine at the Academy in Sorø, Georg Kruck's medical advice, but instead had asked for Worm's. The patient in case was the sixty-two-year-old mayor of Odense, Hans Nielsen Chulenbrun, of a choleric and occasionally melancholic temper. Chulenbrun had fallen down the stairs two years earlier after a feast given by Steen Bille. Moth had been called the following day and found that Chulenbrun had no temperature, but that his right side was black and blue, though without wounds. He had applied plasters and ointments, plus a mild purgation; Chulenbrun had made a quick recovery and been able to attend the coronation in Copenhagen. However, a couple of months later he began to develop piles. This Moth considered 'Nature's own expedient', but because he started to lose his strength Moth had bled him and given him an enema and fortifying remedies. Chulenbrun, who clearly believed in the value of a second opinion, had sought the advice of Georg Kruck when the latter arrived in Odense without informing Moth. Kruck had delivered his opinion in writing, advising sweating treatment and bleeding. Kruck may well have chosen this rather unusual

---

75 *Ibid.*, nos. 1573 and 1574.

approach to appear above board, making it possible for his colleague Moth to see his opinion. Understandably Moth sought out Kruck in order that they might act jointly. They then tried bleeding which resulted in a violent tertiary fever, which found its own way out through a violent nosebleed. Since then Chulenbrun had recovered even if he still suffered from pains and blood in his stools.[76] Worm would undoubtedly have agreed with Moth's and Kruck's treatment of the mayor.

1637 proved a significant year for Worm's medical practice. It was the year he was first called on to treat members of the royal household. Together with the botanist and physician Joachim Burser who had served as professor of medicine and natural philosophy at the Academy in Sorø since 1625 Worm was called on to attend two of Christian IV's many children with his second wife Kirsten Munk. The two young Countesses, Christiane who was ten and her sister Elisabeth Augusta who was fourteen, had caught a fever while residing at Antvorskov Palace in Sealand. Burser based in nearby Sorø was obviously the closest physician of some standing who could attend the two young girls, while Worm was drafted in from Copenhagen. By late February Worm had returned to the capital and Burser informed him that Christiane had been free of fever for four days while Elisabeth had been without fever the day before yesterday, but had suffered a minor attack yesterday. He was optimistic, even if he prescribed the girls purifying pills out of fear of a relapse.[77] The news from Burser became less positive towards the end of March. Burser had been unable to leave Antvorskov Palace while the two girls still suffered from fever attacks. However, he hoped that they would return to full health before the king's expected arrival at Antvorskov within the next few days. Worm thanked him for his report about 'their patients' and declared that if his presence was wanted on the king's arrival, he would return immediately to Antvorskov. However, he pointed out he suffered from the gastric problems which always bothered him that time of year. He bade Burser to draw this to the attention of the Lord Chamberlain in order that it might serve as an excuse for his absence.

By mid-April Joachim Burser had been called back to Antvorskov. The younger Countess was doing fine but the older, who was engaged to get married, had suffered a relapse. He had prescribed sweating treatment and intended to return to Antvorskov in three days. However, when he was about to post his letter a messenger had arrived informing him that Worm's presence was required in Antvorskov.[78] Worm responded immediately expressing his disappointment about the relapse of the young Countess, but he did not think his presence was needed because the patient was not, in his opinion, in any immediate danger. However, he took care to ask Burser to

76 *Ibid.*, no. 1703.
77 *Ibid.*, no. 629.
78 *Ibid.*, nos. 635 and 643.

inform him if his absence was causing offence. The fact that the king had returned to Copenhagen may well have influenced Worm's decision not to go to Antvorskov. Worm emphasised that he was at present tied down by a host of engagements and businesses with the result that he found it extremely difficult to leave home.[79]

This also meant that Worm was unable to attend one of his noble patients at the Academy of Sorø, Axel Skeel. He asked Burser to apologise for him to Axel's mother. Worm had clearly attended Axel Skeel when he had been at Antvorskov Palace in February treating the two young Countesses. By the start of March Burser had wanted to send Skeel to Copenhagen so Worm could look after him. Skeel had requested Worm to attend him again by mid-April, but Burser was of the opinion that had only been done for safety's sake. The young Skeel had evidently injured his head and one of his arms, but he showed signs of improvement. Burser reported that the previous Saturday Skeel had walked around the yard and garden in Sorø and slept well. Even so he had developed a headache in the uninjured side of his head which had been accompanied by a certain lethargy and convulsions, starting gently in the injured arm and then spreading forcefully to the rest of his body. According to Bucer young Skeel might have suffered from what appeared to have been epileptic attacks prior to his injury. Bucer's optimism, however, proved misplaced and Axel Skeel died five days later at the tender age of eighteen.[80]

In May 1644 Worm was back at the Academy in Sorø attending Ulrik Christian Gyldenløve, the son of Christian IV and his mistress Vibeke Kruse, who had caught measles. After Worm's return to Copenhagen the boy's tutor, the historian Jens Dolmer, informed him that the fourteen-year-old Gyldenløve was recovering quickly, especially after his somewhat hysterical mother had left the Academy and no longer disturbed his sleep. Worm was delighted and instructed Dolmer to rub Gyldenløve's blisters with, fresh, sweet almond oil, immediately after they had formed scabs. He agreed with Dolmer that Vibeke Kruse's departure was good news, even if Vibeke herself had developed a painful tumour containing mucous on her wrist. This, in Worm's opinion, had been caused by anxiety and vigils, together with the jolts from her carriage which had stirred her scorbutic juices bringing forth the tumour. By early June the young Gyldenløve was fully recovered and the measles had left no scars only insignificant spots. Dolmer emphasised that he meticulously rubbed the marks on the young man's face with freshly pressed almond oil according to Worm's instructions, but that he found it increasingly difficult to keep the young man indoors. Worm expressed his satisfaction with how matters had proceeded and told Dolmer to stop rubbing the almond oil on the boy's face since Nature could be relied on to do the rest. He also instructed Dolmer to gradually allow

79 *Ibid.*, nos. 643 and 644.
80 *Ibid.*, nos. 622, 644 and 645.

Gyldenløve to be out of doors.[81] It would appear that Gyldenløve's case was part of a measles and small pox epidemic which was affecting Sealand at the time.[82] In the summer of 1644 Worm was summoned to Frederiksborg Palace to treat some courtiers who suffered from a type of epidemic dysentery.[83] 1644 proved a year when Worm found his medical practice extremely demanding. Writing to his friend the historian Stephanius in Sorø on Boxing Day he claimed to have been overwhelmed with visits to patients 'which hardly allowed him to draw breath' and now a nasty fever was spreading rapidly in Copenhagen killing many.[84]

In February 1650 Ludvig Pouch, town physician in Ribe contacted Worm about the treatment of the local mayor Hans Friis, who suffered from colic and kidney pains. Pouch informed Worm that Friis's urine had a red deposit and his stomach was distended and he remained unresponsive to medicine. At the same time he enclosed a drawing of a monstrous head of a girl recently born in Ribe who had lived for only twenty-six hours. Worm responded that he found it difficult to provide advice without seeing the patient, but nevertheless offered detailed advice for appropriate medical remedies.[85]

The French physician, Pierre Bourdelot, who served as royal physician to Queen Christina of Sweden during 1652–53 initiated a correspondence with Worm in the spring of 1652 sending him gifts for his cabinet of curiosity. This resulted in an exchange of letters about how to treat tertiary fever. Worm was recovering from this illness when he responded to Bourdelot's letters. He informed Bourdelot that an infectious fever was spreading rapidly in Denmark. Depending on the physical predisposition of the individual it had all the characteristics of tertiary fever. If it was treated appropriately Worm was of the opinion that it could be cured before the seventh attack, but for those who did not take care and neglected their lifestyle it often degenerated into double that and lasted seven to eight weeks. Worm had used the traditional remedies on himself, even bleeding, which he thought would amaze Bourdelot when he realised that Worm was sixty-five years old. It had, however, proved a useful antidote which caused intense perspiration defeating the evil before the fourth attack. Worm informed Bourdelot that he was waiting to see what would happen that evening, because the fever normally began with a light shiver around eight.

Worm was aware that the Dutch chemist and physician, Johannes Baptista Helmont, did not consider anyone a proper physician who could not overcome any fever on the third day, but he had his doubts that Helmont

81 *Ibid.*, nos. 1205, 1206, 1207, 1210.
82 *Ibid.*, no. 1215: A number of Henrik Motzfeldt's younger relations were ill with measles and small pox. No. 1242: Henrik Fuiren's mother had been seriously affected by a nasty case of small pox, but was recovering.
83 *Ibid.*, no. 1243.
84 *Ibid.*, no. 1264.
85 *Ibid.*, nos. 1678 and 1681.

could even do that himself. He added that likewise the professor of medicine at the University of Montpellier, Lazare Rivière, was known to have boasted of his ability to drive away any fever, even tertiary fever. If Bourdelot had any definite knowledge about this Worm begged him to share it with him. Worm pointed out that he had a colleague who always placed an amulet on the wrists of his patients for them to wear for nine days. This colleague claimed to have cured several hundred patients, but Worm remained sceptical and unable to confirm it. In fact, everyone who had used this treatment had begun by using the traditional remedies which he had greater trust in, especially the antipyretic. He asked Bourdelot to offer him his opinion about this approach at his convenience. Having received Bourdelot's response Worm pointed out that he agreed with him that curing the common tertiary fever through the use of amulets was a method promoted by empirics who shouted loudly about their secret remedies which might work in one case, but failed in thousands of others. However, Worm's experiences from his daily practice forced him to acknowledge that other signs emerged in those cases where Providence played the leading role over and above the normal causes. Speaking from experience he emphasised that if antidotes were not applied immediately the poison would seize the heart and subsequently destroy the patient. At that point frequent bleeding and the use of laxatives, according to the traditional approach, or the use of preventative remedies would have no effect. Worm took care to point out to Bourdelot that the illnesses which were rampant in the Nordic countries were severe and if their evil was not countered immediately those affected would perish. Worm praised Fracastorius's diascordium for evil fevers in particular, adding that when one had broken the power of the complaint all the symptoms became milder and progress could be more safely made with the traditional method. Worm, of course, was aware that Bourdelot was likely to be aware of these points; he therefore apologetically added a much used observation of his: but why bring owls to Athens[86]?

5 The friendship with Henrik Køster and the treatment of the Elected-Prince[87]

The German physician Henrik Køster, Senior, whom Worm had become acquainted with around 1631 when Køster arrived in Copenhagen, became a good friend and a regular correspondent.[88] It may well have been on

---

86 *Ibid.*, nos. 1725 and 1730; for Pierre Bourdelot's stay in Sweden, see O. Garstein, *Rome and the Counter-Reformation in Scandinavia. The Age of Gustavus Adolphus and Queen Christina of Sweden 1622–1656*, Leiden 1992, 580–83.

87 Denmark was an elective kingdom where the king was chosen by the council of the kingdom. Prince Christian was the first prince to be elected king before the death of his father, Christian IV. In effect he became crown prince, when at the age of seven he was elected and given the title elected-prince in 1610.

88 For Henrik Køster see Ingerslev, *Danske Læger*, vol. 1, 308–09.

Worm's recommendation that Køster settled as district physician in Odense a couple of years later.[89] His stay in Odense, however, proved of short duration. It only lasted a couple of years and fell well short of Køster's financial expectations. In July 1635 he accepted the position of personal physician to the Elected-Prince Christian and took up residence at the prince's court in Nykøbing Falster.[90] From then on the correspondence between Worm and Køster grew while Køster became increasingly reliant on Worm's advice. Initially, Køster was concerned whether he had enough experience for his new position, and like in Odense he was disappointed with his income. By 1637 he was evidently well enough regarded within the wider royal household to be able together with Ole Worm to recommend some pills for the use of the king, Christian IV. Their advice was appreciated, and Worm was able to inform him that the king used the pills with great satisfaction.[91]

Henrik Køster found life as personal physician to the elected-prince far from easy.

Prince Christian had long suffered from caries of the bone in one leg, and what Køster described as ruined and crumbling bones. This was likely to have been a consequence of the prince having caught the French pox. He was regularly attended by surgeons seeking to deal with this complaint. Towards the end of 1637 Christian IV had recruited a surgeon cum executioner from Glückstadt who had promised to heal the elected-prince permanently. Køster had his doubts, but had to admit that the start of the treatment looked promising, even if he thought that the executioner had promised more than he could possibly deliver. Not wanting to commit all his views to paper he informed Worm he would tell him more when next they met. By March the surgeon/executioner had been dismissed, but far too well remunerated for his, according to Køster, disastrous treatment, having been rewarded with 200 Reichsthaler and a large gilded silver jug. Køster considered him to be an irresponsible empiric who through his use of strong external remedies had caused gangrene around the wound in the prince's leg, not to mention pains in his chest and diaphragm, because of what Køster diagnosed as retention of fluids. He had been excluded from the surgeon's treatment of the prince. He therefore refused to discuss possible treatment with the surgeon whom he repeatedly referred to as a dangerous empiric.

Even after the dismissal of the executioner Køster found it difficult to control or influence the medical treatment of the prince. Not least because, a German surgeon/physician quickly arrived in Nykøbing Falster, namely,

---

89 *Ibid.*, no. 472. For Køster's involvement in the case against the Paracelsian empiric Hartvig Lohmann in Odense, see O. P. Grell, 'The Reception of Paracelsianism in Early Modern Lutheran Denmark: From Peter Severinus, the Dane, to Ole Worm', *Medical History*, 39, 1995, 78–94, especially 88–89.

90 *Ibid.*, no. 562.

91 *Ibid.*, nos. 622 and 626.

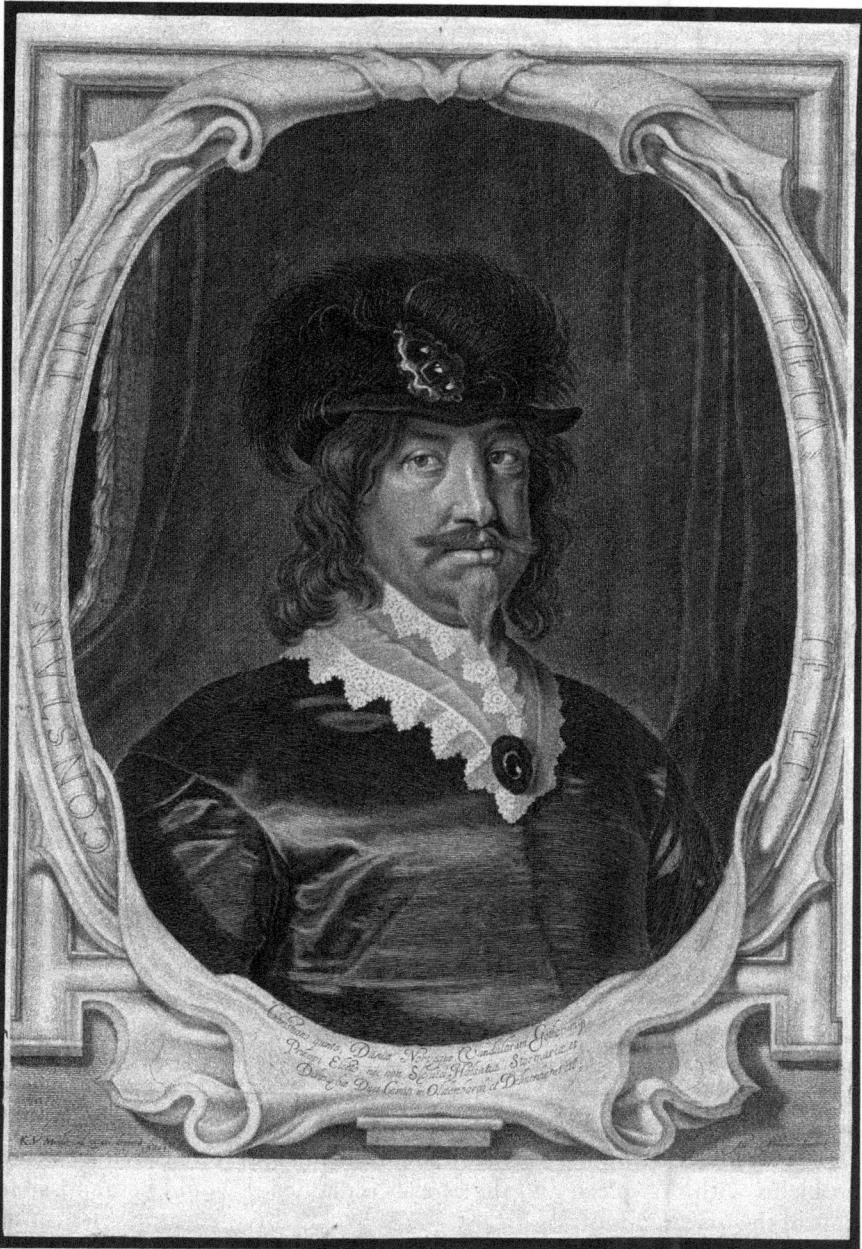

Figure 1.6 The Elected-Prince Christian (1603–47) by Karel van Mander; courtesy of the Royal Danish Library.

the physician to the elector of Brandenburg, Helvig Dietrich. Bearing in mind the fairly close contacts between the court of Brandenburg and that of Christian IV, whose first wife had been Anne Catharine of Brandenburg, Dietrich's arrival in Denmark was hardly surprising. Køster acknowledged that Dietrich was highly competent, but he disliked him because he considered him an 'ambitious and evil man', as he put it. By using a hot iron repeatedly on the prince's shin Dietrich had been able to stop the gangrene, but the treatment initially took its toll on the prince, who had suffered terribly and remained bedridden. However, within a short period the prince had been able to walk around his bedroom using a stick.

Worm shared Køster's disdain for the empiric from Glückstadt, but not his reservations about Dietrich, who happened to have sent a greeting to Worm through mutual friends; and Worm was keen to meet him.[92] Worm's positive attitude to Dietrich was never shared by Køster who found himself isolated and excluded by the Brandenburg physician who appears not to have trusted any of the physicians who had previously been involved in the treatment of the prince. Even so, Køster admired him as a surgeon, as opposed to his abilities as a physician. However, he continued to find Dietrich's pride and rude behaviour intolerable while simultaneously envying him his considerable rewards. He informed Worm that Dietrich had been given a large gilded, silver jug and a gold box containing a priceless diadem, which he had sent back to his wife. According to him Dietrich had also received more than 400 Reichsthaler in travel expenses, and it was rumoured that he had received two solid gold chains with portraits of the prince and his wife, not to mention the very large sum of 2,000 Reichsthaler. This was clearly a major cause of envy for Køster who struggled to obtain what he considered a decent salary at the court in Nykøbing Falster.[93]

Helvig Dietrich left the court in Nykøbing Falster after a brief and successful visit, but the improvement in the elected-prince's condition proved short lived. Køster, still dissatisfied with his own remuneration, informed Worm that the prince's health had deteriorated after Dietrich's departure. However, he had to admit that the leg/foot had improved, even if it was not fully healed, but the prince had developed digestive problems, which Køster thought were rooted in his spleen. This had spoilt his appetite and made sleep difficult, something which was not helped by the presence of two openings or drains in each foot. By then Worm was clearly tiring of Køster's repeated dissatisfaction with his financial situation, recommending him to hope for improvement, but also to accept 'what cannot be changed'. Worm expressed his sorrow for the prince's situation and agreed that as long as the problems with the spleen and the bowels remained it would be impossible to heal the diseased foot.[94]

92 *Ibid.*, nos. 686, 704, and 705.
93 *Ibid.*, no. 708.
94 *Ibid.*, nos. 730 and 733.

By the start of 1639 Køster's financial situation had finally improved, but he was still concerned about the damage done to his reputation as a physician and his standing at the court which he felt had been undermined by Helvig Dietrich. Meanwhile, the elected-prince's health had deteriorated further, and the newly appointed royal physician, Jacob Fabricius, had been sent to Nykøbing Falster by the king. Køster appears to have got on with Fabricius, not least because the latter shared his doubt about whether the elected-prince had been fully restored to health. They agreed that the complaint had been halted rather than cured. Recently, he informed Worm, the previously affected foot had once more become badly inflamed and caused great pain. A festering wound had opened up, not uncommon when the bone below was badly affected, according to Køster. This had been complicated by the skin around the wound starting to rot, something which would have spread rapidly if it had not been dealt with urgently.[95]

By the autumn of 1640 Ole Worm had become directly involved in the medical treatment of the elected-prince, and in early September he was present at the court in Nykøbing Falster. He was back at home in Copenhagen a week or two later only to be ordered back to Nykøbing Falster on 8 October. This may well have been on the order of Christian IV. Worm might well have taken on these duties with some reluctance if his comments to his friend Johannes Cabeljau in Amsterdam a couple of months earlier should be taken at face value. Worm had claimed that he was withdrawing himself from court life with approaching old age and would only become involved again if forced. Instead he would focus on his research when his daily practice and the complaints of his patients would allow him.[96]

The health of the prince had improved enough for him to undertake a lengthy journey through Jutland to Holstein that autumn. By January 1641 the elected-prince and his courtiers were on their way back via Antvorskov Palace. From there Køster reported to Worm that everything had gone well except that the prince still complained about hypochondrial pains every other night. The royal physician, Jacob Fabricius, had advised him to take a stomach powder, containing among other things quercetin and pimpinelle root and some pills fairly similar to what he and Worm had previously prescribed. Køster's advice was to wait and see, but he despaired about the 'impatience of great men', that is, the elected-prince. If the prescribed treatment did not work immediately, they sought help somewhere else. Worm was not surprised that the prince still suffered from hypochondrial pains. It was a case which, in his opinion needed to be treated carefully and demanded the full cooperation of the prince who would have to maintain a modest diet, avoiding eating too much food which was difficult to digest.[97]

95 *Ibid.*, no. 763; for Jacob Fabricius see DBL.
96 *Ibid.*, no. 843.
97 *Ibid.*, nos. 889 and 890

Meanwhile, Worm received further information about Dr Dietrich from his friend and former pupil, the Königsberg physician, Joachim Timmermann. He informed Worm that only two years earlier Helvig Dietrich had discovered a sulphur spring in his neighbourhood which he had convinced the then elector of Brandenburg, Georg Wilhelm, to drink from to the detriment of the latter's health. Rumours even had it, that Dietrich, who now resided in or around Königsberg, was to be charged with having murdered the elector through his prescription of strong emetics and mercury. Furthermore, Dietrich boasted that he had been offered the post of court physician to the elected-prince. By mid-April 1641 Worm was back at the court of the elected-prince on the order of the king. He remained at the court for some days before returning to Copenhagen where he received a report from Køster the following week. By then Helvig Dietrich had returned to Nykøbing Falster trying to secure a position for himself as court physician, pointing out how much he was in demand at other European courts from which he claimed to have received multiple offers of employment. Modesty was evidently not one of Dietrich's qualities. Within a week Dietrich had left again heading for Hamburg and then Dresden with the firm promise of returning after two months.[98] Shortly after Dietrich's departure Worm received another letter from Timmermann claiming that there was no substance to Dietrich's bragging which he, in Timmermann's opinion, shared with charlatans in marketplaces whose empirical methods he also advocated. Only his language abilities impressed Timmermann. By early July 1641 Dietrich was expected to arrive back in Nykøbing Falster to treat the elected-prince's foot which was troubling him once more. Dietrich made a brief visit to see the prince, before heading towards Königsberg via Elsinore. Worm was informed that Dietrich intended to move his family to Nykøbing Falster and act as an independent physician there, but expressed his reservations to Køster. Meanwhile, Dietrich had arrived at Gottorp Castle where he managed to become personal physician to the duke and where rumours had it, that he was also about to be appointed court physician to the elected-prince. Not surprisingly Køster felt somewhat exposed and concerned about his own position.[99]

Worm's medical practice within the wider royal households grew rapidly during the 1640s. In September 1641 he provided remedies for the treatment of Lady Elisabeth Gyldenløve, the king's daughter with his mistress Vibeke, which he forwarded to her tutor, Samuel Scherm. Later that month he travelled to Frederiksborg Castle to treat another of the king's daughters for an epidemic fever.[100] On 22 June 1644 Worm was among the physicians who were summoned to attend Christian IV who had returned to Copenhagen after the naval battle of Lister Dyb where he had defeated a Dutch-Swedish

98 *Ibid.*, nos. 913, 917, 919, 922, and 935
99 *Ibid.*, nos. 960 and 963.
100 *Ibid.*, nos. 966 and 972.

fleet.[101] Meanwhile, the elected-prince had been well enough to undertake a two months journey through the duchies in the summer of 1642. He had been accompanied by Køster who reported to Worm that they had encountered Dr Dietrich at the Ducal Court at Gottorp Castle where Dietrich had been engaged as extraordinary physician to the Duke with the promise of promotion to court physician in the immediate future. To Køster's consternation, the elected-prince had paid no less than 800 Reichthaler to a Jewish, physician and mathematician by the name of Rosales for setting his horoscope during their stay in Glückstadt.[102] Generous payments like that always irked Køster who felt underpaid and undervalued.

Køster continued to be concerned about his position and influence at the court of Prince Christian and his letters to Worm are full of worries about his job security and financial situation. By the beginning of 1643 he started to share the anxiety about his own health with Worm. By this stage he suffered from severe constipation and stomach problems. Worm recognised this as a common problem among 'the learned' and admitted to suffer from the same but in a milder form. Worm disclosed that he used the same pills containing ammonia as Køster, but with a different regime, he then proceeded to quote Crato who recommended not to consult physicians and use medical remedies in such cases. 'It was better if the stomach was well lubricated either by its own doing or through enemas or similar gentle remedies. Much depended on lifestyle which had to be planned correctly including those things which neutralised the dry and sluggish digestion of the bowels'. Worm then went on to provide Køster with a detailed schedule of his daily routine and in particular what he added to his diet. However, he concluded by referring to the fact that Køster in his opinion was too inclined towards worries and depression. As much as those concerns might be a product of his illness they might also be its cause in Worm's opinion. An unhealthy mind always resulted in an unhealthy body according to Worm. He recommended Køster to see more of his friends for lively discussion and good fellowship. Whether Køster followed Worm's advice we do not know, but a couple of month later he informed Worm he was on the mend.[103]

Later that year Køster had further cause to worry. The elected-prince intended to move his residence from Nykøbing Falster to Skanderborg Castle near Aarhus because of the abundance of fish, game and wood there. Køster was concerned about the costs to him personably and the difficulties in finding suitable accommodation in and around Skanderborg Castle. He planned to settle his family in Aarhus and asked Worm to recommend him to the Bishop of Aarhus, Morten Madsen. Meanwhile, the prince was once again on the mend and had travelled to Holstein. This time without Køster, who had managed to excuse himself. The fact that the elected-prince

101 *Ibid.*, no. 1224. See also Hovesen, *Lægen Ole Worm*, 222–23.
102 *Ibid.*, no. 1066.
103 *Ibid.*, nos. 1108 and 1115.

needed surgery while in Rendsburg on the foot he had previously broken
and where the bones were 'eaten away', as Køster put it, proved unfortunate, not least because the prince was attended by Dr Dietrich whom
Køster particularly distrusted and disliked. Even so Køster pointed out that
he felt justified about the doubts he had expressed a couple of years earlier
when Dietrich had first attended the prince and claimed to have healed
him. The roots of the illness had clearly not been properly dealt with, despite Dietrich's boast of having healed the foot. Worm did his best to reassure Køster, pointing out that his expenses on the removal to Skanderborg
might easily be retrieved because there was no physician in Aarhus or any
physician who could serve the nobility in the immediate neighbourhood.
He added that the Bishop was delighted to hear about Køster's immediate
arrival and hoped he would provide him with medical advice for his chronic
illness. Worm was surprised that Køster had not been called to the prince
in Rendsburg. He also wanted to know whether anyone else than Dietrich
had been involved in the treatment of the elected-prince. Worm always a
firm adherent of astrological medicine expressed his surprise that they had
commenced the treatment of the prince during the dog days.[104]

By August Køster informed Worm that the prince's condition was improving even if he had not been totally cured. This was due to the efforts of
Dietrich in particular, but he had been ably assisted by the surgeon who had
arrived from Lichtenburg the previous year, whom Køster described as very
experienced. Evidently Køster had finally improved his relations with Dietrich whom he stood in for when the latter became badly affected by gout
and bedridden. During the elected-prince's recent stay in Glückstadt, when
Køster had been allowed time off, he had been looked after by the two royal
physicians Jacob Fabricius and Jacob Janus. They, however, had been unable to agree on his treatment, but apparently without falling out.[105] Worm
was delighted to hear about the prince's improvement and asked Køster to
greet Dr Janus if he returned to Glückstadt and remind him of his promise
to Worm of a sweet smelling stone for his cabinet of curiosities. Worm
was sorry to hear that Køster once more suffered from serious constipation
and recommended him to try cream of tartar which he remembered had
proved useful against serious constipations. When used in soups it served to
remove the melancholic juice which had attached itself to the guts. Køster
was prevented from trying the remedy recommended by Worm because of
his move to Skanderborg. Instead he complained about heart trouble when
he had gone to bed.[106] The invasion of Jutland by Swedish forces based in
Germany under General Torstensson guaranteed that Køster and the court

104 *Ibid.*, nos. 1129, 1149, and 1152.
105 *Ibid.*, no. 1156; see no. 1079 for the arrival of the new surgeon from Lichtenburg.
106 *Ibid.*, nos. 1161 and 1165.

of Prince Christian only remained in Skanderborg for a few months. By January 1644 they had taken up residence in Frederiksborg Castle.[107]

Later when back in Nykøbing Falster Køster resumed his regular correspondence with Worm inquiring about the physician Otto Sperling, who was supposed to have fallen out of favour with the king; he also wanted to know whether or not plague had broken out in Copenhagen. Here in January 1645 Køster referred for the first time to the artificial sulphur well or spring invented by Dietrich and specifically recommended to the king. He had heard rumours that all the physicians in Copenhagen had rejected Dietrich's invention. In his response Worm commiserated with Køster about his continuing health problems, adding that his own health was as good as his age and frequent visits to the sick would allow. He pointed out to Køster that they were both wearing themselves out in the service of others. Worm was concerned about the dangerous fever in Copenhagen which had already killed a fair number of people even if he had yet to see any signs of plague in the capital. He denied that the Copenhagen physicians had rejected Dietrich's invention. However, the head of the government, Christen Thomesen Sehested, had informed the physicians through the royal apothecary, who had helped Dietrich in constructing the sulphur well, what minerals and braekvinsten had been used. They were, however, alarmed about the effect it had had on some of those trying it, including the king himself, causing dizziness, loose teeth, and other symptoms. Bearing that in mind they had advised the king to refrain from using the well.[108]

That Køster should take an interest in Otto Sperling's troubles with the king was hardly surprising bearing in mind Sperling's prominent position within the medical establishment in Denmark. Sperling, a German like Køster, had until recently had a spectacular career in Denmark. He had been made physician to the Children's hospital in 1637, royal botanist the following year, and city physician of Copenhagen in 1641 with title of royal physician. He had been part of the medical team, including Worm, who had treated Christian IV for his wounds after the naval battle at Colberger Heide the previous year. Worm explained that no decision had yet been made in Sperling's case, but that Sperling hoped the king might be influenced by his patrons to take a more positive view. Køster was delighted that the case against Sperling had stalled, and pointed out that the elected-prince was a supporter of Sperling and hoped that he could disentangle himself from his present difficulties with honour. A week later Worm reported that things looked much better for Sperling. Christian IV had been impressed by Sperling's supporters and a positive outcome was to be hoped

---

107 *Ibid.*, no. 1182.
108 *Ibid.*, no. 1270.

for, even if Sperling's accuser was the royal secretary Otte Krag who had no intention of giving up the case.[109]

Køster, however, was convinced that the rejection of Dietrich's artificial sulphur well by the Copenhagen physicians was of a more formal and serious nature than Worm had indicated, and that it had been issued by the medical faculty. He claimed their verdict had been presented to the elected-prince who had instructed him to find out, who the people were, who claimed to have suffered from loose teeth, not to mention the other symptoms referred to by Worm. Køster and the prince suspected that the loose teeth had been caused by scurvy rather than the sulphur well which contained a significant amount of sulphate, which worked against any easing, unless the faculty referred to the copious amounts of mercury which the sulphur well contained. Køster also wanted to know whether the medical faculty attributed the dizziness to braekvinsten or mercury. He himself attributed it to mercury which when plentifully present in a sulphur well affected the head, filling it and dissolving the liquids. Worm responded by forwarding Køster a copy of the short public advice which the medical faculty had issued against the severe fever outbreak in Copenhagen. This proved a timely publication appearing when the infection was spreading rapidly in the city. Worm also wanted to know whether the apothecary at the court of the elected-prince had originally assisted Dietrich in preparing his artificial sulphur well. If so, he wanted a detailed description of its content to see whether it was identical with what Dietrich had given some of his patients to drink in Copenhagen.[110]

A week later Worm informed Køster that no written verdict about the artificial sulphur well had been submitted. The Copenhagen physicians had been forced to give their advice after an influential, noble person had brought the case before them and had explained that much copper and iron had been added to the well. Having heard that the king and several noblemen had complained about dizziness after having taken the water and some of loose teeth, they had recommended the king to abstain from its use while he took other medical remedies. Because of these symptoms and the lack of clarity about what ingredients were in the sulphur well they had considered it unsuitable for the king.[111]

The issues raised by the artificial sulphur well gave rise to an intense correspondence between Worm and Køster in the first months of 1645. On Worm's request Køster approached the local apothecary in Nykøbing Falster to find out what ingredients were in the artificial well. However, the apothecary had been sworn to secrecy by Dietrich. Whether that made the case more suspicious, Køster left for Worm and others to decide. Even if he

109 *Ibid.*, nos. 1270, 1273, and 1276. For Otto Sperling see DBL.
110 *Ibid.*, nos. 1273 and 1274.
111 *Ibid.*, no. 1276.

failed to obtain the recipe from the apothecary Køster at least managed to find out that braekvinsten, sulphur, and soda had been added while red-hot tin had been cooled in the water. He was, however, not sure whether mercury vapours had been added.

Meanwhile, Worm and his colleagues had convinced a reluctant king to stop using the sulphur well with the result that his condition had improved significantly. The king no longer complained about being unable to sleep – a complaint he had shared with others – nor about suffering from dizziness. A report given by the royal apothecary Samuel Mejer about the use of braekvinsten, mercury, vitriol, and terra sigillata in the artificial well had convinced Worm to refrain from using it. He and his Copenhagen colleagues had also compared the water from Dietrich's artificial well with the water from springs in Prussia regularly imported into Denmark and found they differed significantly in both taste and colour.[112]

A disagreement between Worm and Køster about the composition and effects of Dietrich's artificial well had been brewing for some time before it came to a head in February. Both Køster and the elected-prince were delighted that the king was feeling so much better after he had stopped taking the water from the well. Køster was, however, not convinced that the sulphur well could be the cause of insomnia and dizziness, because dizziness was, in his opinion, more likely to result in sleepiness. Køster also forwarded a second sample of the water from the sulphur well made by their apothecary who continued to deny that mercury had been added. The apothecary, however, still refused to divulge the recipe. Køster had sampled the water a couple of times, but apart from having felt a weight on his chest a couple of hours later, he had recorded no positive or negative effect. He concluded that without knowing its composition he felt unable to recommend it. He could not come to a decision about unknown things except in so far as it was possible to estimate their beneficial or harmful qualities. In other words he was neither for nor against.

Worm was not pleased, pointing out that the symptoms shown by those who had taken the water from the artificial sulphur well were solidly documented and evidenced. All the patients and physicians involved remained alive and would support his diagnosis. The sick were all better after having stopped taking the water, so who, according to Worm, could reach a different conclusion 'unless they were prepared to disregard their senses'. Worm rejected Køster's view that dizziness resulted in sleepiness. This was only the case when someone was intoxicated by alcohol and then the reason for their sleepiness was not dizziness but anaesthesia. Furthermore, if mercury was not included in the water then the royal apothecary had misled them all, because he had personally assured them that a substantial amount of mercury had been added. It was not the differences in taste and colour between the imported sulphur spring water from Prussia and Dietrich's creation which concerned Worm and his colleagues, but the effects. Køster clearly realised that he was in danger of antagonising Worm and apologised. It was on the express order of the elected-prince that he had pursued the case and expressed the views which had displeased his friend. He thought that when Helvig Dietrich returned from Germany he would be vexed about the controversy his well had caused. However, the case appeared to rumble on with enquiries made on the prince's behalf to the king's personal physician Jacob Fabricius who had offered a different interpretation from Worm. Køster thought that Dietrich might try and place the responsibility on the shoulders of the apothecary in order to protect his own reputation. He then added rather peculiarly that Worm and his Copenhagen colleagues were excused because they had judged the case on the basis of reports and did not know more about the components of the artificial well than he himself; and that he would not recommend it until he knew the ingredients.[113] What exactly were Worm and his colleagues excused from? Køster may well by then have known about Christian IV's anger over the unauthorised investigation into Dietrich's artificial sulphur well and the possible fall from royal favour of the physicians involved.

If Worm had been wondering about the meaning of Køster's cryptic remark it all became clear within the next couple of weeks. By then Worm had realised that considerable commotion had arisen around Dietrich's sulphur well and that the crux of the matter had become his letters to Køster which were to be used as evidence in the case. Not surprisingly Worm was deeply unhappy about this development, asking what one was to do, when what had been privately communicated to a friend could be used in such a manner that it might cause danger and loss to them. Who in future would feel that they could safely communicate by letter with a friend he asked. Worm, however, declared that he was convinced that Køster would use his insight to make sure that no unpleasantness would befall Worm and his colleagues. Worm, in other words, applied considerable pressure to Køster to sort out a mess which he considered of Køster's making.

It had the desired effect. Køster was seriously rattled. He explained that his master, the elected-prince, as far as he understood, had demanded a statement from him on the king's order. He sent Worm a copy of the statement he had just made. Køster had read it out to the elected-prince while urgently entreating him to intervene with the king to make sure that Worm in particular should not suffer any negative reaction. Evidently Køster had acted on the elected-prince's instructions when he had questioned Worm about the Copenhagen physicians concern about Dietrich's artificial sulphur

---

113 *Ibid.*, nos. 1282, 1286, and 1291. For Jacob Fabricius, who had been an apprentice to Tycho Brahe and had become Royal physician to Christian IV in 1637, see J. R. Christianson, *On Tycho's Island. Tycho Brahe and His Assitans, 1570–1601*, CUP 2000, 276–77.

well. For this he now apologised. But he had clearly shown a lack of discretion when referring to Worm's letters during a lunch given by Prince Christian to guests and courtiers whereby it had become common knowledge at the court. Having read Køster's statement Worm expressed his satisfaction. However, he pointed out to his friend that the king still remained displeased with him, because he had corresponded with Køster about the matter. He saw no immediate way out of that because he was not given access to the king, so he could explain and apologise. He added that since things had gone that way it was better not to correspond about them in future and avoid the risk of losing the king's favour.[114] Not surprisingly Køster felt guilty and wanted to reassure Worm, informing him that the elected-prince had personally written to the king about the case on his request. As a result he was convinced that Worm would regain the king's favour. He explained that the king's anger had not been aroused by Worm's letters, but by the consultation undertaken by the Copenhagen physicians without royal authorisation. Meanwhile, Prince Christian had decided that the 'mistake' had been the apothecary's, concluding that the water did, indeed, contain mercury.[115]

It would appear that the unfortunate correspondence between Worm and Køster about the artificial sulphur well resulted in an interruption of their regular exchange of letters for around half a year. By August 1645, however, Køster could no longer contain his curiosity about rumours which had reached him in Nykøbing Falster about Christian IV's interest in the water from St. Helene spring near Frederiksborg. Christian IV had been interested in the spring for some time by then. He had visited the spring in 1639 and drunk the water, and at least twice, in 1640 and 1644 he had taken delivery of water from the spring. Despite warnings from the leading Bishop of the Danish Lutheran Church, Jesper Brochmand, about the use of such springs, the Helene Spring had become popular by the middle of the seventeenth century. By 1645 Christian IV wanted clarification about the potential medical benefits from the spring water. He ordered seven physicians, including Ole Worm and Otto Sperling to discover what minerals and metals were contained in the water and to assess its medical value.

Køster had been informed by Otto Sperling that he had received a sample from the spring and after having distilled it, he had found that it contained a small amount of salty soil. Køster wanted Worm to tell him if the sample also contained soda and whether he himself had discovered something different from his sample. Rumours of the wonderful power and properties of the water from the Helene Spring were rife at the court of Prince Christian. Worm informed Køster that as opposed to his six colleagues, who were excited about the water's potential, he had only discovered a variety of marl

---

114 *Ibid.*, nos. 1301 and 1302.
115 *Ibid.*, no. 1315.

mixed with ochre none of which was of any medical use. Worm admitted that rumours about the miracles produced by the water were also plentiful in Copenhagen, but among the people he had encountered who had actually drunk the water from the spring, none could claim to have been healed by it.[116]

A month later Køster wanted to know if Worm had come across a Württemberg physician by the name of Abraham Schopf who recently should have arrived in Copenhagen selling potable gold. Køster doubted that a potable gold, which had been completely dissolved, could be made. He asked Worm if he had experienced such a liquid which was supposed to be especially wholesome for the human body according to the chemists. Worm confirmed he had seen Schopf in public, but he did not know him personally. Worm shared Køster's doubts. He did not believe gold could be dissolved unless he had personally seen it done and tried it himself. He reminded Køster how the famous seller of potable gold, Anthonius Anglus, had fooled everyone. Personally he would only recommend those remedies which their predecessors considered safe, sound, and reliable based on extended experience.[117]

New regulations for the apothecaries were issued in 1645 and Køster wondered whether Worm had been involved. He hoped not, because he had discovered that they were full of mistakes. Worm reported back that he knew nothing about them until the bookseller Joachim Moltke had shown him a printed copy, but he could report that the apothecaries were unhappy about them. Later that year Køster informed Worm that a rumour had reached him that Dr Simon Paulli had demanded large annual payments from the Copenhagen apothecaries. Pauli had been appointed professor of anatomy at the University of Copenhagen in 1639. He was the son-in-law of the royal physician Jacob Fabricius. In 1645 he had become temporary city physician in Copenhagen while Otto Sperling was abroad and clearly saw this as an opportunity to make some easy money. Worm told Køster that not only had Paulli asked for far more money than he had been told – 500 rather than 200 Reichsthaler per annum – but he had also demanded free remedies for his household, plus paper and ink, 'and I know not what' as he put it. Worm clearly agreed with the apothecaries who refused to meet Simon Paulli's demand, pointing out that it was unheard of that a city physician should receive such payment for services the apothecaries neither needed nor had asked for.[118]

116 *Ibid.*, nos. 1338 and 1341; see also J. Chr. V. Johansen, 'Holy Springs and Protestantism in Early Modern Denmark: A Medical Rationale for a Religious Practice', *Medical History*, 41, 1997, 59–69, especially 64–65.
117 *Ibid.*, nos. 1348 and 1351.
118 *Ibid.*, nos. 1348 and 1351 for the regulations of the apothecaries; 1367 and 1371 for Simon Paulli's financial demands of the apothecaries; see also Schepelern, *Museum Wormianum*, 18–21 and 178–80. Paulli had never been shy on promoting himself and

By December 1645 Køster informed Worm that the elected-prince and his wife had decided to travel to the sulphur wells and springs in Langenschwalbe and Wiesbaden in Germany by early spring the following year, unless Dietrich changed their minds. Køster clearly considered Dietrich's influence paramount while he personally had his doubts about the value of such an expensive and dangerous journey at a time when the Thirty Years War was still raging in Germany. He assumed that Worm had been consulted and added that he was not unsympathetic towards the use of sulphur wells and hot baths as long as they could be used regularly. He finished his letter by inquiring about a young physician, Oluf Pedersen, recently returned from Italy and reputedly an excellent chemist who was selling potable gold and had been recommended to the court of Prince Christian. Worm, however, had not been consulted about the prince's planned journey to the German springs and spas, but expressed his best wishes for a fortunate outcome. He was aware of the recently returned Danish physician from Padua, but indicated that his talents might well be overestimated at the court in Nykøbing Falster. A couple of months later Worm had formed a more definite view of Oluf Pedersen. Pedersen had by then treated the king's mistress, Vibeke Kruse, and Worm had heard, that his intervention had not been appreciated by either the king or his mistress. Worm was well informed having lately attended Vibeke Kruse himself on several occasions and discovered that her complaint was not serious, but easy to treat as long as she would listen to sensible advice.[119]

By the end of January 1646 the king had given his consent that the elected-prince could undertake the planned journey to the sulphur wells and spas in Germany. Apart from Helvig Dietrich the prince should be accompanied by the Glückstadt-based royal physician Jacob Janus, who was considered an expert on wells and spas. By then Dietrich would appear to have lost the favour of Christian IV and been dismissed from the position of royal physician he had occupied since 1644. Køster had no doubt that Dietrich's fall from grace was linked to his failed treatment of the king's mistress, Vibeke Kruse, who continued to suffer from scurvy and rheumatism. Vibeke Kruse now relied on Jacob Janus and a Jewish physician from Hamburg, Benjamin Musjafa. Worm already knew of Dietrich's fall from grace, but had no idea why he had lost his position as royal physician, but he demonstrated his awareness of the fickleness of royal favour by stating that 'good fortune had to be treated cautiously and that Courtly favour was as brittle as glass'.[120]

---

exploit opportunities. In 1639 he had attempted to encroach on Køster's position at the court of the elected-prince by being made court physician. He failed, but managed to displease his father-in-law whom he had failed to consult.

119 *Ibid.*, nos. 1367, 1371, and 1399. Ole/Oluf Pedersen from Copenhagen eventually settled as a physician in Bergen, Helk, *Danske-Norske Studierejser*, 344
120 *Ibid.*, nos. 1381 and 1382.

By the start of 1646 some concern about the health of the privy councillor Knud Ulfeldt, who had accompanied Christian IV at the naval battle
at Colberger Heide and like the king had been wounded, was raised at the
court in Nykøbing Falster. Køster had been asked by Princess Magdalene
Sibylle of Saxony, wife of Prince Christian, to seek Worm's opinion on Ulfeldt's illness. Ulfeldt was evidently a favourite of the princess who had
proposed to organise his wedding before he departed for the spas in Upper
Germany.

Worm reported back that he had already been attending Knud Ulfeldt
for three weeks. He had been summoned on the advice of Ulfeldt's other
physicians. He had found him in bed with a swelling of the 'epigastric region' (upper central region of the abdomen), especially in his right side, not
to mention scurvy spots on his lower legs and feet. Ulfeldt had no appetite
and suffered from thirst during the night, but all his wounds had healed.
Worm had diagnosed it as scurvy combined with dropsy. He concluded that
everything had so far been done properly, but recommended that the remedies against scurvy should be used more frequently and in greater doses.
This was agreed to by Ulfeldt's other physicians. It resulted in the swelling abating significantly, the nightly thirst disappearing, and the patient's
calmness and appetite returning. Worm was delighted with the results
which meant that the patient was now so well that he was no longer bedridden, but could walk round in his chamber and attend to business. Only
the swelling of his legs and feet still remained to be dealt with. For that to
happen Worm planned to deploy sweat generating remedies against scurvy
combined with other water generating cures. Worm was so confident that
he informed Køster that he could tell the prince that Ulfeldt would soon
have regained his former health.

When Worm wrote to Køster again on this subject a couple of days later
his optimism had been replaced by some concern not least because Ulfeldt
had been so won over by Worm's treatment of him that he had dismissed
his other physicians and wanted Worm to take sole charge. This had been
done without Worm's knowledge and consent and clearly embarrassed him.
He did not consider Ulfeldt fully cured and still in need of more than one
physician's medical opinion. Worm found himself between a rock and a
hard place. If he refused he would insult a very influential patient and if
he accepted the dismissed physicians might see him as a mendacious colleague. Clearly there was more at stake here than Worm was prepared to
admit. The patient had still to recover fully. His appetite was still missing,
his stomach did not function properly, and he remained severely weakened
even if the disease was waning. If anything went wrong Worm would now
be solely responsible, and bearing in mind the importance of the patient, he
did not find this an altogether comfortable thought.[121] Worm had reasons

---

121 *Ibid.*, nos. 1375, 1376, 1379, and 1382.

to be cautious when attending noble patients who as he knew from his involvement in the case concerning the medical treatment of Tycho [Axelsøn]
Brahe's wife could prove dangerous and career threatening.

Despite his preoccupation with the Ulfeldt case Worm found the time
and space to provide Køster with advice about the treatment of smallpox.
Worm recommended that a vein was opened at the start of the disease.
If plenty of blood and signs of other substances linked to the illness were
found they were to be evacuated and the vehemence of the blood restrained
while the patient's strength remained, not least because such a provident
opportunity was unlikely to present itself again. Furthermore, when Worm
was called to such patients he immediately gave them an enema if they
suffered from constipation, then he offered them diascordium [a laxative]
before he bled them the following day. Finally he continued to offer the
patient antidotes and cordials throughout the illness.[122]

Despite having lost the favour of Christian IV Helvig Dietrich still retained the favour of the elected-prince. Køster reported in early April 1646
that Dietrich had recently returned to Nykøbing Falster on the prince's
order, but for what reason he did not know. Dietrich, however, was preoccupied with arranging a trip to the spas in the Southern Netherlands for
his wife who suffered from a number of illnesses. As often was the case,
Køster wanted Worm to confirm a rumour about a medical colleague, once
again Otto Sperling whom he had heard had regained his position as city
physician and royal botanist. Worm confirmed that Sperling had regained
his position as physician to the royal secretary Corfitz Ulfeldt, but not his
public positions.[123]

In what may well have been his last letter to Worm Køster told him that
Prince Christian had been impressed by Dietrich and his wife's recent, very
successful visit to the spas. Køster was concerned that this report might
hasten a similar trip by the elected-prince next spring which had, as we
have seen, long been in the planning. Worm was delighted with the success
of Dietrich's visit to the spas. He wondered, however, what to make of the
properties of the spas, and whether or not it was true what was regularly
reported, namely that those in Ascherleben surpassed all other springs,
'even Nature itself'.[124] By early autumn Køster had fallen ill and was unable to fulfil his obligations as court physician, eventually dying sometime
in early 1647. Worm was therefore summoned to Nykøbing Falster when
the elected-prince fell seriously ill in September. Shortly before Christmas
Prince Christian fell ill again and Worm was summoned by Helvig Dietrich,
who had been responsible for the prince's treatment together with Dr Jacob
Janus. Both Dietrich and Janus were shortly to leave for Germany and the

122 *Ibid.*, no. 1382.
123 *Ibid.*, nos. 1398 and 1399.
124 *Ibid.*, nos. 1439 and 1441.

services of Worm had been specifically requested by the prince. They hoped
Worm might arrive before their departure so that they could consult about
the patient.[125] Ole Worm spent Christmas and New Year at the court of
the elected-prince unhappy about being away from home. He had been left
in sole responsibility for the treatment of the prince with no idea of when
Dietrich and Janus would return which clearly caused him considerable
anxiety. Even so, Worm felt obliged to stay and treat the elected-prince, not
least because he felt that his work was highly appreciated. He stated that he
would rather act against his own interest than desert the prince and fail in
his public duty. He was, however, concerned about the bad health of Prince
Christian, who suffered continuously from hypochondrial pains, dizziness,
upset stomach and other signs of serious illness.

Furthermore, the elected-prince had repeatedly asked him to make himself available to escort him to the spas. Worm had excused himself, emphasising his age and infirmity, not to mention his large family and his public
obligations and other issues, which he hoped would be accepted. Interestingly Worm was not sure how he would be paid for his troubles.[126] Evidently service at the court offered the promise of generous rewards which
did not always materialise. It proved a long stay for Worm in Nykøbing
Falster. Writing to his nephew Thomas Bartholin in early February 1647
Worm declared that he had developed such a loathing of courtly life that
he would prefer anything to being a courtier. This was not because he had
been badly treated, far from it, but he missed his wife, family, and friends.
He was convinced that the position of court physician was a young man's
job unsuitable for an 'old' man like himself. Worm finally managed to ex-
tricate himself from the court of Prince Christian in late February when
Dietrich returned to Nykøbing Falster. Back in Copenhagen Worm handed
over Dietrich's monthly report about the health of the elected-prince to the
king. This was done through the chancellor, Christen Thomesen Sehested.
The king proved unhappy with Dietrich's report which he refused to accept.[127] At the same time Worm together with Dietrich, and Janus was
asked by Christian IV whether a visit to the spas or sulphur wells would
prove beneficial to the health of Prince Christian. They all supplied detailed
but fairly identical answers, describing the symptoms of the prince's illness
and agreeing that a visit to the spas would serve the elected-prince well, as
long as he did not disregard other medical advice.[128] Dietrich obviously
felt exposed having had his report rejected by Christian IV and contacted
Worm asking him to intervene on his behalf with the king by making sure
that the chancellor was better informed about his activities. Dietrich feared
that his reputation had been damaged by those who actively envied him and

---

125 *Ibid.*, nos. 1453 and 1471.
126 *Ibid.*, no. 1473.
127 *Ibid.*, nos. 1476 and 1478.
128 *Ibid.*, no. 1480.

who sought to turn the king against him. Meanwhile, he informed Worm
that the elected-prince had praised him and asked him to accompany him
on the planned trip to the spas.[129] Worm reported back that he had not seen
the king since his return from Nykøbing Falster, but he had been able to
discuss the case in detail with the chancellor who was far from being hos-
tile to Dietrich or negatively inclined towards the planned trip to the spas.
Worm did not find the present time an opportune moment to discuss the
matter with the king, who was preoccupied with the disastrous fire which
had destroyed the royal armoury. Worm agreed with Dietrich's diagnosis
and treatment of Prince Christian and promised to act as Dietrich's friend
whenever the treatment of the prince was discussed at the court.

Both Worm and Dietrich believed that the repeated treatment of the prince
with antimony and tartar had produced a positive effect and improved his
health. Dietrich, however, remained concerned about the opposition and
defamation of those who envied him. Dietrich was clearly annoyed by the
presence of other medical practitioners at the court of the prince, referring
in particular to someone he described as the 'dual headed Janus' bringing
hundreds of boxes with medical remedies he had obtained in Rome and
Syracuse. He concluded that he hoped to be able to discuss these matters in
greater detail with Worm when shortly they were taking leave of the king
before travelling to the spas.[130] The elected-prince set out for the German
spas on 8 May with Helvig Dietrich in his retinue. Less than a month later
on 2 June 1647 the prince died near Dresden.

Informing Ole Worm about the death of the Prince Christian in a letter
written a week later Dietrich lamented his inability to control the treatment
of the prince. He complained that his medical advice had been continuously
ignored. He claimed that the journey to the sulphur springs in Eger had
been undertaken against his advice. In fact, he was of the opinion that the
elected-prince had been altogether too weak to undertake such a strenuous
journey. However, he had acted under duress to refrain from writing to the
king to have the journey stopped. Evidently Dietrich felt the need to de-
tach himself from the decision to travel to the German spas now the prince
had suddenly died. He claimed that Worm was familiar with the advice he
had given the prince some years back about the use of some of the most
tested sulphur springs. He reminded Worm about the many influential men
who had initially disagreed with him only for them to agree later, but in a
way which disregarded the timing of the treatment, which physicians like
he and Worm attached as much importance to as the patient's strength.
This was exactly what both of them had recommended for some time, and
this more sensible plan had initially been followed by Prince Christian.
But their efforts come to nothing from the moment the prince rejected all

129 *Ibid.*, no. 1481.
130 *Ibid.*, nos. 1484 and 1485.

such suggestions and decided to head directly for Eger. Like Worm Dietrich appears to have been a believer in astrological medicine, but more importantly the letter sought to make sure that Worm would remain a supporter of his in a difficult situation where he could easily find himself blamed for the death of the elected-prince. Dietrich therefore asked Worm to act as his friend by handing his enclosed letter for Christian IV to the chancellor and to offer support for his case. Dietrich was concerned about the possible damage the prince's death might do him.[131] Worm was clearly not exposed to the same degree, but was concerned about the damage the death of the prince might do to his own prospects. He had evidently been hoping 'for greater things' through the prince's favour. He claimed to have lost a generous protector for himself, his children, and his whole family.[132]

Dietrich, meanwhile, remained worried and sent a number of letters to Worm during the autumn of 1647. Deeply concerned about his reputation and apprehensive about his detractors he once again asked Worm to forward a letter to the chancellor. By then he had regained his position as court physician to the duke of Brandenburg, whom he was escorting to Spa. He asked Worm to use his influence with the chancellor to make sure he was granted a 'gracious discharge' by the king whom he claimed was exceptionally and unreasonably angry with him. He repeated his request in late January 1648 having received no response from Worm. He wanted to know if he had insulted or angered Chancellor Christen Thomesen Sehested or others. He emphasised that he had served the elected-prince faithfully until the latter's death and only sought a graceful discharge plus payment of what he was owed at some later date.[133] Worm responded from Frederiksborg where he was attending Christian IV and apologised for the delay to his response, but one of Dietrich's letters appeared to have gone astray and with it his enclosed letter for the chancellor. He told Dietrich that the chancellor was presently away from the court, and that he had heard that the king was, indeed, unfavourably disposed towards him, but he did not know the reason. Worm was unable to help him with his discharge, but promised to take every opportunity to speak honourably about him. Dietrich was grateful for Worm's response and sent him another letter for the chancellor in order to obtain the sought-after dismissal and payment of what he was owed.[134]

Dietrich by then appeared more confident and less desperate for closure on his service to the elected-prince. He even found time to enquire about a wooden flute in Worm's possession which a boy was supposed to have accidentally swallowed after having it pushed down his throat. Worm confirmed the story. Not only did he have the flute, but he also had a statement signed by the young man whom it had happened to. He turned out to be

131 *Ibid.*, no. 1501.
132 *Ibid.*, no. 1505; see also postscript to no. 1508.
133 *Ibid.*, nos. 1547 and 1553.
134 *Ibid.*, nos. 1559 and 1563.

a seventeen-year-old youngster who attended school in Køge on Sealand. He had borrowed a flute from one of his classmates and while playing it his friend had wanted it back. A struggle had ensued whereby the flute had been pressed deep down into his gullet and blood had streamed out. The injured boy had done his utmost to push the flute up, even trying in vain to pull it out with his hands. The flute remained stuck for about a quarter of an hour until it gradually slid down into his stomach. Here it caused severe pain in the right side because, in Worm's opinion, it had torn and damaged the opening to the stomach. This forced the boy to spend the next three days in bed unable to sleep, eat, and drink. On the third day, around four in the afternoon, he passed the flute in his stools without the use of any medical remedy, but suffering excruciating pain; surprisingly the flute was in one piece and not changed in any way. After the flute had been excreted the pains gradually disappeared, but that day the boy was still unable to eat and drink, but he was quickly overcome by sleep. By the following morning he was able to eat a little soup, but not without pain because of the damage to his gullet. Gradually the boy regained his strength and was alive and still attended the same school. This had been certified by the boy himself and the headmaster of the school. Worm even supplied Dietrich with a sketch in crayon showing the size and shape of the flute.[135]

6 Physician to King Christian IV

Ole Worm became closely involved in treating King Christian IV during his final illness and death in 1648.

According to Worm what proved the king's final illness had begun in October the previous year with loss of appetite and a constant, oppressive pain in the stomach, making it difficult for the king to eat and drink. This had all been aggravated by the recent death of Prince Christian and had initially been treated by his 'regular physician', presumably Jacob Fabricius. However, the king's condition had deteriorated further and Ole Worm together with Otto Sperling had been summoned to Frederiksborg Palace to attend the king on 10 February 1648. They immediately realised that the king had very little strength left and that his stools were too loose and frequent; Sperling and Worm managed to deal with that issue, but could do nothing for, what Worm described, as 'the old and by now weakened body of the king' even with the finest medical remedies available. For convenience they finally had the king moved to Rosenborg Palace just outside the capital, where he expired in the arms of Ole Worm on 28 February between five and six in the evening after having taken Holy Communion the previous day preparing himself for his death.[136]

---

135 *Ibid.*, nos. 1563 and 1566.
136 *Ibid.*, nos. 1565 and 1566. In a letter to Thomas Bartholin written the previous day Worm had described how he kept vigil for the king at Rosenborg, *Ibid.*, 1564.

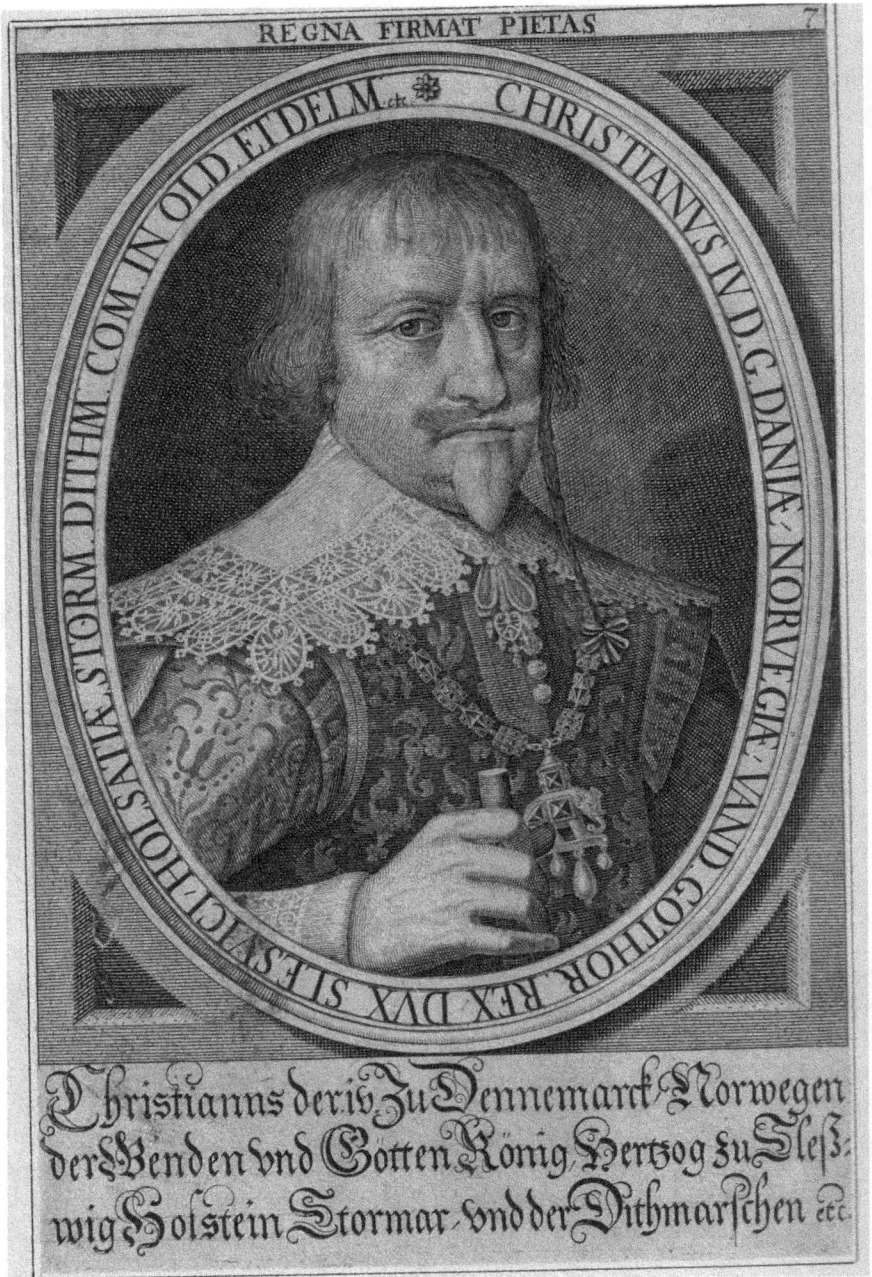

Figure 1.7 Christian IV (1577–1648) ca. 1650 age 60; courtesy of Ole Peter Grell.

Christian IV never fully recovered from the injuries he received at the naval battle at Colberger Heide on 1 July 1644 where he lost the sight in one eye. In a letter written on Christmas Eve 1644 to his son-in-law and Steward, Corfitz Ulfeldt, he requested him to call before him all the leading Doctors of Medicine and ask them to deliberate how he could be restored 'in his head' which continually left him feeling as if he was drunk. He had suffered from this condition since the battle of Colberger Heide when his ear had been blown apart, which had caused blindness in his right eye despite the eye itself having been undamaged. He was able to sleep for four hours at night. If he then got out of bed for a couple of hours he was able to sleep for another hour or two. By day he struggled to stay awake after three in the afternoon and needed a rest of around a quarter of an hour to recover.[137] Corfitz Ulfeldt would appear to have acted immediately for only four days later nine of the country's leading physicians, including Ole Worm and his friend Otto Sperling, gathered at the University of Copenhagen to discuss the king's ailment. Presumably some of the nine physicians would have examined the king on an earlier occasion, but otherwise they based their deliberations exclusively on the king's letter. They agreed that in the first instance the king needed a universal remedy which could bring about a gentle evacuation, such as Vinum Cephalicum Medicatum, which consisted of head-strengthening and purifying herbs. When that had been done bloodletting should be applied by opening either a vein in the leg or Vena Cephalica in the arms or hands. This should be followed by the use of cupping glasses placed on the neck, throat, shoulder blades or arms. When not taking the medical wine the king should be given an enema. They also advised the use of mucous removing remedies.

They then suggested that brain fortifying remedies should be applied in whatever form the king preferred to take them, either in tablets or through a liquid electuary, or as a warm head-fortifying water used internally and externally.

Among other external remedies the nine physicians recommended were Cucuphæ, remedies inhaled through a hood, in particular, combined with head-fortifying plasters and powders to be sprinkled in the hair; similarly head baths with head-fortifying herbs were proposed, as were occasional footbaths to drain off bodily fluids, and incense powders which could bolster the brain.

The king was in other words offered a broad selection of Galenic remedies for his complaint without much of a diagnosis. As Galenists, the nine physicians also provided the king with detailed advice about his lifestyle. In the present winter period they were concerned that excessive heat from stoves would fill the king's head. They were also worried that the king might eat too many smoked products during the winter which they claimed

---

137 Letter cited in Hovesen, *Lægen Ole Worm*, 223.

might have a similar effect on the king's head. After meals they advised the king to take some light laxatives such as his Pulvis Pepticus. They also advised His Majesty to avoid excitement because it generated too much movement of the bodily fluids.

The physicians, however, were not particularly concerned about the king's drowsiness in the middle of the afternoon. They considered this a natural consequence of his age, mode of life, and medical treatment, and they viewed it as a positive rather than negative development. As such they considered it in no need of a medical response.

They recommended their joint advice to the physician who was responsible for the treatment of the king, presumably the royal physician Jacob Fabricius. They had no doubt that what they endorsed would benefit the king as long as it was not spoilt by the use of other medical remedies.[138]

From the correspondence between Ole Worm and Otto Sperling during the middle of February 1648 it is clear that, having been summoned to assist in the treatment of the king less than a week earlier, the two of them found it difficult to work with Christian IV's personal physician, Jacob Fabricius. Worm provided Sperling with detailed reports on the king's health after the latter's departure from Frederiksborg Palace a couple of days earlier. Christian IV's appetite had improved somewhat on the day Sperling had returned to Copenhagen. The king had been given a light laxative (latvaerge) at three in the afternoon and had felt better and slept quite well during the night. When Worm and his colleagues attended him the following day at eight in the morning the king informed them that he had only had one bowel movement during the night and that he felt the light laxative he had been given had improved his condition. The medication was then repeated and Worm had expected to be present while the king ate lunch, but 'their mutual friend', as he put it, had prevented him from being present because he wanted to reserve that honour for himself. This was an oblique reference to Jacob Fabricius, which both he and Sperling deployed in their correspondence, possibly as an insurance against their letters being intercepted.

Jacob Fabricius had subsequently told Worm that the king had been weak and eaten very little during lunch. Worm, evidently distrusting Fabricius, had later found out from General Claus Ahlefeldt, who had been at the lunch, that this had not been the case. The following day the king had risen at five in the morning, but because he suffered serious stomach pains he had been forced to return to bed which had prevented him from following his normal dietary routine. However, he swallowed his normal light laxative and ordered Worm to be present while he had lunch at ten. This happened, according to Worm, despite opposition from Fabricius who clearly, as the king's personal physician, wanted to limit access to the king by other

---

138 The response is cited in full in Hovesen, *Lægen Ole Worm*, 223–24.

physicians. Worm was satisfied with Christian IV's appetite and concluded that he drank and ate well considering his illness. Worm, however, informed Sperling that Fabricius had expressed disappointment that 'their great antidote' – as he condescendingly referred to their 'latvaerge' – had not served to improve the king's health further. Worm had responded that within the forty-eight hours it had been applied it had improved the king's sleep, stopped his diarrhoea, and improved his appetite, while preventing his strength from deteriorating further.

However, on 15 February when Worm wrote to Sperling, the king was much worse. He had spent a restless night suffering from what he himself described as 'colossal flatulence' and complained about pains in the stomach. After having received his normal medication around three in the afternoon the king felt somewhat better. But Worm was far from satisfied with how things were progressing and prayed that God would give him and his co-physicians some healing advice which could help the king defeat 'this extremely difficult illness'.[139]

Otto Sperling shared Worm's distrust of the king's personal physician, Jacob Fabricius, and having returned to Copenhagen he made sure that the apothecaries Samuel Mejer and Esias Fleischer, kept him informed about what medical remedies Fabricius ordered for the king. Worm evidently felt the need to keep Sperling fully informed about developments at Frederiksborg Palace not least because of his distrust of Jacob Fabricius, and he wrote again to Sperling the following day. He reported that he and Fabricius had attended the king as normal at eight in the morning. Christian IV informed them that he had slept well and he found it easier to swallow his medicine and appeared more cheerful. He had had bowel movement sometime during the morning and his faeces was firmer and better digested; his urine had a plentiful and satisfying deposit. Worm had been cheered up by this and thought that the danger was receding. However, at lunch the king was feeling unwell again and ate hardly anything. When the physicians attended the king at three they found him in bed. They gave him his normal remedy and he seemed a little better. The king was also attended by the Stadtholder Corfitz Ulfeldt to whom Worm and Fabricius explained the king's illness. Worm was deeply concerned. He thought everything about the king's illness was unpredictable. The moment they had cause for optimism they were quickly disappointed by sudden changes which destroyed all hopes.

Worm informed Sperling that the light laxative they had prescribed was coming to an end, and that he had argued that the amount of theriac should be doubled in the new portion of 'latvaerge' to be prepared. He wanted Sperling to check that his prescription was followed by the apothecaries in Copenhagen, because their 'friend' (Fabricius) had insisted on taking

139 *Ibid.*, no. 1555.

control of the order. Worm finished his letter by recommending Sperling to discuss the case with the Stadtholder whom Sperling served as personal physician.[140] Sperling was grateful for Worm's detailed description of the king's condition. He agreed with Worm that Fabricius could not be trusted. He provided Worm with a copy of the prescription for the 'latvaerge' with added theriac which he had seen at the apothecary Elias Fleischer. The remedy had been made more liquid, to make it easier for the king to swallow. Sperling promised to visit the other apothecary Samuel Mejer the next day to find out what remedies he had been ordered to send. Sperling, on the Stadtholder's recommendation, encouraged Worm to remain at Frederiksborg until he arrived, in order that Fabricius should not slander him.[141] Evidently the level of distrust between Fabricius and his medical colleagues was considerable and growing.

Writing on 19 February Worm expressed his confidence that Sperling would keep him as well informed as he had Sperling. He was convinced that Sperling had already been informed by the Stadtholder, Corfitz Ulfeldt, about the king's loss of memory on the morning of the 17th. His urine sample had shown reasonable deposit and his stools were digested. However, despite Worm's repeated reminders to Jacob Fabricius to have a new portion of 'latvaerge' prepared nothing had been delivered to Frederiksborg. Worm suspected that Fabricius wanted their 'latvaerge' replaced with his own pills. The king felt slightly better at lunch and ate well and drank half a glass of wine. Everyone present attributed his cheerfulness to his conversation with the Stadtholder and wished he might have remained longer. Worm had no doubt that if the king always had such a man around him with whom he could negotiate necessary business it would improve his health considerably. When the physicians returned at three they found the king in bed, but no weaker than normal; because the 'latvaerge' had run out Christian was offered Fabricius's pills instead. He took three and drank some wine afterwards as normal.

The night of the 18th passed quietly even if the king got out of bed three times; he had digested stools and his urine was yellow-red without deposit. He was offered Fabricius's pills but refused them pointing out he wanted the 'latvaerge' which finally arrived from Copenhagen correctly reinforced with theriac. At three when he normally received his medication he was offered the choice between the pills and the 'latvaerge' and chose the latter, evidently to Worm's satisfaction. The king had complained in the morning about the presence of a heavy and tough slime in his throat which he struggled to cough up. A gargling remedy was prepared by the physicians which was administered the next day with some success. The king had a quiet night on the 19th and he only rose once, and had no bowel movement. His

140 *Ibid.*, no. 1557.
141 *Ibid.*, no. 1558.

urine at eight o'clock was ticker than normal, yellow in colour and with bubbles.

Worm pointed out this was his last report because the court was about to move to Copenhagen and take up residence at Rosenborg Palace. Apparently Fabricius was now seeking to befriend Worm who, however, had little faith in his sincerity. He told Sperling that he would co-operate with Fabricius for as long as his conscience would allow him.[142] Christian IV died only nine days after his transfer to Copenhagen, as we have seen, in the arms of Ole Worm. The fact that Worm appears to have played an increasingly central role in the treatment of the dying king speaks highly of his ability as a physician with an excellent bedside manner. Perhaps the appreciation of the Stadtholder, Corfitz Ulfeldt, mentioned by Sperling, of Worm's 'modesty, wisdom, and amiability' was not just flattery.[143]

7 Ole Worm's health

In the spring of 1635, when he had turned forty-seven, Worm began to worry about his own health. In May that year he had been affected for three weeks by what he referred to as a serious illness and later in July he struggled for a fortnight with an illness he described as a tertiary fever. This was a disease which appears to have affected all the physicians in Copenhagen at this particular time. The following year Worm found himself bedridden for a further three weeks with what he diagnosed as a liver obstruction and hypochondrial pains, all of which he linked to the start of his grand climacterium which in this particular case he dated from his 48th birthday.[144] The concept of the climacterium or climatic years was rooted in astrological medicine which claimed that people during those years were exposed to great bodily changes and serious risks of death. The first climacteric would occur in the seventh year of a person's life; the rest were multiples of the first, with the particular important years being 21, 49, 56, and 63. The grand climacterium usually referred to the 63rd year where the dangers were supposed to be particularly prominent.

In the summer of 1641 Worm had a nasty accident falling down the stairs. Initially he was bedridden having injured his left side and suffering pains in the adjoining regions and his diaphragm. It took him a considerable time to recover and he claimed that he was only able to breathe freely a couple of weeks later.[145] Four years later he contracted a horrible catarrh that had slid down his right side and caused serious coughing and pain for several weeks.[146] By the summer of 1645 Worm was exchanging letters

---

142 *Ibid.*, no. 1560.
143 For Ulfeldt's remarks see *ibid.*, no. 1558.
144 *Ibid.*, nos. 558, 564, and 592.
145 *Ibid.*, nos. 957 and 960.
146 *Ibid.*, no. 1304.

with his friend Henrik Køster about their failing health. Køster continued to suffer from serious and unpredictable digestive problems mainly constipation which he tried to tackle solely by changing his lifestyle and diet, apparently with only moderate success. Worm admitted that his own health was precarious. He had been suffering from a chest infection with a painful cough which had proved fairly pervasive within Copenhagen. However, he had now made a full recovery. Worm had taken the traditional remedies for this complaint, but they appeared to have had little beneficial effect. He added that his many patients prevented him from looking properly after his own health.[147]

Writing to his nephew Erasmus Bartholin in Leiden in April 1650 Worm complained that he had been suffering from a serious catarrh for nearly a month which had entered his chest giving him headaches and from which he struggled to recover. He was concerned about his health in general and added that he hoped no greater evils would threaten him in his grand climacterium. A week later, when he wrote a number of letters to his Icelandic friends, he remained pessimistic about his health. Evidently he found it difficult to recover from the catarrh. This led him to worry about the prospects for his general health during his grand climacterium [sixty-third year].[148]

By early May 1650 Worm had failed to recover. He was low on energy having suffered from a chest infection for more than a month, and he was concerned that his illness would prove ominous for his approaching grand climacterium.[149] Worm was still struggling with the remnants of his infection three weeks later, when writing to Lady Birgitte Thott of Thureby. He apologised for his late response, but explained that he still suffered from headaches and a cold which hampered his writing and caused him considerable anxiety about greater inconveniences in the year of his grand climacterium.[150] Worm had given his nephew Erasmus Bartholin who was studying in Leiden a similar pessimistic view of his health and expectations of what he clearly considered a significant year for his future health. Erasmus responded by expressing his hope for his uncle's speedy recovery, stating that he hoped God would confirm the view of the Leiden classics professor Claude Saumaise, and prove it through the example of Worm.[151] Erasmus was referring to the recently published work by Claude Saumaise, *De annis climactericis et antiqua astrologia diatribae*, Leiden 1648. Here Saumaise refuted two popular, humanist notions about the value of prognostic astrology and the validity of the concept of the climacteric years,

---

147 *Ibid.*, nos. 1338 and 1341
148 *Ibid.*, nos. 1685 and 1687–90
149 *Ibid.*, nos. 1687–90.
150 *Ibid.*, no. 1693.
151 *Ibid.*, no. 1694.

especially the significance of medical astrology for the grand climacterium or the sixty-third year. Worm, a strong believer in astrological medicine, would have been unlikely to have been convinced by Saumaise. That is, if he ever read the work.

1650 proved a difficult year for Worm struggling, as he did, to recover from his catarrh. When Worm wrote to his friend Johan Rhode in Padua in August that year he pointed out that this was the year both of them had reached their grand climacterium and he wanted to know how Rhode was faring. He added that for him the year so far had not proved promising. He referred to the severe catarrh and fever he had contracted which he claimed had caused a 'disturbance of most of his internal as well as external senses'. He had yet to recover fully from the effects and doubted that he would succeed because old age had debilitated his strength causing him concerns about the outcome of the year. By April 1651 Worm was recovering, but he was not yet back to his old self. The experience of what had been a difficult year in health terms lingered on throughout 1651 as can be seen from Worm's letters.[152] The following spring Worm caught the tertiary fever which was spreading rapidly across the country while attending an engagement party in Scania, but he appears to have recovered quickly.[153]

8 Epidemics

A number of epidemic diseases affected Copenhagen in particular and Denmark in general in the first half of the seventeenth century. In March 1619 Worm was concerned that plague had broken out in Copenhagen affecting a number of houses in the city. He expressed the fear that the whole kingdom might be infested 'unless God stopped this evil', which had yet to affect the university and the leading citizens.[154] By April that was no longer the case and plague had spread across the city, and writing to his 'old' tutor in Basle, Caspar Bauhin. Worm reported that the university was in a grievous state. Plague had hit the city from all directions and forced the closure of the university. By then Worm had moved his residence to Roskilde after having lost his eldest daughter to the epidemic.[155] Worm was right, and this proved a major outbreak. It has been estimated that around 7,000 people died in Copenhagen alone. The epidemic was serious enough for the medical faculty to publish its medical advice in a pamphlet entitled, *A short Instruction of how to conduct yourself in these dangerous Times*. It was the first such publication since the plague advice issued nearly a century earlier by the then professor of medicine at the university, Christen Thorkelsen

152 *Ibid.*, nos. 1698 and 1711, and 1712–14.
153 *Ibid.*, no. 1726.
154 *Ibid.*, nos. 55–56.
155 *Ibid.*, nos. 62–63.

Morsing in 1546, and it drew heavily on that publication.[156] Plague was still lingering in Copenhagen in the summer of 1622, but proved only a minor inconvenience compared with the disastrous outbreak in 1619.[157] Writing in February 1625 to his friend Peder Schelderup, who had been minister at Our Lady's Church in Copenhagen until 1622 when he was promoted to Bishop of Trondheim, Worm offered a detailed view of the health situation in Copenhagen:

> In the past summer dysentery has killed a number of people here; at present the plague germs have been expelled; they only wiped out a few families, but then totally. Even if the evil now appears to be yielding it must be feared that it may gain ground again in the unsettled spring weather. Smallpox and measles greatly are rife among infants; they have recently carried off the youngest of Plum's children. Our children are still in good health – as long as it pleases God![158]

Worm's forecast proved correct and plague returned to the city even earlier than expected. By early 1626 a growing number of people in Copenhagen were killed by the plague. This proved another serious epidemic and by May Worm and his family had once again sought sanctuary in Roskilde.[159]

During the next major plague epidemic in the summer of 1629 Worm lost his father, his sister, and his brother-in-law Caspar Bartholin. The epidemic continued into the autumn and Worm promised his brother-in-law Jacob Fincke to look after his family while the latter was away in Germany. He also informed Jacob that many of their friends had fled Copenhagen while he himself remained in the city. Times were clearly desperate and Worm was on the lookout for a remedy to fight the plague. A friend had recommended pills made to the recipe found in Paracelsus's Alkahest, but after having read it Worm was not convinced. Furthermore, he was obviously badly affected by the death of so many relations and friends. Briefly at the beginning of November he had thought that the plague was finally coming to an end when only eight deaths were reported in Copenhagen. But his optimism proved premature and by the end of November when many more family members including his wife and his brother-in-law Jørgen Fuiren had died from the plague Worm reached a new low, declaring that they were 'totally surrounded by the plague and had yet to identify a dawn. The University was dissolved, the professors spread, some of whom have been carried away by the plague'.[160] Despite the seriousness of the epidemic and

---

156 See section on 'Pestskrifter' in *Cista Medica Hafniensis*, 105–25.
157 *Ibid.*, no. 104.
158 *Ibid.*, no. 173.
159 *Ibid.*, nos. 189 and 198.
160 *Ibid.*, nos. 280, 282, 295, 313, 324.

his personal loss Worm remained in Copenhagen throughout the outbreak looking after his patients.[161]

Eight years later, in June 1637, Copenhagen was once more hit by a major plague epidemic and once again the medical faculty issued its advice in the form of a revised edition of the 1619 pamphlet. Worm informed his friend Bishop Wegner in Stavanger that he had advised Wegner's son who was a student at the University of Copenhagen to return home. A number of their mutual friends were affected. Christen Sørensen Longomontanus's wife died and Jesper Brochmand's family was infected, but had left the city. A week later Worm informed his colleague in Lund, Niels Foss, that around 189 people had died of plague during the previous week, adding that he felt unable to travel to Lund because, as he put it, 'Who would dare leave their wife, children, and family when it is uncertain if they shall ever return'.[162] Worm's own wife died from the plague in August, an event which shattered him and caused him great sorrow for an extended period. Writing to Henry Spelman in London in May 1638 Worm informed him that the plague had killed his beautiful wife and filled his household with great grief and affliction, and depressed him to such an extent that he hardly managed to fulfil his normal obligations. By January 1638 the epidemic was coming to an end, but the university still remained closed, and more than 5,000 people had died.[163] The physician and botanist Otto Sperling praised Worm for the medical advice he had given him when he had caught the plague and most of his friends and relations had given up on him. He claimed to owe Worm his life, having followed his advice and opened a vein and bled four ounces of blood, whereby the poison had been purged.[164]

In December 1644 Worm reported that a nasty fever was spreading rapidly in Copenhagen killing a fair number of people. It continued into January 1645 and would appear to have spread across the whole country since the medical faculty was ordered by the king to publish a pamphlet in Danish offering medical advice.[165] In June 1649 Worm reported to his nephew Erasmus Bartholin in Leiden that the country was threatened by plague because of the death of livestock and scarce crops. This proved a pessimistic forecast, but by September 1652 a nasty fever together with dysentery had been prevalent for some time in Copenhagen and the university had been closed for two months.[166] Copenhagen was hit by another major outbreak of plague in April 1654. By May Worm was deeply concerned about 'the terrible plague which lays waste to us and kills people on the third day of the illness'. As a consequence the meeting of Parliament was moved to

161 *Ibid.*, no. 342.
162 *Ibid.*, no. 663.
163 *Ibid.*, nos. 654, 663, 668, 673, 674, 692, 713, and 719.
164 *Ibid.*, no. 676.
165 *Ibid.*, nos. 1264 and 1270.
166 *Ibid.*, no. 1731.

Kolding in Jutland and the medical faculty once again published its advice in a revised and augmented form. Worm remained in Copenhagen having been elected vice chancellor for the year, but worried that he was not up to the job in such dangerous times. By the beginning of June more than 180 people a week were dying and the better off professors and students had left the city. A couple of weeks later the number of weekly deaths had risen to 279. The number of casualties kept growing and by 1 July the university was disbanded and all the professors had left the city apart from Worm and two colleagues. Despite the fact that the plague claimed increasing numbers each week Worm thought that it did not make sense to leave Copenhagen at this stage. Experience had taught him that such a change could not be undertaken at this point without danger. A view he appears to have changed a couple of weeks later when he sent his son Matthias to 'safety' in Bergen.[167]

By late July 1654 the plague was claiming more than 600 deaths a week as Worm reported to his son Willum in Leiden:

> What can I say about the plague which rages here. The Medical Faculty has published a guide in Danish, and I would forward it if I could. It is a most violent illness which during the fourth day suffocates the infected. The signs are not the same for everyone, but differs according to temperament, loss of strength, pressure in the heart, most are possessed with fear and cold from the start; then they get tumours and buboes and towards the end black and yellow spots. Most of those who die make the mistake at the start of disease by undermining their strength by bleeding or purgation. If you do not take measures against the disease within six hours you are lost. The moment you feel a change in your body an antidote must be given so you can be prepared for a spell of sweating, which should be repeated every six hours until you feel a significant change and the poison has been expelled. You can see it all in our guide.

Under these extreme conditions Worm decided to halt his medical practice.[168] Little did it help him and five weeks later, on 31 August 1654, Ole Worm died, possibly a casualty of the plague having remained in Copenhagen as vice chancellor of the university.[169]

9 Conclusion

Ole Worm started practising medicine as a young man of twenty-two while studying in Paris, a couple of years before he was awarded his

---

167 See *Ibid.*, nos. 1569–72, 1774, 1777, 1779, 1780, 1784, 1788, 1793.
168 *Ibid.*, no. 1789.
169 It has been suggested that Worm died from an urinary disease, see Bruun and Loldrup (eds.) *Cista Medica*, 98.

MD. After he had received his MD in Basle he served for a year and a half as personal physician to the English nobleman and later earl of Warwick Robert Rich, before he took up a professorship at the University of Copenhagen in 1613. Within a few years of having taken up his professorship Worm had established a thriving medical practice in Copenhagen, where his services were much in demand among his academic colleagues. By the 1620s Worm had also become physician to a number of prominent noble families and his growing reputation meant that his advice was often sought in difficult cases, as can be seen from that of Jytte [Birgitte] Brok.

By the 1630s Worm's reputation as a physician and his prominent position within the medical establishment as a leading professor of medicine within the university meant that his advice and presence was increasingly in demand by the wider royal household. Initially he was called on to provide medical treatment for the offspring of Christian IV and his second wife Kirsten Munk, but at the same time he had the opportunity to recommend the use of some pills to the king which were much appreciated. A few years later Worm became directly involved in the medical treatment of the ailing elected-prince, spending considerable time at the prince's court in Nykøbing Falster.

Christian IV never recovered from the injuries he suffered at the naval battle at Colberger Heide in July 1644. Worm was among the physicians whom the king consulted in the aftermath. He was eventually summoned on 10 February 1648 to assist the royal physician Jacob Fabricius in what proved Christian IV's final illness. From that date Worm remained in constant attention of the king who eventually died in his arms eighteen days later on 28 February at Rosenborg Palace.

There was in other words a clear upwards social trajectory in Ole Worm's medical practice, even if the majority of his patients always were and remained wealthy burghers in and around Copenhagen. Sadly we know little or nothing about those patients whom Worm regularly attended, because they have left little or no trace in the sources.

From 1629 Worm remained in Copenhagen during major epidemics looking after his patients and students despite the obvious dangers. From his letters written during these outbreaks one gets the sense of a physician who was driven by both a moral rectitude and a deep sense of responsibility towards his patients and the university. That he died during the major plague epidemic in 1654 was hardly a coincidence.

Not surprisingly Worm was a strong advocate of learned medicine and a believer in the need for medical regulation. As such he was negatively inclined towards all lay practitioners be they barbers, women, or charlatans. He was highly regarded within his profession and repeatedly provided advice to colleagues be they good friends such as the physician to the elected-prince, Henrik Køster or former students such as Poul Moth, or physicians such as the Aarhus based Johan Christoph Creuzauer and Ludvig Pouch in Ribe. Likewise Worm treated his medical colleagues with respect and sought to behave in a collegiate manner whenever possible. Thus, he was uncomfortable with the dismissal of the Copenhagen physician Tancred Leyel after he had been called on to assist him in the treatment of Jytte [Birgitte] Brok. Likewise he was uneasy with the dismissal of the physicians who had attended the Privy Councillor Knud Ulfeldt until he had been summoned.

Ole Worm took an unusually high number of consultations by letter. Even if he was conscious of the limitations of this approach, it was not something he discouraged. Most of these cases were with patients based on Iceland or the Faroe Islands where no physicians or apothecaries were available, and with whom Worm had become acquainted during their earlier residence in Copenhagen, more often than not as students at the university. Due to the infrequent contacts with these islands, caused by their geographical distance from Denmark and the harsh weather conditions, considerable time often lapsed between letters seeking medical advice arriving in Copenhagen and Worm being able to forward medical advice and remedies to his patients on Iceland and the Faroe Islands. In some cases nearly a year would slip before medical assistance became available. Added to that, Worm was seriously concerned about the long sea voyage needed to deliver his medical remedies, often damaging them in the process, even if he sought to prescribe remedies which, in his opinion, were particularly robust and durable.

Ole Worm was in some ways a typical Galenic physician who adhered to the humoral system. His patients' lifestyles and diets were important starting points for Worm as were bloodletting and evacuations of other bodily fluids such as urine and faeces. He was, however, also influenced by the revived Hippocratic ideas which emphasised that the seeds of disease were to be found both within and without the human body, and that the roots of diseases which affected large numbers of people were to be found in the local environments. Worm also drew on Paracelsian, alchemical ideas and developed his own chemical remedies for some of his patients. He was undoubtedly attracted to the occult and it is in that context that his firm belief in astrological medicine should be seen. He considered astrology of paramount importance for his own health as we have seen in the concern he demonstrated for having reached his grand climacterium. Likewise he considered it important that the medical treatment of his patients should be guided by astrology, and he was convinced that the right timing of their treatments determined their effectiveness. Together with his empirical observations about what remedies worked in some situations and for some patients astrological medicine proved a central plank in Worm's medical approach.

2 The Professor

In July 1613, at the age of twenty-five, Ole Worm returned to Denmark to take up a professorship in pedagogy at the University of Copenhagen a few months later. At the time of his appointment Worm had sampled the best medical education available at the leading universities in Europe. He had been educated by some of the most prominent medical men of the age, having often participated in their private colloquia and classes. Through this varied experience Worm quickly developed a hands-on, observationally based, experimental approach to natural philosophy and medicine, happily mixing a Hippocratic approach with aspects of Paracelsianism, and sound scepticism with an open-minded inquisitiveness. Furthermore, by then Worm had also practised medicine in some of the larger European cities, mastering several languages, while simultaneously finding time to benefit from the company of some of the leading intellectual figures of the age. By the time he returned to Copenhagen Ole Worm had established a comprehensive network of friends and contacts across Europe that would prove particularly important for a man who was to spend the rest of his life at the University of Copenhagen. Without it, Worm's entry into the international republic of letters would have been extremely difficult, as would his attempts to keep abreast of the new discoveries and challenges to established knowledge in the first half of the seventeenth century. However, from the outset, the driving force behind Worm's thirst for knowledge lay in his hope of obtaining true knowledge and understanding of the natural world as created by God.

1 Early university career

For an MD, like Worm, to accept a professorship of pedagogy within a faculty of philosophy was a fairly common route to eventually obtain the desired chair in medicine. It provided a first step on the academic ladder. Worm gave his inaugural lecture on 10 September 1613, De Dignitate ac Præstantiatia Literarum, and the following Monday he began a lecture series on Cicero, Cato Major, which lasted six months. Worm's lectures were

DOI: 10.4324/9781003290940-3

fairly standard stuff and, as one might expect, occasionally had a medical flavour.[1] Taking the advice by Cato that wisdom was to be guided by Nature, and that one should obey it as a God, Worm defined Nature, as the by God created power and order, or all-commanding spirit of God, which permeated all parts of the created world. Therefore he, who followed Nature, followed God, as Nature obeyed God, being essentially the spirit of God. Worm then proceeded to discuss the different issues surrounding the concept of Nature, often referring to medicine in the process. It is noteworthy that Ole Worm when discussing whether Nature intended to produce monsters, referred to the newly published work, *Physica Christiana*, by his colleague, the professor of theology Cort Aslaksen, which emphasised that God's power of creation generated everything and God in his wisdom also produced monsters. Aslaksen, who had served as an assistant to Tycho Brahe on the island of Hven, was a forceful exponent of a Melanchthonian philosophy and theology and sought to synthesise Tycho Brahe's natural philosophy with the biblical version of the creation.[2]

Before Worm had finished his first lecture series on Cato Major in March 1614, he had already started another series on grammar, entitled 'A collection of controversial questions about grammar, especially testing the truth of the teachings of Phillip Melanchthon'. Worm may well have lectured on another, major Latin text after March 1614 when he had finished Cato Major. He clearly more than fulfilled his teaching obligations at the university, and later that year was promoted to the senior chair in pedagogy. The fact that he was also made university secretary in 1614 demonstrate the trust and esteem in which he was held.[3] His two years as professor of pedagogy did not result in any printed disputations, possibly because the issues discussed were too basic to merit publication.

The following year, in August 1615, Ole Worm was promoted to the chair in Greek, which he was to occupy until September 1621 when he was awarded the chair in natural philosophy. His marriage on 26 November 1615 to Dorothea Fincke, the third daughter of the influential professor of medicine at the university Thomas Fincke, undoubtedly served to enhance his career, connecting him with one of the most powerful men within the University of Copenhagen, while making him brother-in-law of another

---

1 For the manuscript for Worm's lectures on *Cato Major*, see Royal Library, Rostgaard 269, quarto, nr. 25 and Rostgaard 195, quarto, 35–110. The lectures are discussed in some detail in Schepelern, *Museum*, 100–03.

2 See Cort Aslaksen, *Physica et ethica mosaic, ut antiquissima, ita vere christiana duobus libris comprehensa*, Hanau 1613, Chapter 5, problem 1. For Aslaksen, see A. Mosley, 'After Tycho: Phillipist Astronomy and Cosmology in the Work of Brahe's Assistants', 60–81 in O. P. Grell and A. Cunningham (eds.), *Medicine, Natural Philosophy and Religion in Post-Reformation Scandinavia*, New York 2017 and O. Garstein, *Cort Aslakssøn: Studier over Dansk-Norsk universitets- og Lærdomshistorie omkring år 1600*, Oslo 1953.

3 Schepelern, *Museum*, 104–06 and Hovesen, *Ole Worm*, 127–30.

two prominent physicians, Jørgen Fuiren and Caspar Bartholin, the latter, professor of medicine, and a leading figure within the university.[4]

Worm began his teaching as professor of Greek by lecturing on, Work and Days, by the poet Hesiod, followed by a lecture series from Easter 1618 until May 1619 on Aristotle's *De Mundo*, concluding with lectures on two works by the rhetorician Isocrates, Evagoras and Busiris. The last lectures do not appear to have resulted in any disputations, whereas two disputations in July 1616 and July 1617 around the Hesiod lectures were published, as were two of the four on Aristotle's *De Mundo*. The Hesiod disputations primarily tackled logical and philological issues, but they also dealt with medical and natural philosophical questions. Worm's first student-respondent, Bjørn Sørensen Drachard, eventually ended up as a professor in theology at the Academy in Sorø. Worm corresponded with him in 1618 while he studied in Germany, recommending him to apply himself to the study of the classical languages. Worm considered them essential for making progress not only in theology but also other 'sciences'. He also instructed Drachard not to forget philosophy, especially if he could get access to private classes. Drachard had clearly complained about the costs he had incurred during his studies in Germany and Worm sought to cheer him up by stating that life in Wittenberg might be cheaper.[5]

Ole Worm's university career was progressing well until May 1616 when it was his turn to take over as dean of the Faculty of Philosophy for the coming year. To his consternation he was passed over because some of his colleagues in the Faculty objected to his appointment, claiming that he could not grant degrees in philosophy while not holding a master's degree in the subject himself. His opponents within the Philosophy Faculty were being led by the professor of logic, Hans Jensen Alanus, who had been dean in 1610, when Worm briefly had been back in Copenhagen before resuming his travels. That Worm had not felt obliged to obtain an MA at the university on that occasion may have been taken as a slight by Alanus and caused his animosity. Worm was furious and it may well explain why he gave up the position as university secretary in May 1616. Realising that in spite of his objections, he was about to be passed over as dean once more in 1617, Worm wrote to his friend, the professor of theology, Jesper Rasmussen Brochmand, who had recently been appointed tutor to the elected-prince and was residing at court, asking him for his assistance by presenting his case to Christen Friis, the newly appointed chancellor.

---

4 Hovesen, *Ole Worm*, 266–67, a fourth daughter of Fincke later married the professor of theology at the university Hans Rasmussen Brockmand; see also *DBL* articles on Caspar Bartholin, Thomas Fincke, Jørgen Fuiren.
5 See Schepelern, *Museum*, 106–09; see also *Breve fra og til Ole Worm*, nos. 77 and 78 for Worm's plans to have the Hesiod disputations published in Frankfurt rather than Copenhagen where they were eventually published; for the letter to Bjørn Sørensen Drachard, see *Ibid.*, no. 39.

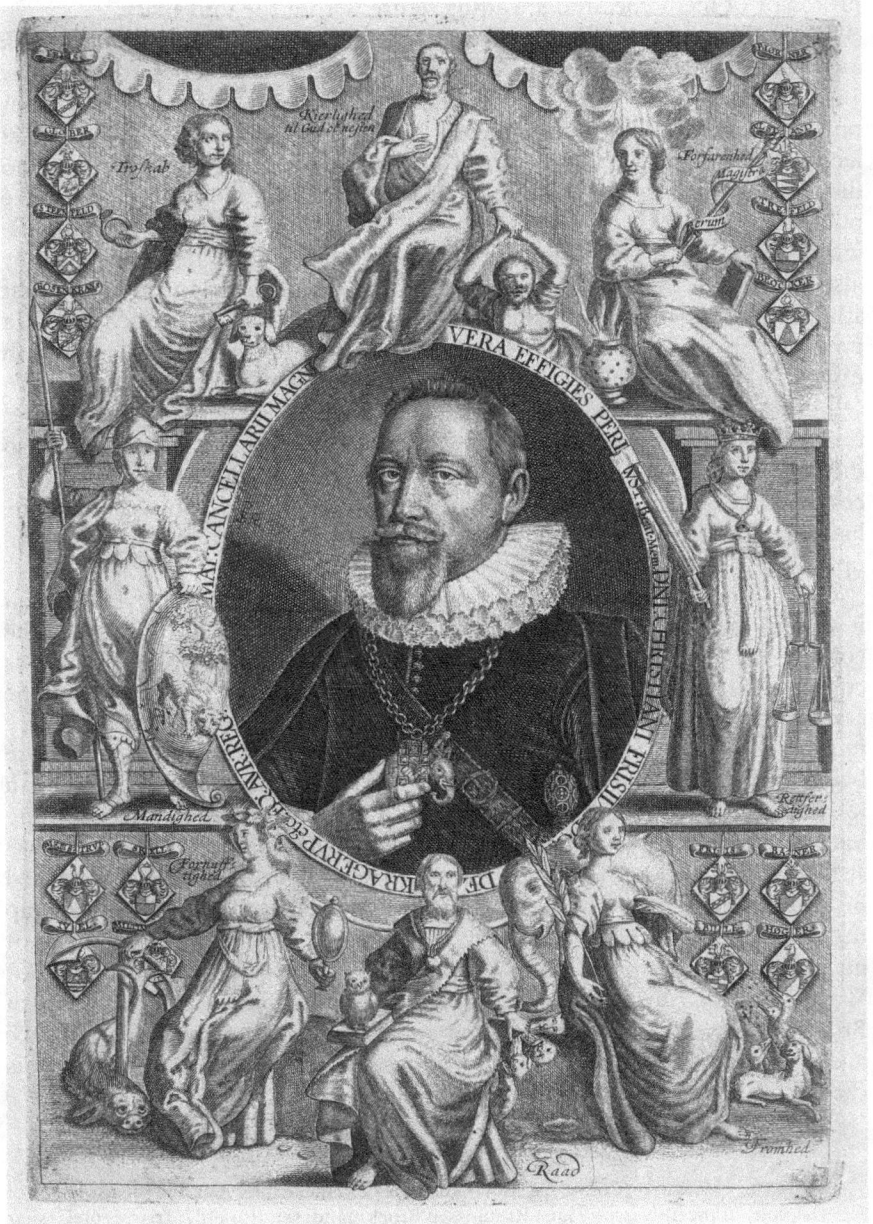

Figure 2.1 Chancellor Christen Friis (1581–1639) by Simon de Pas; courtesy of the Royal Danish Library.

Worm included a copy of the statement he had provided for the professors in the Academic Council. Here Worm claimed that nothing could be found in the university's instrument of foundation or statutes which excluded an MD legally appointed as professor in the Faculty of Philosophy from any honour within the university. Worm was keen to have his case dealt with before the new vice chancellor elected for 1617 began his term of office on 29 June 1617, especially since he was convinced that the new vice chancellor was less positively inclined towards him. The person in question, the professor of theology, Hans Paulsen Resen, an advocate for Lutheran uniformity, was clearly not a friend of Ole Worm.[6]

Meanwhile, Worm was advised by Christen Friis to write to the University of Basle asking them for confirmation that his MD simultaneously awarded him a degree in philosophy. Worm did not expect this to prove straight forward, since he had already received proof of his degree from Basle. Furthermore, he was not allowed to reveal why he needed further evidence of what his degree incorporated, because the University of Copenhagen had forbidden him to disclose his case to outsiders. Worm was also concerned that if he received the desired document, it would arrive too late to affect the upcoming year's choice of dean. He was therefore keen for Jesper Brochmand to ask the chancellor to find a different way of resolving the conflict. Even so Worm sent off the desired letter to the medical faculty in Basle asking them to provide the evidence needed, but also making it clear why it was needed.

When the new dean of the Faculty of Philosophy was to be elected in June 1617 Worm realised that he was about to be passed over once again, but this time he was intent not to let it pass quietly. When the outgoing dean, Hans Jensen Alanus, attempted to hand over the keys for the deanship to Christen Longomontanus, professor of mathematics, without a vote, Worm took the opportunity to intervene against his antagonist. He objected to what he described as an illegal procedure in the election of the dean. A decision, which should depend on a vote within the faculty, had been commandeered by an individual at a time when an unresolved difference of opinion about the deanship remained. Furthermore, Worm pointed out that the faculty had recently decided that new deans needed to provide evidence publicly that an MA in philosophy had been properly conferred on them. This had been demanded of Worm at the previous year's election and he therefore insisted it was done now before an election could take place, while demanding that the case be brought before the Academic Council of the

---

6 Similarly, when Worm's brother-in-law and close friend, Caspar Bartholin, was offered the Chair in Theology in 1624 Resen was far from keen on his candidature. It would appear that Resen was doing what he could to make the promotion of protégés of Holger Rosenkrantz difficult for both religious and political reasons, see M. Fink-Jensen, *Fornuften under troens lydighed. Naturfilosofi, medicin og teology i Danmark 1536–1636*, Copenhagen 2004, 241–44 (who does not draw the same conclusion).

university. Worm received the support of a number of his colleagues within the Faculty and the meeting was dissolved.

Worm then had a meeting with the new vice chancellor, Hans Poulsen Resen, who promised to call a meeting of the Academic Council when it could be conveniently convened. Resen confirmed Worm's concerns about him as not being helpful to his cause, when he informed him that he had already discussed his case with the chancellor, who had declined to intervene in an affair which he considered partly decided. Worm informed Jesper Brochmand that he was missing his support in the Academic Council. He suggested that Brochmand expressed his views in a letter to the professor of theology, Cort Aslaksen, in order that the latter could refer it to the Academic Council, if and when the issue was brought up. Clearly, Worm associated himself with the Melanchthonian, open-minded wing within the university and its most prominent exponent, Cort Aslaksen, who was opposed to Resen and his drive towards Lutheran uniformity.

At the subsequent Academic Council meeting Worm was allowed to present his view previously expressed to his colleagues in the Faculty of Philosophy. Hans Poulsen Resen then informed the council that the chancellor had advised him that Christen Longomontanus should be made dean because he had previously held the post, while the other controversial issue should be left to be decided at a later date. At that point the two professors of medicine, Thomas Fincke and Caspar Bartholin, Worm's in-laws, intervened, arguing that this was something which concerned the Faculty of Medicine and that they intended to confront Worm's antagonists. Vice Chancellor Resen promised to bring this to the chancellor's attention. Even so Worm was deeply disappointed with the outcome, contemplating personally to bring his case before Christen Friis.[7] Rather than the testimonial from the Faculty of Medicine in Basle, it probably proved the intervention of the Faculty of Medicine in Copenhagen through his relations, Thomas Fincke and Caspar Bartholin, that proved decisive.

Having made Worm's case their own Ole Worm finally became dean of the Faculty of Philosophy in 1618. Even so, Worm had to accept a compromise and reluctantly apply for degree of MA in philosophy in 1617, even if he used the occasion, giving the speech on behalf of the candidates, to insist that such a degree, in his opinion, was already included in the higher degree of doctor. It resulted in a somewhat bizarre event at the graduation in May 1619 when Ole Worm as dean had finished his address to the new candidates and was about to confer their degrees. In stepped the previous year's dean, Christen Longomontanus, and conferred the MA in philosophy on Worm, who then proceeded to award the degrees.[8]

7 For these events see, *Breve fra og til Ole Worm*, nos. 26–31.
8 For this, see Schepelern, *Museum*, 112–13.

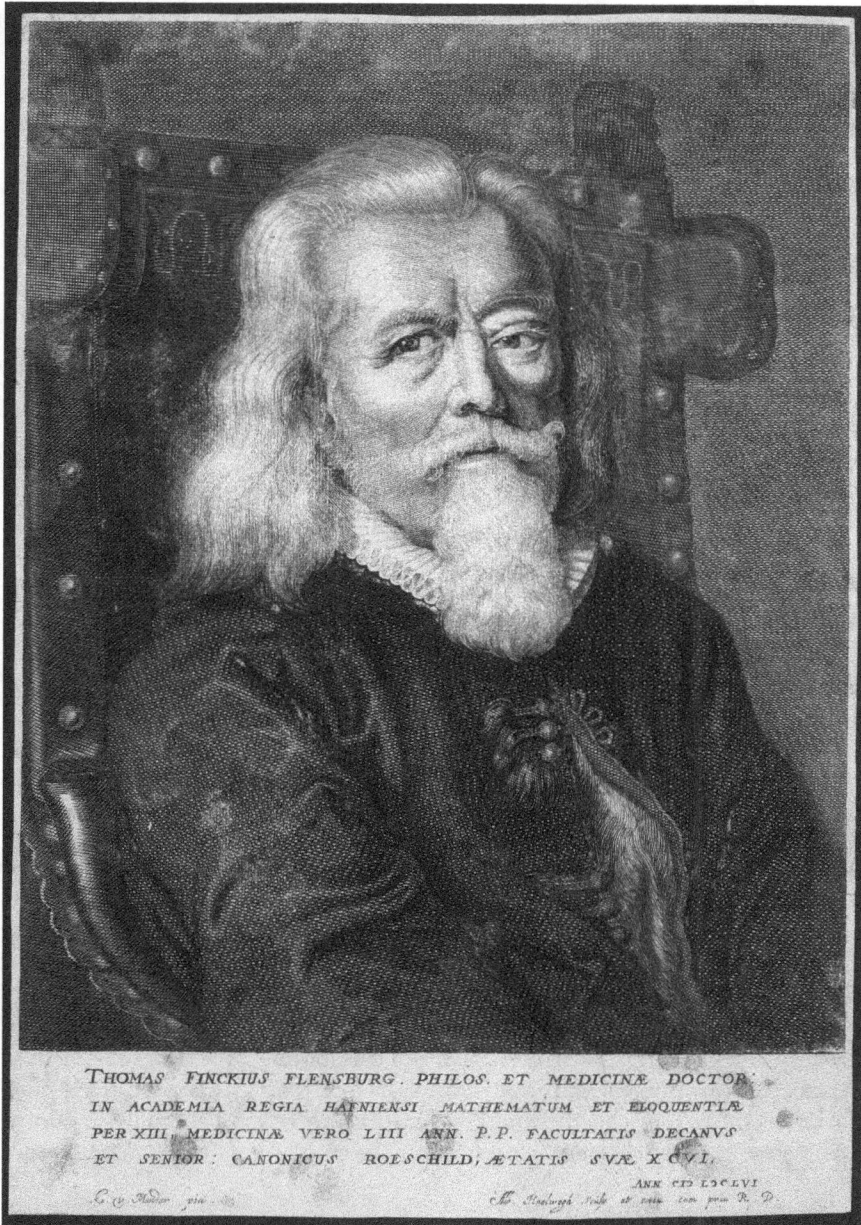

THOMAS FINCKIUS FLENSBURG. PHILOS. ET MEDICINÆ DOCTOR:
IN ACADEMIA REGIA HAFNIENSI MATHEMATUM ET ELOQUENTIÆ
PER XIII, MEDICINÆ VERO LIII ANN. P.P. FACULTATIS DECANVS
ET SENIOR: CANONICUS ROESCHILD; ÆTATIS SVÆ XCVI.

ANN CIↃ IↃCLVI

Figure 2.2 Thomas Fincke (1561–1656) by Albert Haelwegh; courtesy of the Royal Danish Library.

2 The Rosicrucians

In his inaugural address, Oratio Inauguralis de Fratrum R.C. Philosophiam Reformandi Conatu, Ole Worm congratulated the students on their achievements, but more importantly he warned them against the teachings of what he considered a dangerous sect which had published two treatises, *The Fama* and *The Confessio*, under the name *Fratres Rosæ Crusis*. These Rosicrucian brethren had according to Worm embraced Hermetic medicine many years before they published *The Fama* in 1614.[9] Worm provided a brief survey of the writings for and against Rosicrucianism, before rejecting the claim that the teaching within the university was too dependent on the works of Aristotle and Galen and 'obstructed the splendid radiance of truth'. Worm referred to J.C. Scaliger as the inspiration for his critical approach. Like Scaliger he believed that disputations were the vehicle by which rare and unusual subjects and views could be brought forward and cleansed of doubt and uncertainty. Worm may well have been inspired by Scaliger in his critical approach, but his reliance on observation and inductive reasoning went beyond what Scaliger had envisaged by pointing towards the importance of the activities of physicians, the role of anatomical theatres, botanical gardens, chemical laboratories, the calculations of astronomers, and the observations and experiments of natural philosophers. The true philosopher, Worm argued, did not exclusively follow one man's teachings.

According to the Rosicrucians a new philosophy drawn from the Bible was needed. Worm admitted that philosophy was the servant of theology, but not to the extent that philosophical reasoning – ratio – was subject to faith – fides theological. On that basis Worm praised the achievements of contemporary explores, astronomers, anatomists and their discoveries. The Rosicrucians' appeal to the learned to accept their wonders was meaningless as long as they remained hidden and unexplained. It was noteworthy that Worm in his rejection of Rosicrucianism also took the opportunity to deny theology the right to control and determine research into natural philosophy, medicine, and natural history.[10]

Apart from personally having developed serious reservations about Rosicrucianism over a number of years while retaining his fascination with the phenomenon, Worm may well have had good political and religious reasons for publicly rejecting Rosicrucianism at this point. The fact that he had taken a serious interest in the Rosicrucians and read and owned their publications might have been enough to put him at risk by May 1619. Worm had, as we have seen, opponents within the university among whom were

9 The fame of the brotherhood of R. C., *Fama Fraternitatis R. C.*, was published in Germany in 1614; the confession of the brotherhood of R. C., *Confessio Fraternitatis R. C.* was published in Germany in 1615; it is interesting that Worm does not refer to the third of the Rosicrucian manifestos, *The Chymical Wedding of Christian Rosicross anno 1459*, which was published in 1616. See Frances A. Yates, *The Rosicrucian Enlightenment*, London 1972, especially chapters IV and V.
10 See Schepelern, *Museum*, 115–17.

the professor of theology, Hans Poulsen Resen, the leading advocate of Lutheran uniformity. A couple of years earlier Resen had played a prominent part in having his own brother-in-law, H. K. Vejle, deposed as Bishop of Funen for his perceived Calvinism. Vejle had stood accused of having encouraged his ministers to read books which did not correspond with the Danish Church Order. Publicly washing his hands in 1619 of any connection with Rosicrucianism undoubtedly served Worm well. His timing would appear to have been impeccable. Shortly afterwards Hans Poulsen Resen dismissed the Rosicrucians as dangerous religious fanatics, while continuing to seek out dissenters in his drive for uniformity.[11] This was demonstrated by the fall of the royal mathematician Christopher Dybvad, who had been deeply opposed to Resen and his quest for religious uniformity and had settled in Bergen, where he had carelessly voiced his criticism of Resen. In March 1620 a royal order was issued to collect evidence against Dybvad for having used 'strange words and loose talk'. Subsequently the court of the university convicted him of religious heterodoxy. Dybvad lost his position for what he had 'expressed against God and the Christian religion'.[12]

Significantly, however, in 1622 Worm's patron and main religious influence, Holger Rosenkrantz, the Learned, found himself accused of being a Rosicrucian by his former teacher, the Stettin professor of theology Daniel Cramer. According to him, Rosenkrantz had become the mouthpiece of Spiritualists and Rosicrucians. Bearing in mind how difficult it proved for Rosenkrantz to disassociate himself from these accusations, it is obvious how politically and religiously opportune Ole Worm's public rejection of Rosicrucianism in May 1619 had been.[13]

Worm admitted in his 1619 oration that he had become seriously interested in the Paracelsian- inspired Rosicrucian phenomenon which swept across northern Europe in the years leading up to the Thirty Years' War. In 1611 Worm had been shown a 'secret', manuscript version of *The Fama Fraternitatis* by a 'famous iatrochemist' at a German university. This was undoubtedly Johannes Hartmann, professor of chemistry at the University of Marburg. Worm claimed that initially he had considered Rosicrucianism to be pure fantasy and totally obscure, but that Hartmann had convinced him of its value through weighty arguments. Consequently Worm had remained fascinated by Rosicrucianism until shortly before his speech on 10 May 1619.[14]

---

11 See, O. P. Grell, 'The Acceptable Face of Paracelsianism: The Legacy of Idea Medicinæ and the Introduction of Paracelsianism into Early modern Denmark', 245–67 in O. P. Grell (ed.) *Paracelsus. The Man and His Reputation, His Ideas and Their Transformation*, Leiden 1998, especially 260.

12 *Den danske Kirkes Historie*, ed. Hal Koch, vol. IV by Bjørn Kornerup, Copenhagen 1959.

13 Grell, 'Acceptable Face', 264–65

14 O. P. Grell, 'In Search of True Knowledge: Ole Worm (1588–1654) and the New Philosophy', 218 in Pamela H. Smith and Benjamin Schmidt (eds.), *Making Knowledge in Early Modern Europe. Practices, Objects, and Texts*, 1400–1800, Chicago 2007; for the identification of Johannes Hartmann as Worm's source, see H. Hotson, *Johann*

Back in August 1616 Ole Worm had asked his brother-in-law, Jacob Fincke, then studying in Giessen, to pass on reliable information about the Rosicrucian Brethren. He wanted to know who they were and where they were located, and whether or not the local prince, as rumoured, belonged to their society. Especially, Worm wanted to know anything which was *not* known from their published tracts, which he already possessed. He was particularly excited by the prospect of receiving the second part of *Nosologia Harmonica Dogmatica*, by the professor of medicine at the University of Marburg, Heinrich Petraeus. Petraeus, whom Worm had befriended while in Padua, was son-in-law of the famous chemist Johannes Hartmann and was seeking to find a unifying principle between Galenic medicine and chemical/alchemical medicine inspired by Paracelsus.[15] The following spring Worm asked his friend, Niels Foss, then in Strassburg to inform him if he had heard anything definite about the Rosicrucians. He was clearly fascinated even if he acknowledged that people differed fundamentally in their judgement of this phenomenon. However, the publication of Georg Molther's response to the Rosicrucians, *Antwort, der Hochwürdigen und Hocherleuchten Brüderschafft dess Rosen Creutzes* (1617), published at the latest Frankfurt Book Fair had convinced him that the movement could not be 'pure fabrication'. Molther, a recent graduate in medicine from the University of Marburg, managed to produce one of the most highly rated pamphlets in the rapidly growing literature on Rosicrucianism. His publication described the impressive exploits, learning, and eloquence of a traveller who had recently passed through the town of Wetzlar near Herborn, claiming to belong to the Rosicrucian Society.[16]

Worm, however, continued his search for reliable information about the Rosicrucians. Once again, in January 1618, he contacted his brother-in-law, Jacob Fincke, still in Giessen, asking him for information about the fraternity, pointing out to him that 'weird things' in print and rumours were circulating about them in Copenhagen. By the beginning of 1618 Worm still remained convinced that the Rosicrucians merited serious consideration. He had broached the matter with his good friend, the professor of theology, Jesper Rasmussen Brochmand, who served as tutor to the elected-prince. He even lent some of his Rosicrucian pamphlets to Brochmand for an extended period. When Brochmand returned them he side-stepped the issue by pointing out that 'to explain the new things, about which you have enigmatically written to me, an Oedipus would be required'. It is likely that Worm was by then already developing some religious reservations about Rosicrucianism and therefore sought the advice of Brochmand, in his capacity of professor of theology.

Alsted, 1588–1638: Between Renaissance, Reformation, and Universal Reform, Oxford 2000, 99.

15 *Breve fra og til Ole Worm*, no. 20; see also Grell, 'True Knowledge', 218–19.
16 *Ibid.*, no. 25; see also Grell, 'True Knowledge', 219 and *Hotson*, Alstedt, 100–01.

Writing to his student Laurits Scavenius in Strassburg in March 1618 Worm had revealed some reservations about the Rosicrucians when he described them as a sect. By then he had clearly realised the potential dangers of religious heterodoxy linked to Rosicrucianism. Even so, his interests in them had been reawakened by Scavenius's description of a busybody (ardelio) who had declared himself a supporter. Worm therefore wanted to know more about him or others who claimed to belong to them. A couple of months later Worm concluded that the Rosicrucians were lunatics who would eventually manage to disquiet even their own supporters after having for so long put off the credulous with empty promises. 'They had only produced tall tales and some sheets smeared with sweet visions' having promised with much bragging a total renovation of language and knowledge. It would all go up in smoke if they did not fulfil their promises'.[17] Worm, however, continued to be fascinated by the Rosicrucians, even if he remained deeply ambivalent about the phenomenon. On one hand he considered the Rosicrucians to be lunatic sectarians while on the other he sought as much information as he could possibly obtain about them.

The University of Giessen where Worm's brother-in-law, Jacob Fincke, studied was evidently a centre for Rosicrucian activity. Fincke informed Worm about the undertakings of 'the mad king of Jerusalem', Philip Ziegler, in the spring of 1618. Worm was delighted and had no doubt that if Ziegler was considered one of the pioneers of the Rosicrucians then one could easily conclude what to think about the others. Even so, he was keen to know what had happened to Ziegler and what he had done. Worm also wanted to know what Ziegler had declared, where the new Rosicrucian college had been established and whether he had succeeded in encouraging certain people to join his Society.[18] When Worm eventually received further news about Ziegler more than two years later, in August 1620, it was through his friend, Anders Jacobsen Langebæk, studying at the University of Jena. Philip Ziegler, an itinerant self-declared prophet had arrived in Jena on his travels and was clearly causing a stir. Worm had himself encountered Ziegler while in Heidelberg in January 1612. Then as now, Ziegler pandered his 'sweet melancholy' to impressionable people who, according to Worm, needed to be given 'stinking hellebore' so they could recover their senses.[19] Langebæk had also drawn Ole Worm's attention to a Rosicrucian pamphlet about whether the host was the true bread. Worm already knew and possessed this work. From that he had deducted that the whole Rosicrucian brotherhood, if it was anything at all, was a confluence of all sects.

17 *Ibid.*, nos. 44 and 48; see also Grell, 'True Knowledge', 219.
18 *Ibid.*, no. 49.
19 *Ibid.*, no. 78; for Worm's presence in Heidelberg in 1612, see V. Helk, *Dansk-Norske Studierejser fra reformationen til enevælden 1536–1660*, Odense 1987, 429; for Philip Ziegler, see R. Heisler, 'Philip Ziegler: The Rosicrucian King of Jerusalem', *The Hermetic Journal*, 14, 1990, 3–10.

He acknowledged that in some writings they declared themselves to be Lutherans, but their accounts were tainted by fanaticism and Anabaptism mixed with Paracelsianism. Even so Worm was still eager to be notified if anything new about them materialised, adding that he was convinced that the Rosicrucian Society had dissolved into nothing.[20] Despite his rejection of Rosicrucianism in his oration to graduating student in May 1619 Worm remained fascinated by the Rosicrucian furore until 1620, despite having serious doubts about their religious orthodoxy, and realising that they had promised much and delivered little.

In the summer of 1622 Worm wrote a letter to the itinerant patrician from Hamburg, Joachim Morsius, then residing in Rostock. He had met Mosius during the latter's visit to Copenhagen in 1617 and signed his album amicorum. Morsius was a leading Rosicrucian sympathiser who was one of the most assiduous collectors and editors of Rosicrucian and Hermetic manuscripts. Worm thanked him for the many manuscripts he had received from him over the years, but for which he had been unable to thank him until now, because of his itinerant life style. There can be no doubt that these manuscripts were copies of the Rosicrucian and Hermetic writings that Morsius had collected.[21] A year later in July 1623 Ole Worm asked his student Hans Andersen Skovgaard in Wittenberg to obtain a copy of the Rosicrucian associate and Paracelsian Henning Scheunemann's *Hydromantia*.[22] Worm, in other words, found it difficult to let go of his fascination with Rosicrucianism and retained his interest into the 1620s.[23]

3 The centenary of the reformation

Worm's brother-in-law, Caspar Bartholin, contributed to the celebrations of the centenary of the Reformation which had begun in Wittenberg in 1617, by giving a memorial lecture about Luther at the University of Copenhagen on 18 February 1618, the day of Luther's death. The oration, *De Luthero Panegyrius*, a Melanchthonian comparison of Elaijah with Luther, was published the following year.[24] It was part of an eight day celebration of the

20 *Ibid.*, no. 78.
21 *Ibid.*, no. 109; see also Schepelern, *Museum*, 117–18; for Joachim Morsius, see Hotson, *Alstedt*, 102 and 119–20.
22 *Ibid.*, no.142; see also H. Scheunemann, *Hydromantia Paracelsica seu de fonte circa Annabergam repetition*, Frankfurt 1613.
23 Not only did Ole Worm retain some interests in Rosicrucianism post 1619, but his interests in Paracelsianism remained strong and unaffected throughout his life. That the Rosicrucian debacle should have resulted in Worm rejecting Paracelsianism, as claimed by Jole Shackelford, 'Rosicrucianism, Lutheran Orthodoxy, and the Rejection of Paracelsianism in Early Seventeenth-Century Denmark', *Bulletin of the History of Medicine*, 70, 1996, 181–204, is not correct. See also Fink-Jensen, *Fornuften under troens lydighed*, 206 note 15
24 See Fink-Jensen, *Fornuften under troens lydighed*, 241–45.

centenary of the Reformation with sermons and speeches across Denmark and Norway. One is left with the impression that Worm was convinced that less might have been enough. Even if he appears to have been disappointed that no commemorative medals had been coined as they had in Strassburg. However, Worm was delighted with Bartholin's oration which had been well received by a large gathering of professors and ministers.[25] Bartholin having subsequently been elected vice chancellor in June 1618 then encouraged his brother-in-law, Ole Worm, to give another memorial lecture on 31 October 1618, celebrating the centenary of the Reformation. This was evidently an act meant to endorse and promote his brother-in-law, offering Worm and opportunity to show his Lutheran orthodoxy. As a newly elected dean who, like Caspar Bartholin, had studied theology before he had dedicated himself to medicine, Worm was also a reasonable choice for such an honour. His oration entitled *Jubilum Evangelicum*, was a forceful attack on the Jesuit Adam Contzen who had recently published his *Jubilum Jubilorum* in Maintz which sought to undermine the centenary celebrations of the Protestants. The frontispiece of Contzen's publication was a picture of the medal issued in 1617 by the Catholic Church. It had an image of the sun on one side with the inscription: 'The constant age of the church. It shines still after 1,617 years without changing'. On the other a picture of the moon, a symbol of perpetual change and the text: 'The inconsistent novelties of the heresies as they change their form 16,000 times in 100 years. Below the illustration Contzen quoted Ecclesiastes 27:12, 'The conversation of the pious is constantly wise, but a fool is as changeable as the moon'. In his tract Contzen traced the continuing disagreements among Protestants which confirmed his thesis that heresy destroyed itself, so after 100 years only the Catholics had anything to celebrate. Contzen and his tract in order words constituted an excellent polemical target for a Lutheran oration celebrating the centenary of the Reformation. Included in Worm's oration was a criticism of the Roman medal used by Contzen. In his manuscript for *Jubilum Evangelicum*, which was published in 1619, Worm included the design for two Protestant medals celebrating the centenary, clearly inspired by the Catholic medal from 1617, which were, however, never minted. One entitled Evangelical Splendour showed on the front an open Bible shone on by the sun and on the back the figure of Christ carrying a lamb. The other entitled Papal Squalor depicted lit candles under a bushel with reference to Matt.5:15 and Luc.11:33, indicating the secrecy and darkness in which the Bible was held by the Catholics while the back portrayed the Pope as Antichrist.[26] On publication in March 1619 Worm forwarded a copy to his patron, Holger Rosenkrantz the learned, to whom he had dedicated his

---

25 *Breve fra og til Ole Worm*, nos. 43 and 44; see also B. Kornerup, 'Reformationsjubilæet i Danmark 1617', *Kirkehistoriske Samlinger*, IV, R. 2, 1936, 33–83.
26 See Royal Library, Gl. Kgl. Saml. 3113, f. 251–52; see also Schepelern, *Museum*, 111–12

oration. The letter confirmed Ole Worm's close association with Rosenkrantz as a regular member of a group who were invited to attend Holger Rosenkrantz's theological lectures.[27]

4 Worm's university career takes shape

Worm, had as already mentioned, begun his lectures on Aristotle's *De Mundo* after Easter 1618. They resulted in four disputations of which two, II and IV, have survived. Disputation II took place on 29 July 1620 and the student-respondent was the later minister Anders Pedersen Hegelund. Disputation IV took place on 14 April 1621 and the respondent was the Icelandic student Thorlak Skulason who became a life-long friend and correspondent of Worm. Since Chapters 2 and 4 of Worm's published commentary *De Mundo* are based on the two surviving disputations, we can assume that the two lost disputations provided the material for Chapters 1 and 3.[28] The lectures most likely came to an end when Worm was made professor of natural philosophy in April 1621, while the plans for publishing the commentary on *De Mundo* would appear to have taken shape a year later. Worm used Bonaventura Vulcanus's edition from 1591 and agreed with him that Aristotle was the author of *De Mundo*. Worm's commentary incorporated new and recent discoveries in astronomy, geography, and medicine. Always the patriot Worm took the opportunity to point out, that if Aristotle had known about the fertile and glorious islands in the Danish sea he would rightfully have labelled this kingdom 'Europe's larder, inexhaustible barn and the wet nurse'. Worm claimed that if strangers had not been able to fetch so many thousands of oxen, such myriads of fish, and an abundance of crops, many would have perished because of famine. Denmark had been the richest store-room for all things necessary for life. That did not include the vast number of the finest horses which were in strong demand for warfare by the Germans, the French, the Spaniards, and the Italians, which were exported annually. Nor had any kingdom or empire produced a greater amount of gold and silver coins than the Danish custom house at Kronborg Castle. A fair assessment, Worm claimed, would recognise that the Danes were more necessary to other nations than they were to the Danes.[29]

Ole Worm's *De Mundo* was eventually published in Rostock in 1625 after a long and difficult publication process. It proved an experience which came to shape Ole Worm's attitude to publishers and printers as

---

27 *Breve fra og til Ole Worm*, no. 57; see also J. Glebe-Møller, 'Holger Rosenkrantz, 'the learned' (1574–1642)', 99–116 in O. P. Grell and A. Cunningham (eds.), *Medicine, Natural Philosophy and Religion in Post-Reformation Scandinavia*, New York 2017.

28 Schepelern, *Museum*, 123–24; see also Ole Worm, *Liber Aureus Philosophorum Aqilæ Aristotelis de Mundi Fabrica*, Rostock 1625; for Thorlak Skulason see below Chapters 2–4.

29 *Breve fra og til Ole Worm*, no. 104.

being generally unreliable and solely interested in short term profit. In 1622 Worm informed Joachim Morsius that he had included an honourable reference to him in his *De Mundo*, but that the printer Ferber through his carelessness and failure to keep his promises had forced him to recall this work in order to hand it to a more reliable printer either in Copenhagen or Rostock. Ferber had by then been sitting on Worm's manuscript for about a year. Worm was evidently hoping that Morsius might help him arrange for another Rostock printer to take on his work, such as Johann Hallerfort who eventually published it. Worm claimed he would be happy if he received only fifty copies of his book, as reward for his work.[30]

Johann Hallerfort published *De Mundo* in 1625, but early proofs of part of the book reached Worm in the summer of 1624. Worm was far from impressed with what he had received as he made Hallerfort understand. The book had not been properly proof read and was full of mistakes, and Aristotle's text had not been included, leaving Worm's commentaries on their own. Worm also disliked the ostentatious title Hallerfort had given his work. He felt particularly aggravated by Hallerfort's description of his commentaries as being 'highly erudite', which in his opinion amounted to boasting. It contained so many misprints that Worm was reluctant to accept the book as his own. He sent Hallerfort a long list of errata which should be added and told him to take greater care with the rest of the book and make sure it was provided with an index. Worm also informed Hallerfort that he wanted a hundred copies on fine paper since he was to receive no payment for his efforts.[31] Worm's intervention did little to improve the quality of the publication and he remained deeply disappointed with it, claiming that it had been mangled by the publisher whom he would never trust again.[32]

Shortly after his promotion to the chair in natural philosophy in April 1621, Ole Worm was elected dean of the Faculty of Philosophy for the second time. Having been chosen unanimously by his colleagues for this chair Worm's career prospects had improved considerably.[33] The inaugural address Worm gave when taking up the chair in natural philosophy was of particular significance and laid out his approach to the subject. Worm adhered to the same Melanchthonian methodology in natural philosophy which had been advocated by his predecessor, Jens Sinning, three generations earlier in a speech from 1545, *Oratio de Studiis Philosophicus*,[34] emphasising the significance of natural philosophy for other disciplines

---

30 *Ibid.*, nos. 109 and 111.
31 *Ibid.*, no. 158.
32 *Ibid.*, nos. 163, 167, and 489.
33 *De physics Præstantia et Utilitate*, fol.2r in Royal Library Copenhagen, Rostgaard 269, quarto, nos. 28–29
34 *Oratio de Studiis Philosophicis* was published with an introduction by Anders Sørensen Vedel in Ribe in 1591. See Jens Andersen Sinning, *Oration on the Philosophical Studies Necessary for the Student of Theology 1545*, ed. E. Jacobsen, Copenhagen 1991; see also Fink-Jensen, *Fornuften under troens lydighed*, 112–21.

such as theology and medicine. However, in a number of significant aspects Worm offered a different interpretation.

Worm's oration, *De physics Præstantia et Utilitate*, provided a programme for how the true natural philosopher should gather knowledge. In each case he had to 'analyse in depth the object or case in hand, describe in detail on what plan or reasons he depended, determine what qualities it had, in order that he could explain as perfectly as possible what it could do, and what it was useful for, and to what extent it was created and nurtured by the Highest and Almighty God'.[35] According to Ole Worm natural philosophy was introduced by God, who at the time of the Creation gave it to Adam in Paradise, the father of all mankind, as if to couch him in a unique sign of innate divinity. Because, when he had countenanced all species of animals which had just been created for his glory, he gave them different and distinctive names while carefully considering, weighing, and illuminating the nature and relationship of each specie.

Worm then described how Adam had transferred his knowledge of natural philosophy to his children and their descendants from whom it had reached the Egyptians. Even if Moses picked it up from the Egyptians, Worm was convinced that he had received the foundation for this divine, natural philosophy from God himself and God's people after the Creation. King Salomon had proved particularly knowledgeable about Nature, and his reputation had attracted the Queen of Sheba, who having received this knowledge, had it written down in hieroglyphs. If God through his Grace had shared this knowledge with his own age, Worm was convinced that they would not now be stuck in this great haze, like the fox in Aesop's fable restricted to liking the glass jar without touching the porridge.[36] Instead early modern scholars were forced to retrieve this knowledge through Plato and Aristotle. Despite the fact that these Greek philosophers were heathens, scholars were allowed to seek out the knowledge which God had given Man at the time of the Creation. Thus, natural philosophy made it possible to recognise God's omnipotence through Nature, his Creation.[37] Worm had no doubt that by the early seventeenth century the guardians of the secrets of Nature were the physicians who had become the true natural philosophers who had helped recover them.[38] This history of natural philosophy, its loss and retrieval, was one which Worm shared with Paracelsians and those who held the Hermetic writings in high regard.

Ole Worm began his lectures dealing with the natural philosophy of Aristotle under the title Epitome Physices Aristotelicæ. This was followed

35 *De physics Præstantia et Utilitate*, fol.1r.
36 *Ibid.*, fols 3r–3v.
37 *Ibid.*, fols. 3r–4r; see also Schepelern, *Museum*, 126.
38 *Ibid.*, fol. 8r.

by an analysis of Aristotle's *Parva Naturalia* and his *De Anima*, which he finished in September 1623, only to start once more with Epitome. Dealing with De Anima we can safely assume that Worm used Philip Melanchthon's *De Anima*, in its revised edition from 1552.[39] More significantly Worm gave an introductory speech to his exposition of Aristotle, dated 6 June 1621, which demonstrated his considerable interest and attraction to Hermeticism and Paracelsianism. Referring directly to the supposed Ancient, Egyptian priest, Hermes Trismegistus, he informed his audience that Hermes had emphasised that Man raised himself above other creatures through his soul and reason. Through the guidance of soul and reason Man could, according to Hermes, achieve knowledge of everything created, and gradually reach a perfect understanding of the Creator. Through divine grace Man had been granted a natural philosophical insight which in accordance with traditional religious customs could be used to contemplate everything created. However, if one considered this to be the theory about God's creation, or natural theology, one would totally miss the point. Because it did not consist of a simple contemplation of everything created, but of a profound scrutiny of the causes in Nature, their essence, and their special characteristics, without missing anything which appeared 'in the theatre of the world'.[40] Evidently Worm depended heavily on both Hermeticism and Paracelsianism in his natural philosophical outlook. His rejection of natural theology as a way of achieving detailed knowledge about Nature and the Creation is also significant. For Worm only natural philosophy with its analysis, observation, and description could provide the necessary and reliable knowledge about Nature

However, Ole Worm did not accept Paracelsianism uncritically. One of the two disputations, Qvæstionum Miscellarum Decas (1622), from his three-year stint as professor of natural philosophy, demonstrate that he had issues with Paracelsianism. Worm was particularly critical of what he considered a totally unnecessary construction of a new Paracelsian terminology which only served to obscure the meaning, making Paracelsus's works inaccessible. Likewise, Worm was not convinced of the value of the three Paracelsian principles of salt, sulphur, and mercury promoted by Peter Severinus, the Dane, in his *Idea Medicinae Philosophicae*, and he failed to see that they could make any improvement if they were to replace the four elements.

In June 1620 Ole Worm, on the encouragement of Chancellor Christen Friis, had written to Peter Severinus's son, Frederik Severinus, a friend of

39 See Schepelern, *Museum*, 126 and Fink-Jensen, *Fornuften under troens lydighed*, 180–81; especially 181, note 63 where Fink-Jensen correctly points to the disputation from 1631 and Worm's insistence that the physician should pay attention to the soul, because it was the physician's duty to care for the whole animated body of Man.
40 See Royal Library, Copenhagen, Rostgaard 269, quarto, nr. 39.

his, who had settled as a physician in Flensborg. Christen Friis had been told that Frederik was in possession of his father's manuscripts. Bearing in mind his father's European fame the chancellor wanted Frederik to publish them, and Worm held out the prospect of significant rewards if Frederik Severinus undertook this work.

Frederik Severinus had made some of his father's comments on Aristotle's work on natural philosophy available for Worm to use in his lectures on Aristotle. The chancellor on hearing that had encouraged Worm to edit and publish them under Petrus Severinus's name as an encouragement to Frederik to publish the manuscripts he held. Worm, however, wanted Frederik to take responsibility for publishing all the manuscripts, because he considered him to be in a much better position to undertake the work. Only if Frederick Severinus specifically wanted him to undertake this work would Worm go ahead. Meanwhile, Frederik Severinus's sister had forwarded a list of her father's manuscripts in her brother's possession to Christen Friis. The chancellor had then marked the items on the list he personally wanted to see and asked Worm to forward it to Frederik, reminding him of how much he wanted him to publish these manuscripts. Nothing came of the chancellor's plans most likely because of Frederik Severinus's lack of interest in the enterprise.[41]

5 Professor of medicine

Ole Worm was promoted to a chair in medicine in March 1624. It had become vacant after the promotion of his brother-in-law, Caspar Bartholin to the vacant chair in theology following the death of Cort Aslaksen. In his inaugural address on 23 March 1624, *De Dignitate et Præsentia artis Medicae*, Worm referred to this chain of events, describing Cort Aslaksen as 'once this university's brightest torch and light', while voicing his own concerns about taking up his new position. Aslaksen, a Melanchthonian, who had served as an assistant to the astronomer, Tycho Brahe on the island of Hven in the mid-1590s, was as we have seen much appreciated by Ole Worm and other scholars influenced by Holger Rosenkrantz, the Learned, such as his brother-in-law Caspar Bartholin.[42]

After a brief discourse about ancient medicine Worm took the opportunity to emphasise that the roots of Christian medicine should be found in

---

41 *Breve fra og til Ole Worm*, nos. 73 and 74; there is nothing in these two letters to indicate that Worm wanted to disassociate himself from the Severinian form of Paracelsianism as claimed by Schepelern, *Museum*, 128.

42 The Royal Library, Copenhagen, Rostgaard 269, quarto, no. 31, fol. 1r. For Cort Aslaksen, see above and J. R. Christianson, *On Tycho's Island. Tycho Brahe and His Assistants, 1570–1601*, Cambridge 2000, 252–53

the *Book of Genesis*. God had created medicine to care for both the body and soul.

> There was nothing in botany, nothing in anatomy, which God had not created, but also taught. He invented physiology, created pathology, gifted us semiotics, and transmitted hygiene to us. That only left pathology which provided us with a way to recover poor health. Before the Fall there was no need for this, since God provided our first forefather with total health.[43]

Worm, as a follower of Melanchthon, concluded that Christian medicine differed significantly from that of the ancients because it dealt with the body as well as the soul as opposed to being exclusively focussed on the body. He underlined how medicine, having been given to Adam, passed via Noah, to Moses and Egyptians, who had been the guardians of true medical knowledge after the Fall, while emphasising the divine origin of medicine. He also pointed to the significance of medicine in spreading the Gospel, claiming that apostolic history showed how healing complemented the spread of Christianity.[44]

Ole Worm also took the opportunity to praise Christian IV for what he had done for education and learning in his realm. Medicine in particular had been of importance to the king in strengthening his kingdoms and Worm took the opportunity to thank him and the chancellor, Christen Friis, who had recommended him for the chair in medicine.[45] Eleven years after he had been given his first chair in pedagogy Worm was finally able to take up the position he had always wanted. Giving the inaugural address on taking up his chair in medicine was a major event noted not only by the leading lights within the university but also by the king and his most prominent councillors.

Worm concluded his oration by pointing out that there was plenty to do for those who dedicated their lives to medicine. So far no one knew the extent of botany, nor for that matter had anyone explored the 'deepest layers' of anatomy. An understanding of the composition, behaviour, and capacity of the soul of all humans was still missing. 'The labyrinth of complicated illnesses' which were spreading daily could not be ignored. To deal with all that time was short. In order to properly understand and practice medicine much time and effort was needed in order to comprehend what Worm described as an 'extensive art'.[46]

---

43 *Ibid.*, fol. 3v (marginal addition).
44 *Ibid.*, fols. 5r–6r.
45 *Ibid.*, fol. 8v.
46 *Ibid.*, fol. 11r. Schepelern considered Worm's inaugural address disappointingly bland and offering little new in terms of research, see Schepelern, *Museum*, 160. That misses

Ole Worm was to occupy his chair in medicine for the next thirty years until his death in 1654. Despite all his other engagements as a physician with a large practice, as an antiquarian, and as a collector, he proved an extremely diligent and hard-working professor. Furthermore, he also served the university as its vice chancellor no less than five times, in 1628, 1636, 1642, 1648, and 1654.[47] As professor of medicine Worm was obliged to arrange and set up an annual disputation. He held twenty-four in his thirty years tenure. We have eighteen printed disputations from the period 1624 to 1652, all with the title *Controversiarum Medicarum Exercitationes*, and published annually, and another five from the years 1636 to 1640 which were published together under the title *Institutionum Medicarum Epitome*, and finally a disputation from 1653, *Assertiones Medicæ De Febribus in Genere*. The five disputations published together in 1640 were intended to serve as a textbook for new medical students. Worm undertook no disputations in the years 1625, 1628, 1629, 1635, 1647, 1650, 1653, and 1654. In most cases he was prevented from holding the disputations for a variety of reasons. In 1625 Denmark had entered the Thirty Years' War while the country was still struggling with an outbreak of dysentery, measles, and smallpox. Worm was concerned that 'plague, war, and famine was hanging over their heads'. In 1628 he had become vice chancellor for the first time and his first wife died in November. The following year, 1629, Denmark was hit by a serious outbreak of plague and the university was dissolved. In 1635 Ole Worm was seriously ill in May, but when explaining why he did not deliver his annual disputation that year, Worm excused himself by referring to his extraordinary involvement in Ambrosius Rhode's disputation on scurvy, and his role in inspecting the apothecaries.[48] The next gap in 1637 occurred when he once again became vice chancellor and his second wife died. Ten years later, in 1647, Ole Worm had been obliged to spend two months away from the university, providing medical treatment for the elected-prince at his court in Nykøbing Falster. Finally, in 1654 Worm had been appointed vice chancellor again during the outbreak of another serious plague epidemic of which he himself became a casualty in August that year.[49]

Only a minority of the respondents of the eighteen disputations from 1624 to 1652 became physicians and took medical degrees. The first was Christen Stougaard, who was the respondent at Worm's second disputation in 1626. He was granted a royal bursary from 1627 to 1633 and undertook

---

the fact that it was an occasion of considerable social and political importance, where the major figures had to be acknowledged.

47 Hovesen, *Ole Worm*, 134.

48 *Breve fra og til Ole Worm*, no. 579.

49 See Hovesen, *Ole Worm*, 157–58. The content of the disputations are covered in detail in Chapter VIII, 157–208. See also Schepelern, *Museum*, 160–61; for 1625 see *Breve fra of til Ole Worm*, no. 173; for 1647, see *Ibid.*, no. 1483.

an extensive educational journey abroad before becoming professor of eloquence in Copenhagen in 1639, obtaining his MD from the University of Copenhagen in 1640. Worm remained in close contact with his former pupil until the latter's death in 1645.[50]

The German, Caspar Ringelmann, was the respondent at Worm's sixth disputation in 1632 which was primarily concerned with the circulation of the blood as put forward by William Harvey. Ringelmann, who originated from Osnabrück later became personal physician to the Duke of Oldenburg.[51] In 1645 the respondent was Henrik J. F. Fabricius, son of Christian IV's royal physician Henrik Fabricius. Worm recommended him the following year as a medical student to his friend, Herman Conring, professor of Medicine in Helmstedt.[52]

The last respondent of the Controversiarum Medicarum Exercitationes series was Ole Worm's son Willum, who obtained his MD in Padua in 1657 and was appointed professor of natural philosophy at the University of Copenhagen in 1662.[53]

The *Institutionum Medicarum Epitome* which Ole Worm published in 1640, consisting of five disputations, was clearly intended to form a coherent volume suitable as a textbook for new medical students. The book was dedicated to Worm's father-in-law Thomas Fincke, who was also dean of the medical faculty. Three of the five disputations involved students who held the royal bursary while studying medicine abroad. The respondent of the first disputation in 1636 was the young Thomas Bartholin, then only twenty years old, Worm's nephew, who became professor of medicine in Copenhagen in 1649. The second respondent six years later, in 1638, was Hans Leyel who died while abroad in 1641. Finally in 1640 the respondent was Christen Stougaard, who had been appointed professor of eloquence the previous year. This was his second disputation and served to secure him his MD in December 1640.[54]

Worm's last disputation took place in November 1653 dealing with the role and significance of fevers. The respondent was Henrik a Mønichen, who had served as Thomas Bartholin's assistant in his anatomical dissections. Mønichen left Copenhagen to study abroad shortly after the disputation and eventually returned to become royal physician to Frederik III in 1660.[55]

50 *Ibid.*, 161–62 and 205.
51 *Ibid.*, 185.
52 *Ibid.*, 192–93
53 *Ibid.*, 201–03
54 For these disputations, see *Ibid.*, 203–05; see also Helk, *Dansk-Norske Studierejser*, 162, 298, 391.
55 Hovesen, *Ole Worm*, 207–08; see also Helk, *Dansk-Norske Studierejser*, 321 and *Cista Medica Hafniensis*, 196, 215.

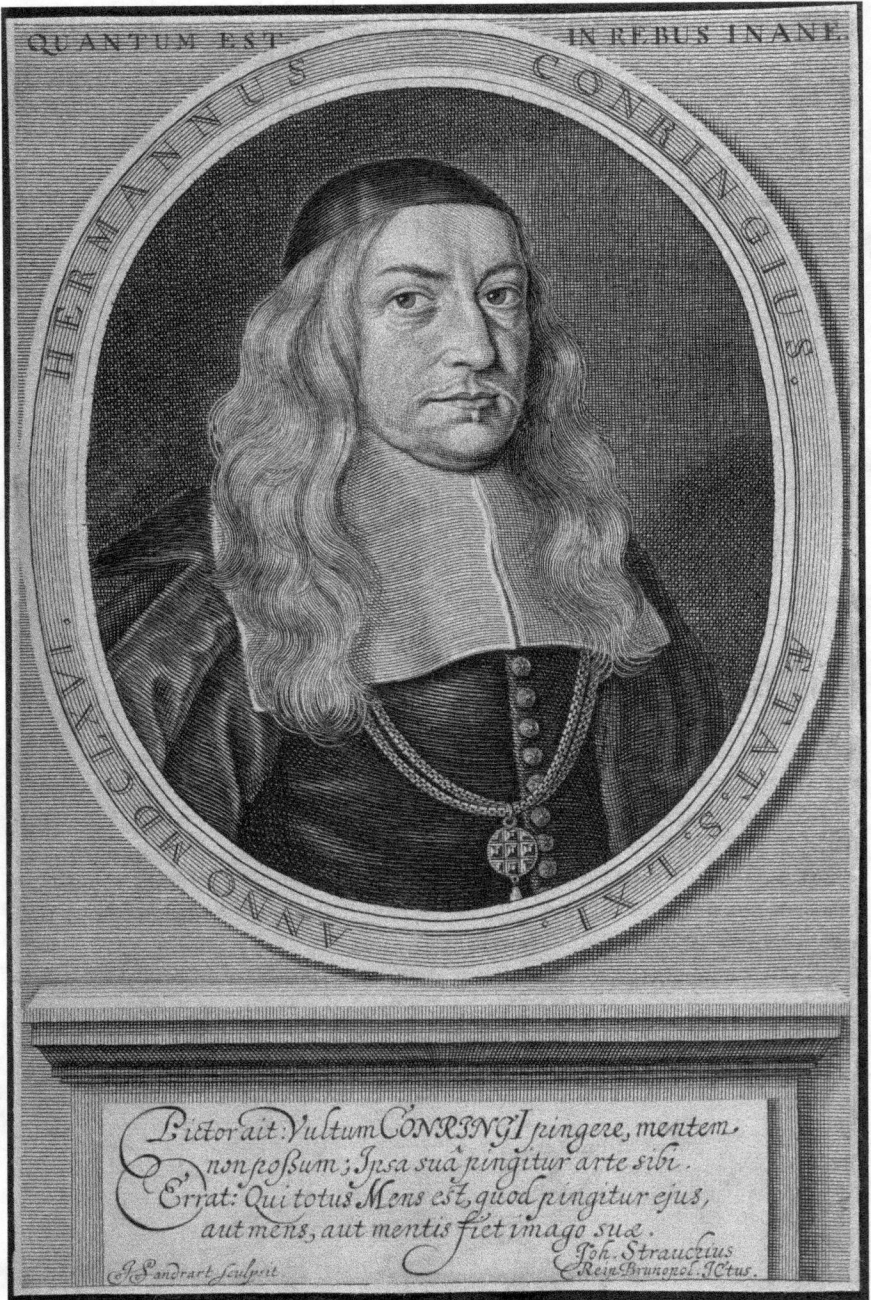

Figure 2.3 Herman Conring (1606–81); courtesy of the Royal Danish Library.

6 The scholar

Despite his disappointment about Rosicrucianism Ole Worm retained his interest in Paracelcianism throughout his life. In March 1618 he recommended one of his students in France, Niels Foss, to travel via Orléans and seek out the iatrochemist, Guillaume de Trogny, and befriend him. Worm had clearly met De Trogny while in France in 1610 on his peregrinatio academica, describing him as 'a fine man extremely experienced in the chemical art'. While in Orléans Worm had been given the opportunity to copy one of De Trogny's chemical works, but having been unable to finish it, he was keen for Niels Foss to obtain this work for him.

Guillaume de Trogny was a prominent member of the alchemical circle around the famous French Paracelsians, Theodore de Mayerne and Joseph du Chesne. He was a Huguenot, a physician and an alchemist, working closely with De Mayerne and known within the French alchemist circle as 'Hermes'.[56]

When Niels Foss reached Paris Worm wanted him to seek out Jean Béguin, whose book *Tyrocinium Chymicum* (1610) Worm considered an excellent beginner's introduction into chemistry. He also encouraged Foss to meet Etienne de Clave, 'a well-bred man, exceedingly experienced in chemistry and a superb practitioner' from whom Foss would not depart without having learned a lot.[57] Both were prominent Paracelsians and Jean Béguin was a protégé of Theodore de Mayerene. Worm had most likely made the acquaintance of both of these men while in Paris in the spring of 1610.[58]

Niels Foss succeeded not only in meeting Guillaume de Trogny in 1619 but also in gaining his confidence. Worm was delighted and told Foss that he should not be too concerned that De Trogny was reluctant to share his views with him, pointing out that scholars in this field were well-known for their discretion. Worm had no doubt that De Trogny would prove more informative when he had discovered what Foss was capable of, not to mention his view of Paracelcianism and iatrochemistry.[59]

Worm was delighted when in 1623 his student Hans Andersen Skovgaard informed him that he was studying iatrochemistry in Wittenberg under the guidance of Daniel Sennert, and that Skovgaard had joined a small group of students who had taken up the offer of private laboratory exercises under Sennert's guidance at the cost of ten thalers each. Skovgaard informed Worm that together with Johannes Hartmann Daniel Sennert

---

56 H. Trevor-Roper, *Europe's Physician. The Various Life of Sir Theodore de Mayerne*, New Haven 2006, 93.
57 *Breve fra og til Ole Worm*, no. 43.
58 For Jean Béguin and Etienne de Clave, see A. G. Debus, *The French Paracelsians. The Chemical Challenge to Medical and Scientific Tradition in Early Modern France*, Cambridge 1991, 80–82, 70–71.
59 *Breve fra og til Ole Worm*, no. 55.

was considered the leading light of iatrochemistry and sent him a copy of Sennert's *Institutiones Medicinae*. Worm encouraged Skovgaard to keep him informed about the experiments he undertook under Sennert's guidance, and asked him to provide him with an example of how Sennert went about curing a specific disease. Worm declared that he greatly admired everything Sennert had written and that everyone praised him for his clarity and honesty.[60]

Worm's students were encouraged to seek out iatrochemists when studying abroad and to get directly involved in their experiments. In 1638 Worm's nephew, Henrik Fuiren, studying medicine in Paris, informed him that he had been taught chemistry by the Scotsman, 'Dr. Davidson'. This was a reference to the Paracelsian iatrochemist and later first professor of chemistry at the Jardin Royal des Plants in Paris, William Davidson. From Davidson's textbook, *Philosophia Pyrotechnia seu Curriculus Chymiatricus*, published between 1633 and 1635, it can be seen that he was strongly influenced by Rosicrucians, neo-Platonists, and Paracelsus, and advocated a mystical chemistry.[61]

Another Parisian physician influenced by Paracelsian iatrochemistry, was the botanist, Guy de la Brosse, who had founded the Jardin Royal des Plantes. His work, *De la nature, vertu et utilité des plantes* (1628), had dedicated one out of five books to a discussion of chemistry. De la Brosse was keen on iatrochemistry and admired both Paracelsus and Peter Severinus, the Dane. He complained, however, that most iatrochemical works were too focussed on theory rather than practice. Instead, De la Brosse encouraged laboratory experiments, pointing out that too many physicians were reluctant to get their hands dirty.[62] He was sought out by Ole Worm's students when in Paris in this period. In January 1639 Worm asked his student Niels Bertelsen Wichman to obtain a copy of *De la nature, vertu et utilité des plantes* for him. Having received and read this book by May 1640 Worm, clearly impressed, wrote to his nephew Thomas Bartholin, then in Paris: 'There is in Paris a certain De la Brosse who is an excellent botanist and chemist; I owe his work on plants, where he promises to publish a book on both the natural and methodological art of medicine'. Worm wanted Thomas to send him a copy the moment it was published.[63]

Ole Worm made a concerted effort to keep himself abreast of new developments within iatrochemistry and Paracelsianism throughout his career. By January 1646, having become aware of the writings of Jean Baptiste van Helmont through his many Leiden contacts, Worm wrote to his nephew Thomas in Paris, referring to Van Helmont as 'a peculiar paradox-monger' who claimed that a physician did not merit his name if he was unable to cure a fever patient within four days. Apparently Van

60 Grell, 'In Search of True Knowledge', 220.
61 *Ibid.*; see also Debus, *The French Paracelsians*, 124–25
62 Debus, *The French Paracelsians*, 82–84.
63 Grell, 'In Search of True Knowledge', 221.

Helmont claimed he could remove the cause of all fevers with a cut, and boasted that he had cured hundreds of tertiary fevers using plasters without any relapses occurring. Worm had been informed that Van Helmont lived near Brussels and he was keen for Thomas Bartholin to travel back to Leiden via Brussels so he could discover whether there was any truth behind his 'bombastic statements'. Evidently the fact that Van Helmont had died a couple of years earlier had yet to reach Copenhagen. Worm, had clearly read some of Van Helmont's work when in 1647 another Bartholin nephew, Erasmus, informed him that the collected works of Jean Baptiste van Helmont were being printed by Elzevier (*Ortus Medicinae*, 1648); this edition would contain all Van Helmont's published works, including 'his excellent books on fevers and the stone which Erasmus knew that Worm was familiar with', but also much new material by his son Franciscus Mercurius van Helmont.

Later that year Worm was asked for his opinion of the treatments advocated by Jean Baptiste van Helmont by the son of his old friend, Henrik Køster, who had just begun practicing medicine. Worm had little positive to say. He began by pointing out that the personal physician to Elector Ferdinand of Bavaria, Henrick van Heer, had labelled Van Helmont 'the Empiric from Brussels', in other words a charlatan. Worm admitted that he had read Van Helmont's pamphlets, but had discovered nothing but empty words. He considered it 'a Paracelsian folly which sought to subvert the foundations of medicine that had been confirmed through extensive experience, together with slander'. Because Van Helmont wanted to appear deeply pious he, according to Worm, drew a veil over the remedies he had used for healing, or shrouded them in riddles to such an extent that they could not be of any use to those who sought to understand them. Worm could not comprehend that Van Helmont's experiments were extolled when he avoided passing them on in a form which made it possible for others to try the same investigations. Unless some clarification was provided Worm thought that Van Helmont and his cures were better ignored.[64]

From this statement one would expect Worm to have abandoned any further interest in the ideas of Van Helmont by 1647, despite the enthusiasm for Helmontian medicine among his students studying in Leiden. However, the impact of Van Helmont's ideas proved significant within the medical schools of the Dutch universities in general, and the University of Leiden in particular.

Thus, it was his Leiden based medical student, Christen Foss who forwarded him a copy of the royal physician Walter Charleton's first published work, *Spiritus Gorgonicus* (1650), offering an account of the formation of stones in the human body, rooted in Helmontian and Paracelsian sources.

---

64 *Breve far og til Ole Worm*, nos. 1536 and 1543. For Van Helmont, see G. D. Hedesan, *An Alchemical Quest for Universal Knowledge. The 'Christian Philosophy of Jan Baptist Van Helmont (1579–1644)*, New York 2016.

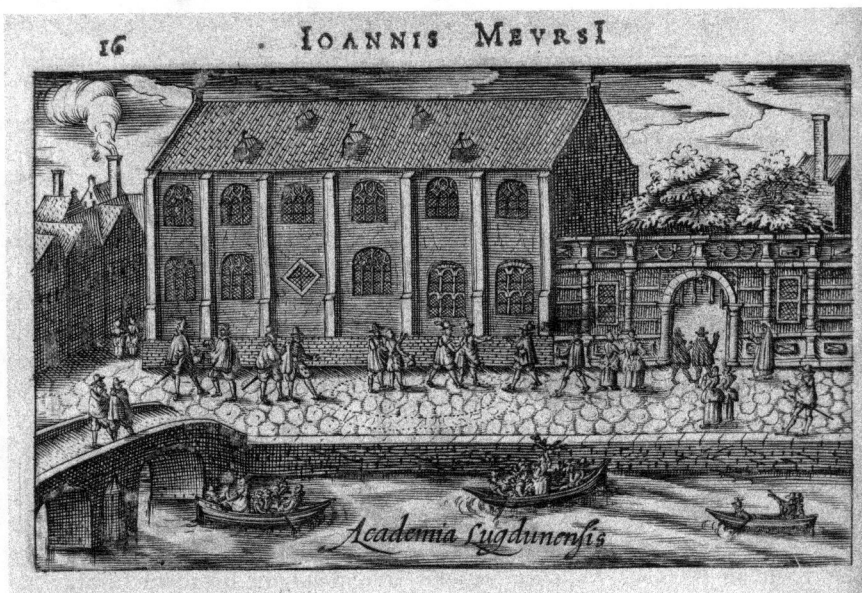

Figure 2.4 Leiden University 1614; courtesy of the Wellcome Collection.

Having read it Worm wanted his nephew, Erasmus Bartholin, to tell him what the stone was like, which Charleton labelled Ludus and claimed could be found in Antwerp. Worm expressed a burning desire to find out what it was, and would be very grateful if Erasmus could obtain a piece of this stone through a friend and send it to him. Worm had always shared the opinion 'of other Paracelsians' that Ludus meant a small stone secreted from the human body or removed by a cut. He added that he would be delighted if Erasmus could find out more about Charleton's Ludus.[65] Bearing in mind the fascination with the ideas of Van Helmont around 1650 within the European medical community Worm's enthralment with the publication of a leading proponent of Helmontianism is understandable. Furthermore, the period had also witnessed a growing obsession within medicine to find a cure for the stone, and Van Helmont's remedy, the so-called Ludus helmontii, promised to be the sovereign cure for that disease and was much sought after by physicians.

Accordingly, Ole Worm encouraged his nephew Erasmus Bartholin to seek out the Helmontian physician Walter Charleton and his associates on his planned visit to London in 1650. Erasmus failed to make contact with Charleton or any of his friends, but on his return journey the physician Joel

---

65 *Ibid.*, no. 1685; for Christen Foss, see *Helk, Dansk-Norske Studierejser*, 211. For Walter Charleton, see C. Webster, *The Great Instauration. Science, Medicine and Reform 1626–1660*, London 1975, 276–78.

Langlot had shown him a small piece of the Ludus. It would appear that Langlot had obtained it from Charleton himself, who had originally been given it by Van Helmont's son. It was a type of flint found on the banks of the river Schelde coloured like clay. It was called Ludus because all those stones looked like dice and had a cubic shape. Erasmus had personally tried to find similar stones walking along the Schelde, but had been told that they were only found deep down in the banks.[66]

Worm eventually managed to obtain some of the Helmontian Ludus from the Netherlands. It was a hard yellow flint shaped like small dice, confirming what he had been told by Erasmus Bartholin. Having been sent a sample of what young Henrik Køster considered to be Ludus, Worm concluded that if Ludus was a type of flint, then the stone, Køster had sent him, which could be scraped with a knife was too soft. It would appear that Køster's stone originated from Van Helmont's son Franciscus, who, according to Worm, had little learning and could not be relied on.[67]

In 1646 Worm had recently re-read *Unheard-of Curiosities* by Jacques Gaffarel, originally published in 1629,[68] and noted that Gaffarel mentioned a method whereby plants could be resurrected from ash in a glass. This phenomenon, known as palingenesis, had been widely discussed among Paracelsians since the sixteenth century, who believed plants could be calcinated to ashes, and then, when heated in a hermetically sealed glass container, the plant's original shape would reappear in a gaseous form in the vessel. It had been advocated by Paracelsus himself and a number of his prominent followers such as Joseph du Chesne and Athanasius Kircher, to mention only two. From his reading Worm had discovered that palingenesis had been demonstrated daily to an audience in Paris by a learned chemist, Etienne de Clave. Worm had therefore contacted the millenarian scholar and diplomat, Isaac La Peyrére, whom he had recently befriended during the latter's visit to Copenhagen to find out more about this man and if possible to obtain the ash from one of his calcinated plants. As it turned out not only was Isaac La Peyrère a good friend of Jacques Gaffarel, but he also knew Etienne de Clave and had seen him produce flowers in a glass, and he was convinced that he could obtain some ash from a variety of plants for Worm.[69]

Having received La Peyrére's response and read Gaffarel's statement Worm was convinced that the resurrection of plants was possible, even if he admitted that he had previously harboured some doubts. Many scholars had written extensively about palingenesis, but Worm had so far remained unconvinced, unless they had personally witnessed the process. So

66 *Ibid.*, no. 1694.
67 *Ibid.*, no. 1751.
68 J. Gaffarel, *Curiosités inouïes sur la sculpture talismanique des Persans, horoscope des patriarches des étoiles*, Paris 1629.
69 For Isaac La Peyrére and his friendship with Worm see below Chapter 4.

far Worm had been unable to bring it about himself having used methods recommended by friends. He referred specifically to the Leipzig professor Philip Müller's work *Miracula chymica, et mysteria medica*, which described the whole process. Despite following it closely Worm had failed to achieve anything. What he wanted was an example from someone who had mastered the art and carried out the 'mystery'. Because of the pettiness which was typical of people who communicated such secrets to others they tended to conceal the most important details. The result was that those who followed their instructions wasted their time.[70]

In April 1648 Worm received an inquiry from his Leiden based nephew, Erasmus Bartholin, asking him if he had managed to obtain the herb which grew in a bottle of water, as described by Athanasius Kircher, which Erasmus knew he wanted. According to Erasmus the Paracelsian physician, Joel Langlot, who had accompanied him on his recent trip to England, and who had recently taken up the post of court physician to the Duke of Gottorp, knew this secret. On Erasmus's insistence he had promised to share it with Worm. However, Worm had heard nothing from Langlot, but was prepared to contact him if Erasmus was certain that he possessed the right method. Worm pointed out that many people had offered descriptions and ways to produce 'such salts'; he personally owned two, but when he had attempted them, they had failed. Meanwhile, Worm felt obliged to clarify a few things for Erasmus. He was not looking for the herb which Kircher referred to in his work on the great art of light and shadow (*Ars Magna Lucis et Umbrae*, 1645), drawing on the work of Andreas Libavius. This plant had grown accidentally and not through art. Worm was looking for what Joseph du Chesne referred to in his work on Hermetic medicine. It was concerned with the ash or salt of plants which a certain Polish gentleman kept in different bowls, and from which, using gentle heat, he was able to produce spirits of plants in life-like colours, which, when cooling down, became salt again. Worm emphasised that he was not interested in whether Langlot had a description of the method, but only if Erasmus Bartholin had seen him successfully conduct such an experiment. He informed Erasmus that he knew that a certain De Clave had regularly demonstrated such experiments for a wider audience in Paris. When in France he encouraged Erasmus to make an effort to seek out De Clave or at least see his show.[71]

Despite not receiving confirmation from Erasmus that he had witnessed a successful experiment by Langlot, Worm wrote to Joel Langlot asking

---

70 *Ibid.*, no. 1483. See also P. Müller, *Miracula chymica, et mysteria medica*, Wittenberg 1611.

71 *Ibid.*, Nos. 1572 and 1575; see also A. Kircher, *Ars magna lucis et umbræ in X libros digesta*, Rome 1645 and J. du Chesne, *Pharmacopea dogmaticorum restituta pretiosis selctisque hermeticorum floribus illustrate*, Paris 1607.

him to share the secret with him which Joseph du Chesne had referred to, namely, 'how plants could be awakened in a gaseous state with bright colours and all its parts from philosophical ash by the use of heat'. Worm emphasised that he already possessed a number of methods of how to produce such plants, given to him by friends, but the ones he had tried had failed, possibly because he was unable to implement them correctly. Worm pointed out that he relied on the assistance of Langlot, having been unable to contact Etienne de Clave who had recently demonstrated palingenesis to a wider audience in Paris.

By the end of the summer 1648 Ole Worm finally put aside his quest for palingenesis. By then he had received no response from Joel Langlot, but his nephew, Thomas Fuiren, who had visited Langlot in his laboratory on Gottorp Castle, had reported back that Langlot had yet to perform such experiments, nor had he been able to produce the necessary salts or ash. Thomas's report appears to have ended Worm's immediate hunt for such ashes or salts.

Five years later, on his way to Leiden, Ole Worm's son Willum visited Joel Langlot in Gottorp, bringing a letter from his father. As a result, Langlot finally responded and sent Worm an account of his proposed method for palingenesis. Worm pointed out that it differed significantly from the methods he had received from friends. Thomas Bartholin had recently shown Worm some manuscript pages from the Athanasius Kircher protégé Hieronimo Bardi's *Theatrum Naturæ Iatrochymicæ Rationalis*, which was published in Rome in 1654. Worm was excited, claiming that

> It indicates a praiseworthy quest for knowledge to investigate the rarities, which both the Indies and other alien people produce, and publish it for the common good, as truly as the treasures of undiscovered Nature has yet to be found by any mortal and put forward in respectable writing. Since Mr. Bardi has recommended himself in these areas and has promised to reveal a number of rare and secret things he cannot be praised enough. Bardi will undoubtedly find a way to subtract the quintessence of plants, so that they with the assistance of mild heat can be reproduced gaseously in glasses whereby the same plants from which they are extracted become visible with real colours, leaves, and flowers.[72]

However, Worm was less concerned with the theory than the outcome, as he pointed out to Langlot. In other words he wanted to know whether or not palingenesis was possible, especially since he was aware that many

---

72 *Ibid.*, no. 1734; see also O. P. Grell, 'In Search of True Knowledge: Ole Worm (1588–1654) and the New Philosophy', 221–22 in P. H. Smith and B. Schmidt (eds.), *Making Knowledge in Early Modern Europe. Practices, Objects, and Texts, 1400–1800*, Chicago 2007.

people denied it. Should he eventually receive details of the successful method used by De Clave in Paris he was happy to send it on to Langlot if the latter remained keen on trying the experiment. Langlot proved interested, and Worm encouraged him further in September 1653, pointing out that he considered it one of the most important issues in chemistry. Worm also thought that Langlot was particularly well positioned to undertake the necessary experiments being under the Duke of Gottorp's protection. Worm, having been asked for his advice, told Langlot that no less than three experiments, conducted simultaneously in separate vessels, were needed in order to spare time. He sent Langlot a recipe he had just received from a friend which was supposed to be 'a unique secret', Worm thought it appealed to common sense, even if he had been unable to try it himself because it demanded far too much time and care. Likewise, he found the approach described by Philip Müller reasonable. Worm was also convinced that most plants would be suitable for the experiments, and because marigolds, carnations, and Christmas roses were flowering, he recommended them for Langlot's experiments as long as the latter agreed.[73]

Ole Worm retained a lifelong interest in Paracelsianism and iatrochemistry. This was in evidence in the advice he gave to his son Willum while studying medicine in Leiden in 1653. He praised his son for having enrolled in 'a chemical college' and particularly encouraged him 'to learn Glauber's method'.[74] Evidently Worm was familiar with the works of the German Paracelsian, Johann Rudolph Glauber, one of the leading practical chemists of the seventeenth century. Like Paracelsus, Glauber was a self-taught controversialist, strongly immersed in the artisanal and practical aspects of iatrochemistry. He had settled in Amsterdam around 1640 after an itinerant existence and quickly acquired a considerable reputation among the so-called Hartlib circle and Worm might well have heard about him from members of that circle. Shortly before his death, in July 1654, Worm received a copy of Glauber's book *Menstruum universal oder Mercurius philophorum genannt*, published in 1653, from Willum.[75]

Ole Worm became fascinated by Paracelsianism and iatrochemistry during his peregrinatio academica. He made a considerable effort to become acquainted with leading Paracelsians such as Joseph du Chesne and Theodore de Mayerne and sought out Johannes Hartmann in Marburg in order to be introduced to the practical applications and experiments needed in iatrochemistry. Worm was clearly affected by the Rosicrucian craze which engulfed Europe in the second decade of the seventeenth century, but his public rejection of Rosicrucianism in 1619 did not diminish his interest in Paracelsianism and iatrochemistry. He kept abreast of

---

73 *Ibid.*, no. 1738, 1747.
74 *Ibid.*, no. 1740.
75 See Grell, 'In Search of True Knowledge', 224; for Johann Rudolph Glauber, see J. T. Young, *Faith, Medical Alchemy and Natural Philosophy: Johann Moriaen, Reformed Intelligencer, and the Hartlib Circle*, Aldershot 1998, 183–216.

developments within the field through books and correspondence with academic colleagues and information from his students studying abroad. Worm, however, was never an uncritical adherent of Paracelsianism and iatrochemistry. They were only one of his many interests prominent among which was anatomy.

Worm never stopped emphasising the importance of human anatomy and regular dissections of animals and humans. He would have been delighted to know that the small supernumerary bones in the sutures of the skull – his only anatomical discovery – are today known in English as Wormian. With his interest in opening up bodies, both animal and human, and observing them, Worm was very much at the cutting edge of the early seventeenth-century's search for better anatomical knowledge.

Two major anatomical discoveries, both published in the 1620s, were to preoccupy Ole Worm and many of his academic colleagues across Europe for an extended period: Gasparo Aselli's discovery of the chyliferous vessels of the intestine, which Aselli labelled lacteals (white veins), and William Harvey's discovery of the circulation of the blood. The former was significant and vigorously debated; the latter was truly revolutionary and remained deeply controversial for decades. Harvey, who had already made his discovery around 1618, was aware of its controversial nature and accordingly refrained for a decade from publishing his results, which contradicted the reigning medical orthodoxy on the functioning of the body and the movement of the blood. Finally, in 1628 Harvey published his results in a short tract, *Exercitatio Anatomica de Motu Cordis et Sanguinis in Animalibus* (Anatomical Exercises on the Motion of the Heart and Blood in Animals). Sometime before April 1631 news of Harvey's discovery had reached Ole Worm in Copenhagen. Writing to his student Jacob Svabe, pursuing his medical studies in Leiden, Worm enquired,

> Because you write that you have seen three dissections of the human body this winter, I would like to know whether your anatomists have demonstrated Aselli's lacteals in the mesentry? Likewise, what do they think of the circulation of the blood in the body according to the opinion of this Englishman? This winter I have for the first time observed it myself in a dog, following the author's instruction. The matter is certainly of great importance and benefit.[76]

It was undoubtedly on Ole Worm's advice that Jacob Svabe had matriculated in medicine in Leiden in May 1630 after having spent three years at the University of Copenhagen. Worm had repeatedly advised young Svabe to focus on anatomy and it was therefore with some pride that he reported back on having attended three public dissections of humans by Otto Heurnius and Adrian van Valkenburg in February 1631.

---

76 *Breve fra og til Ole Worm*, no. 401.

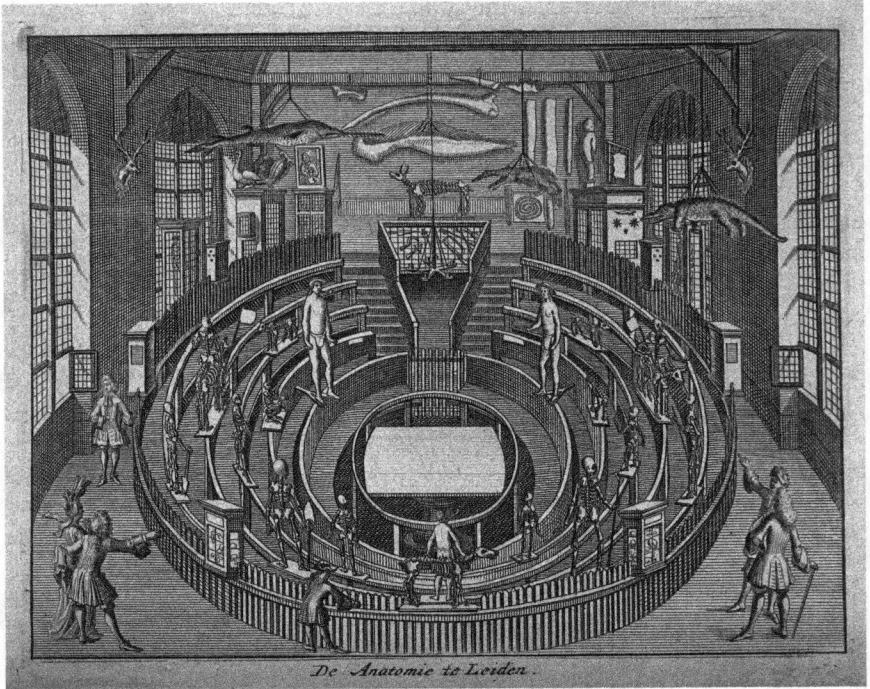

Figure 2.5 Leiden, Anatomical Theatre 1610; courtesy of the Wellcome Collection.

Svabe added an observation clearly meant to please his mentor in Copenhagen:

> Truly, it cannot be denied that the immediate view of an ingeniously dissected corpse is much to be preferred to the beautiful and detailed drawings that a considerable number of people consider to be the alpha and omega of anatomical training. However, they should not be dismissed, since they inspire the eye and the mind through a shadow figure.[77]

Despite his constant advocacy of practical anatomy, Worm appears to have been unable to conduct any human dissections in Copenhagen. Whenever he referred to his own anatomical experiences he always returned to events while he was a student in Basle and Padua from 1607 to 1609. The University of Copenhagen did not acquire an anatomical theatre until 1644, and public dissections did not begin until 1645. This might explain Svabe's qualified acknowledgement of the usefulness of anatomical drawings.

77 *Ibid.*, no. 396; see also nos. 384 and 386.

Worm, as we have seen, dissected animals and performed vivisections, emulating Aselli's vivisection of a dog.

Considering Ole Worm's constant endeavour to obtain new books as quickly as possible through his many excellent contacts with major booksellers across northern Europe, and at the Frankfurt Book Fair, it is surprising that he had not managed to obtain a copy of Harvey's work nearly three years after its publication. This is even more surprising when borne in mind that Worm had managed to obtain Gasparo Aselli's *De lactibus sive Lacteis venis*, which had been published in 1627 only a year before Harvey's tract. Instead, Worm waited until Jacob Svabe returned from Leiden in the summer of 1632 before he borrowed Svabe's copy together with his copy of Adrian Spiegel's *De Humane Corporis Fabrica* (1632), which supported Harvey's views. In other words Worm did not read Harvey's tract in full until the summer of 1632, more than a year after he made his first inquiries about the circulation of the blood.

Jacob Svabe responded with enthusiasm to Worm's inquiry about the circulation of the blood. Despite having spent nearly a full academic year in Leiden studying medicine Svabe had heard nothing about Harvey's ideas before receiving Worm's letter, informing him 'about this new and unheard of conception ... concerning the return-run of the blood'. He had spent a week considering the matter on his own, 'ardently absorbed', as he put it, before he consulted his more experienced friend and fellow-student Hermann Conring. Conring not only possessed a copy of *De Motu Cordis*, which he showed Svabe, but also expressed himself so 'excellently and intelligently about the circulation of the blood' that Svabe was convinced he was in agreement with Harvey. Hermann Conring then got somewhat concerned that he might have converted Svabe to Harvey's 'heretic views'. He quickly backtracked, adding that, even if Harvey's ideas at first glance looked very attractive, his inability to prove them through observation and anatomical demonstration made them less convincing. Then Svabe, still deeply engrossed in the issue, consulted the Leiden anatomists Otto Heurnius and Adrian van Valkenburg, who both agreed with Conring, adding the proviso 'that, concerning questions that change the old and accept the new, we should rather show care and hesitation than be daring and improvident'. Worm declared himself in agreement with Conring and the Leiden anatomists, pointing out that in medicine, 'especially where it is concerned with the connections between the different parts of the human body, we need an eye on every finger in order that we believe only what we observe'.

Unlike Herman Conring, who became a follower of Harvey and the first to defend the theory of the circulation of the blood in Germany as early as 1632, on taking up the chair of medicine in Helmstedt, Worm remained sceptical, not least because he insisted on the necessity of being able to observe the unobservable. Even so, the question of circulation remained central to Worm's interests. In his annual disputation for 1632, which Worm in his role as professor of medicine was obliged to present to the Medical Faculty with a student as respondent, the issue of the circulation of the blood loomed large. From that we can determine that Worm had read Harvey's De Motu Cordis sometime after Jacob Svabe's return to Denmark in June 1632 and the disputation which took place in November that year. Worm quoted Harvey's tract at length in the second and fifth controversy in the disputation. First he dealt with whether or not blood was formed in the parenchyma or in the veins of the liver, then Worm discussed whether the function of the heart is to pump the blood synchronously with the pulse from the arteries to the veins so it can circulate through the body. Worm raised a number of objections to Harvey's work, mainly in terms of the missing observational proof, but admitted that the short form of the disputation did not allow an in-depth analysis of Harvey's views. By the end of 1632 having finally read *De Motu Cordis* Worm felt able to reject Harvey's account of the circulation of the blood.[78]

Gasparo Aselli's discovery of the lacteals, whose vivisection on a dog Worm had been able to copy and observe himself, was another matter, as can be seen from his letter in February 1634 to his nephew and student, Henrik Fuiren, who was studying medicine at the University of Leiden. When in Copenhagen Fuiren had been present when Worm had emulated Aselli's experiment. Worm now wanted to know whether the Leiden anatomists had observed anything relating to the lacteals in the mesentry. Worm was deeply disappointed with Fuiren's response, pointing out,

> I am profoundly surprised that your anatomists treat their subjects with such carelessness, that they dare, contrary to the evidence of every spontaneous observation, to deny or hide those vessels, which are so necessary and useful, and which have been observed and demonstrated not only by so many and precise anatomists but also by students and beginners. Such a thing was never done formerly by Pauw, nor by others, who established the fame of this university.[79]

Thus, Ole Worm was prepared to accept Aselli's discoveries, which he could replicate and observe (even if he sought further confirmation from other scholars), but he rejected Harvey's findings about the circulation of the blood, which ultimately rested on calculation. Worm would appear to have taken little further interest in Aselli's and Harvey's discoveries until another of his nephews and students, Thomas Bartholin, matriculated in Leiden in 1638.

Thomas Bartholin proved an excellent correspondent for his uncle, providing him with a steady flow of information about his anatomical

---

78 Grell, 'In Search of True Knowledge', 226–27.
79 *Breve fra og til Ole Worm*, no. 520.

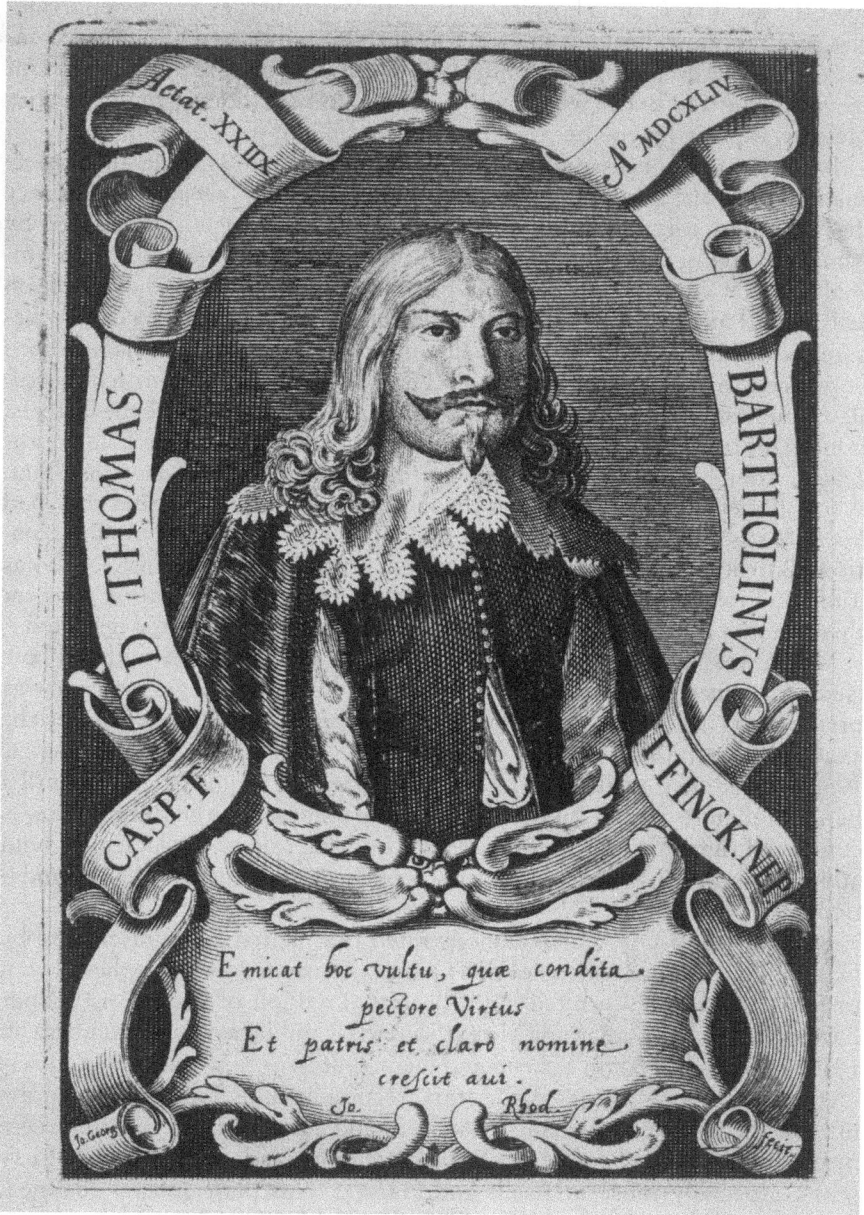

Figure 2.6 Thomas Bartholin (1616–80) age 35, print after Karel van Mander; courtesy of the Royal Danish Library.

undertakings in Leiden, especially the dissections he regularly participated in at the local St. Cecilia hospital in Leiden. Worm was extremely appreciative and reminded him not to forget to keep him informed about new anatomical discoveries. In that connection Worm emphasised how important it was for him to know what the Leiden anatomists thought about Aselli's lacteals, especially whether they had successfully observed them.

Bartholin did not disappoint his uncle providing him with detailed information about the views of the Leiden anatomists on the lacteals. In February 1639 Bartholin had been a member of a group of students, supervised by Van Valkenburg and Johannes Walaeus, who had been engaged in an animal vivisection to demonstrate the presence of the lacteals. The dissection had proved inconclusive, because the lacteals had disappeared from view before they could be properly observed, and only Johannes Walaeus had been convinced. A couple of months later Thomas Bartholin and his fellow students undertook the dissection of a dog in order to demonstrate the lacteals, which this time were clearly seen. Among those present was the Leiden professor, Adolph Vorstius, 'a defender of the old', as Bartholin described him, who still denied the existence of the lacteals despite the fact that they had been clearly shown, arguing that it had all been 'a figment of the imagination'. Bartholin added that the celebrated Amsterdam anatomist, Nicholas Tulp, had told him that he had been able to observe the lacteals at a recent dissection of a hanged man less than five days after he had been executed.

Worm was far from impressed by Vorstius's reaction and wondered how 'such a learned man' could doubt 'his own senses and eyes'. Worm was prepared to accept that one might still harbour some queries about the exact role of the lacteals, but only the blind could doubt their existence. Worm stated that Aselli had more than satisfied the inquisitive mind until a better and more certain knowledge could be obtained in the future. He was convinced that further, careful research into the role of the lacteals would add new and precise observations and conclusions to the excellent foundations laid by Aselli.[80]

By April 1640 Ole Worm demonstrated that he remained fascinated by Harvey's circulation of the blood. This was occasioned by his nephew's plan to issue a new, 'well-printed' and illustrated edition of his father, Caspar Bartholin's famous anatomical textbook first published in Wittenberg in 1611. Thomas Bartholin's friend and mentor, Johannes Walaeus was closely involved in this project from the start, recommending appropriate engravings for the volume and telling Thomas to add a few sections here and there in the book about the new medical discoveries made over the last thirty years, especially those of Aselli and Harvey. This plan quickly changed, however, not least because Walaeus, who had initially had doubts about Harvey's circulation of the blood, had come to accept it by late March

80 *Ibid.*, nos. 768 and 773.

1640. Thomas Bartholin had been part of a group of medical students who had assisted Walaeus in a number of vivisections on animals which had produced supporting evidence for Harvey's view. By the beginning of April Thomas informed his uncle that together with Walaeus he was daily engaged in in vivisections on different animals, all focussed on the circulation of the blood. They had made many discoveries that supported Harvey, and Walaeus had publicly announced his conversion to Harvey's view during a disputation. The other Leiden professors of medicine, according to Bartholin, remained uncertain who to support. Initially, Walaeus had wanted Bartholin to summarise his results in support of Harvey for him, but Bartholin had managed to convince his mentor to summarise his results himself in a letter to be appended to the new edition of his father's anatomy.

From Worm's reaction to Bartholin's news it is evident that he had maintained his interest in the circulation of the blood and that he still remained unconvinced by Harvey's account. Worm admitted that he was aware that Harvey's observations were applauded by some scholars, including Descartes. If Worm had not already read Descartes's *Discourse on Method*, published three years earlier, he was at least familiar with the section on the heart and the motion of the blood, even if the differences between Descartes and Harvey had escaped him. But, as he pointed out to Thomas, there were many other scholars who rejected Harvey's observations. He specifically referred him to James Primrose's recently published tract against Walaeus and Harvey, *Johannis Wallaei Medicinae apud Leydenses Professoris Disputationem Medicam Quam pro Circulatione Sanguinis Harveana Proposuit* (Amsterdam 1640), asking him whether or not he had seen it. Worm had obtained a copy through his contacts in England, and emphasised that he was not drawing Primrose to Bartholin's attention in order for him to reject Harvey's observations, but only to make him aware of what Primrose had found deficient.

Meanwhile, Worm was keen to obtain everything Johannes Walaeus had written about the circulation of the blood. Even so, by May 1640 Worm still had reservations about the circulation, and as he explained, his doubts predated his reading of Primrose. Worm diligently sought to obtain all relevant books and tracts discussing the circulation of the blood, while complaining to his nephew in Leiden that he had been unable to obtain a copy of the Venetian physician Emilio Parigiano's refutation of Harvey published in 1635; for information he sent Thomas a copy of his disputation from 1632 where he had raised his objections to Harvey. Thomas obliged him by forwarding a copy of Walaeus's disputation supporting Harvey and informed his uncle that he had shown his disputation to Walaeus. Thomas Bartholin, however, added that he had already raised similar objections to Worm's some months back when he was directly involved in Walaeus's vivisections. Walaeus had answered them convincingly back then, but had added new 'assumptions' of greater weight in his disputation that needed to be considered.

Eighteen months lapsed before Ole Worm and Thomas Bartholin resumed their discussion about the circulation of the blood. It was occasioned
by a visit made to Thomas Bartholin in Padua by Fortunio Liceti, professor of medical theory, who had just finished his tract on the circulation of
the blood. Liceti rejected Harvey's account and promoted his own double-
circulation, apparently designed to make it possible to integrate the idea of
circulation with Aristotelianism. Thomas Bartholin informed his uncle in
Copenhagen that he had raised some objections to Liceti's account based
on common sense, as he put it, but wondered if Worm had anything to add.
Worm was delighted that 'the learned Liceti, with all his excellent acute-
ness, had examined the still undecided controversy about the circulation
of the blood'. He expressed the hope that Liceti would be able to settle the
matter and bring an end to the controversy. Personally Worm still felt unable to make up his mind, not least because the objections he had originally
raised in his disputation of 1632 had yet to be dealt with by either Walaeus
or Harvey. From what Worm could gather Fortunio Liceti's concept did not
raise similar problems, but, as Worm put it, his sound reflections' would
be considerably more convincing if they had been supported by precise
observations.

Thomas Bartholin had clearly hoped to convince his uncle and mentor
through his letter and Walaeus's disputation. His letter of 3 August 1643
to Worm expressed considerable exasperation, dismissing Liceti's account
of circulation as indefensible, totally lacking any experimental basis relying
solely on speculation. The issue could only be resolved, according to Bartholin, through vivisection on animals.

On this Worm would have agreed with his nephew, namely, that only
observation and experiment could settle the controversy. However, it seems
to have been a book, *Tractatus de Sanguinis Generatione, et Motu Natu-
rali*, published in 1643, by one of Harvey's earliest supporters, the Helmstedt professor of medicine, Herman Conring, which finally managed to
convince Worm about Harvey's account of the circulation of the blood. By
December 1643 Worm had just finished reading this book when he recommended it to Thomas Bartholin, telling him that he would discover 'many
surprising things which go against the common assumptions of the anatomists'. A couple of years later, Worm had occasion to write to Herman
Conring, when Conring's Danish student Frederik Arsinæus, whose father
had been a close friend of Worm, visited him in Copenhagen. Worm informed Conring that he had read his learned work on the circulation of
the blood, adding that he had found the book most engaging, 'not so much
because of the novelty of the content – for this has already preoccupied me
in different ways – but because the truth of this new discovery has been
confirmed with solid proofs'.[81]

81 *Ibid.*, no. 1373; see also Grell, 'In Search of True Knowledge', 231.

Thus, fifteen years after Worm had first become aware of Harvey's account of the circulation of the blood' one can truly say that the Worm had turned. That it happened to be the work of Herman Conring, one of the earliest converts to Harvey's ideas, who had featured so prominently in Worm's earliest inquiries about the circulation, which finally managed to change the mind of Worm, adds a poignant twist to this story. Unfortunately, Worm did not specify what 'the proofs' were that finally convinced him.

It is also noteworthy that Ole Worm would appear to have been aware of Harvey's work before it had come to the attention of the Leiden professors of medicine. Worm's extensive network of contacts established during his prolonged peregrinatio academica, which had also afforded him a prolonged stay in England, made sure that major new undertakings in medicine reached him quickly. News of Harvey's tract about the circulation may well have reached him by the same English contacts who drew the work of James Primrose to his attention. That, together with his many students studying abroad at the best European universities, made it possible for him to stay alert to new developments in Copenhagen. Their letters to their mentor, along with Worm's wide-ranging contacts within the European republic of letters, not to mention booksellers and printers, made it possible for him to acquire new knowledge rapidly.

7 The teacher

As we have seen Ole Worm meticulously fulfilled his teaching obligations at the University of Copenhagen in terms of lectures and disputations throughout his career. A number of students lodged with him and his family. Thus, many of his Icelandic friends and contacts had stayed with him during their time in Copenhagen, such as the later Bishop of Holar, Thorlak Skulason. Worm was also diligent in supplying former students with testimonia in their search for employment. A typical example is the testimonium he supplied in July 1629 for Søren Fridlev from Viborg, who had matriculated at the University of Copenhagen in 1623 and lodged with Worm until 1625. Fridlev was seeking a position after having served as a tutor to the children of Tycho Brahe.[82]

Many of Ole Worm's best students began their studies by spending a couple of years at the University of Copenhagen before they, as their mentor had done, set out on an extensive perigrinatio academica. Worm undertook a considerable correspondence with most of these students, some of whom were also close relatives, providing them with guidance and advice. Among the first to benefit from Worm's experience and knowledge was the physician Niels Foss, who was studying medicine in Marburg in 1615–16. Worm

---

82 *Ibid.*, no. 285.

was delighted that medicine was still thriving at the University of Marburg, but he warned Foss against joining the iatrochemist, Johannes Hartmann's private 'college' before he had reached a firm agreement about what fees to pay. Worm pointed out that Hartmann might still be selling what he himself had paid excessively for. If Hartmann offered something new of great value and significance Worm forewarned Foss that it would not come cheaply. More than anything else, however, Worm advised Foss to make contact with a local apothecary so he could observe and learn what was done in an apothecary's shop and see what remedies physicians ordered.[83] From the outset Worm wanted his students to focus on practical experiences and observations. A couple of years later when Niels Foss had arrived in France Worm specifically advised him to seek out the Paracelsian iatrochemists, Guillaume de Trogny, in Orleans, and Jean Béguin, and Etienne de Clave in Paris, especially the latter who was a skilful artisan from whom Foss, in his opinion, could learn a lot. At around this time Worm also advised Foss against obtaining his MD in Padua, despite the fact that it could be obtained at little expense and with a clear conscience, as long as he could be excused from making the written oath to the Pope. If Foss went down this route, he might still find himself under suspicion of being a crypto-Catholic. Instead Worm advised him to obtain his degree from one of the larger German universities or from Montpellier in France.[84]

Among the first of Worm's students to go abroad was Hans Andersen Skovgaard, a curate's son from Elsinore who had matriculated at the University of Copenhagen in 1620. Two years later Skovgaard was studying medicine at the University of Wittenberg, attending the lectures of Daniel Sennert. In November 1622 Skovgaard sent Worm a couple of recently published book asking him to support his application for the royal bursary for a medical student which had just become vacant. Despite supporting Skovgaard's successful application for the royal bursary, Worm was not particularly pleased with him, accusing him of writing infrequently, with considerable delay, and then not with much information. A few months later, in May 1625, Worm alerted Skovgaard that some of the professors at the University of Copenhagen had objected to the fact that he had yet to obtain his MA, which had then become a prerequisite for recipients of the royal bursary. This clearly rattled Skovgaard, and he responded with urgency and in some detail to Worm's rather sour note. He deplored his loss of favour and pointed out that he had posted no less than five letters recently, which evidently had got lost on the way. Skovgaard claimed that he had followed Worm's instructions to the letter. He had reported back to his tutors in Copenhagen regularly, informing them about his academic progress. Not only had he kept Worm informed, but he had also written to Caspar

83 *Ibid.*, no. 16.
84 *Ibid.*, nos. 43, 47, and 55.

Bartholin and Thomas Fincke about his studies. Skovgaard also claimed that he would have obtained his MA when he had been back in Copenhagen if he had been invited to do so. He would, however, try to obtain a degree in philosophy in Wittenberg in the spring. His winter term would be fully occupied with anatomical studies and Daniel Sennert's iatrochemical exercises. Skovgaard also expected to be able to take his meals at Daniel Sennert's table in the near future. Sennert had promised Skovgaard and a few other students to teach them iatrochemistry privately for a moderate fee of ten thalers each. Hans Andersen Skovgaard was convinced it would prove extremely beneficial, not least because of Sennert's fame, but also because of his honesty. Sennert had not promised them that they would discover great secrets, but only knowledge and experience of the practical laboratory processes. After having covered 'the first four parts of medicine' Skovgaard declared himself ready to focus on iatrochemistry, adding that Sennert was lecturing on the method of medicine, presumably based on Galen.

Skovgaard also took the opportunity to tell Ole Worm that another of his students in Wittenberg, Niels Eilersen, whom Worm had encouraged in his studies in late 1622, had been ill with a fever and deliriousness for three weeks, and was being treated daily by Daniel Sennert. Worm was saddened by the news of Niels Eilersen's illness. Worm considered him a talented young man, but unfortunately Sennert proved unable to help Eilersen, who died a few days later.[85]

Worm, in other words, received the detailed letter he had long desired from Skovgaard only to inform him that 'a letter, as well as being too short, can be too long'. Despite Worm's attempts to show his support through statements such as 'slaps from your friends are better than kisses from your enemies' Skovgaard might well have been left with the feeling that his mentor in Copenhagen was not exactly forthcoming with his support. Worm, however, was full of praise for Skovgaard's iatrochemical undertakings and encouraged him to get directly involved in the experiments and not worry about getting himself dirty, because everything depended on the right artisanal skills. Worm was keen to hear more about the experiments and asked Skovgaard to provide him with an example of how Sennert went about curing a specific illness. He also took the opportunity to remind Skovgaard to convey his greetings to Sennert whom he was not acquainted with, but admired greatly, not least because he was praised for his lucidity and honesty.

By November 1623 Worm had become far more positively inclined towards Skovgaard, informing him how much he had enjoyed his most recent

---

85 *Ibid.*, nos. 131 and 133; O. P. Grell, '"Like the bees, who neither suck nor generate their honey from one flower": The Significance of the 'perigrinatio academica for Danish Medical Students in the Late Sixteenth and Early Seventeenth Centuries', 180–81 in O. P. Grell et al. (eds.), *Centres of Medical Excellence? Medical Travel and Education in Europe, 1500–1789*, Farnham 2010; for Niels Eilersen, see also *Breve fra og til Ole Worm*, no. 120 and Helk, *Dansk-Norske Studierejser*, 203.

letter and how impressed he was with the progress he had made in his medical studies.[86] In May 1624 Hans Andersen Skovgaard enclosed a copy of his recent medical thesis in his letter. Worm praised it and Skovgaard's progress in his medical studies. He wanted to know how much progress Skovgaard had made in Hartmann's chemical 'college', and where he intended to continue his studies. Worm also told him not to worry about the MA, as long as he obtained the degree at a convenient occasion.

Skovgaard, realising that his royal bursary was coming to an end, had asked Worm whether he could continue his perigrinatio academica while financing it by acting as a tutor to young noblemen. While emphasising his continued support for Skovgaard, Worm informed him that this had recently become more difficult, since tutors were now expected to have taught at the newly established Academy for the nobility at Sorø (1623), prior to their appointments. Even so, Worm was not convinced that such a position would serve Skovgaard well. Regarding Skovgaard's worry about the growing costs of his residence in Wittenberg due to inflation and shortage of grain, Worm advised him to move either to France or Italy. In January 1625 Skovgaard finally obtained his MA in Wittenberg. He posted a number of copies of his disputation to Ole Worm for distribution among his professorial colleagues. Subsequently Worm fulfilled his promise of support, when Skovgaard became one of the first recipients of the bursary for medical students studying abroad which Thomas Fincke had established.

Shortly afterwards Hans Andersen Skovgaard returned to Copenhagen, but his sojourn proved a brief one. By January 1626 Skovgaard had arrived in Padua from where he wrote to thank Worm for all the assistance the latter had given him during his time back home, deploring the fact that Worm's many obligations as physician and professor, combined with his own need to make preparations for his journey to Italy, had conspired to prevent them from discussing matters of mutual interest in any depth.

Skovgaard was delighted to have made it safely to Padua, even if he pointed out that the medical faculty was no longer as excellent as it used to be. Only three exceptional professors remained, namely, the Swiss Nicolaus Prævotius and Benedictus Sylvaticus and Johannes Domenico Sala both from Padua. The decline had, according to Skovgaard, started with the death of Adrian Spigelius the previous year which had caused all anatomical and surgical dissections to cease in Padua. It had proved impossible to replace Spigelius who had been a master of both anatomy and surgery. Consequently, Skovgaard had been forced to find private instruction, especially in anatomy. The close contacts between Worm and Skovgaard faded somewhat during the latter's stay in Italy. Skovgaard only managed to write to his mentor in Copenhagen every six months which Skovgaard thought was enough to stay in contact with his former teachers back in

---

86 *Breve fra og til Ole Worm*, no. 139.

Copenhagen. However, his last preserved letter to Ole Worm from October 1627 indicated that he was feeling increasingly isolated and out of touch with his mentor in Copenhagen. Clearly, the negative effect of the Thirty Years' War on regular communication was being felt by Skovgaard. Even so, he provided Worm with a detailed description of his studies in Padua. He gave a detailed report on his extended stay in Pisa, where he had been able to explore the splendid botanical garden belonging to the Grand Duke of Tuscany. He gave details of his journey via Siena and Volterra to Rome, where he had befriended the German physician and natural philosopher Johannes Fabricius, not to mention his trip to Naples, where he had spent considerable time in the company of the botanist Fabio Colonna. Finally, he had returned to Siena in November 1626 to rest before his planned return to Padua. While there, he had been approached by courtiers of the Grand Duke of Tuscany offering him a salary of 200 thalers for conducting public dissections in the anatomical theatre in Pisa during January and February 1627. Skovgaard had accepted the offer after some hesitation and eventually given twenty-four lectures and anatomical dissections for a large audience of 400 people. His performance had been so well received that he was eventually offered a permanent position at the University of Pisa, which he politely declined, pointing out that he was obliged to serve the king of Denmark, having benefited from the royal bursary. Furthermore, as Skovgaard pointed out to Worm he had also had serious religious reservations, fearing for the salvation of his soul if he settled in a Catholic country. Such religious qualms were most likely raised to impress his mentors back in Copenhagen rather than a true reflection of Skovgaard's own views when borne in mind that he eventually settled in an Islamic country.

Having returned to Padua, Skovgaard undertook a trip to Verona in the company of, among others, Worm's friend, the Padua based Danish physician, Johan Rhode, where they visited the museum of Johannes Pona. While in Padua, Skovgaard befriended the physician and natural philosopher Fortunio Liceti, who became his mentor and whose publications he warmly recommended to Worm. Despite the delights of Italy Skovgaard expressed a wish to return home as soon as possible despite the difficulties war had created in Denmark. His actual plans, however, were vague; he might spend a month or two in France; the Thirty Years' War made any firm decisions difficult for him, and as he pointed out, despite his better judgement he might be forced to obtain his MD in Padua in order that he could sustain himself as a physician if need be. Meanwhile, Skovgaard was keenly awaiting Worm's advice, seeking to fend off repeated offers of professorships in anatomy and medicine at the University of Pisa. He was clearly hoping that Worm would be able to help him to an attractive post either at the court or the university, by emphasising how much he was in demand in Italy.[87]

---

87 *Ibid.*, no. 233 and Grell 'Like the Bees', 181–83.

This may well have been the last letter Worm received from Skovgaard who most likely never obtained his MD. When Ole Worm wrote to his friend Johan Rhode in Padua some eight years later, in 1637, asking him when he intended to return to his home country, he also asked for any news about Hans Andersen Skovgaard. Worm added 'that he had heard that he lived in the Greek manner with a Greek woman, which might explain why Skovgaard had forgotten all his friends'. The rumour cannot have been far from the truth, for Skovgaard eventually settled in Constantinople where he appears to have served successive sultans as a physician until his death in 1656.[88]

By 1630 a fair number of Ole Worm's students were studying medicine in Leiden. Among them were Jacob Svabe who had matriculated in May 1630, and, as we have seen, played an important part in Worm's initial inquiries into the lacteals and the circulation of the blood. That year Worm repeatedly told Svabe to take a particular interest in anatomy. Svabe complied by attending no less than three human dissection that winter, conducted by Otto Heurnius and Adrian van Valkenburg, from which he claimed to have learnt a lot. Svabe also attended the public lectures in medicine regularly, and daily attended Adolph Vorstius's class on the foundations of medicine.[89] In 1636 Jacob Svabe found himself in Angers in France, now trying to combine his own studies in medicine with the needs of the young noblemen he was tutoring. This proved difficult in Angers where he found little to interest the medical student. Svabe, however, had compensated by befriending the leading, local physicians, enjoying their learning and practical approach. There is an echo here of Worm's warning to Skovgaard about the difficulties of trying to combine personal studies with tutoring abroad.[90]

Ole Worm's nephew, Henrik Fuiren, who had matriculated at the University of Copenhagen in 1628, began his medical studies in Leiden in October 1633. Fuiren was an exceptionally wealthy student who needed no financial support. His grandfather, Henrik had been among the wealthiest merchants in Copenhagen. Worm praised Fuiren's diligence and the fact that he had received no reports about him being either lazy or misbehaving. He was delighted that Fuiren had stayed clear of 'depraved friends'. Interestingly, Henrik Fuiren was attending botanical exercises under the supervision of his former tutor, Poul Moth, who had matriculated in medicine in Leiden a year earlier. Poul Moth, who had been trained as a surgeon by his father, had from 1628 until he left for Leiden served as a tutor to Worm's nephews, Thomas Bartholin and Henrik and Thomas Fuiren, for whom Worm acted in loco parentis after the deaths of their fathers. Worm also took the

88 *Ibid.*, no. 630 and Grell 'Like the Bees', 183.
89 *Ibid.*, nos. 386, 388, and 396.
90 *Ibid.*, no. 578.

opportunity to ask Henrik to remind Poul Moth to learn to heal hernias through 'golden puncture', something which Worm was convinced would prove extremely beneficial not only to him but also to Henrik.[91]

Before he left for Leiden Poul Moth had studied for a couple of years at the University of Copenhagen where Worm had been among his teachers. Nor surprisingly Moth informed Worm that he particularly enjoyed anatomy in Leiden, a fairly obvious choice for a trained surgeon. In December 1633 Poul Moth had been fortunate enough to be able to dissect a still-born foetus which he had obtained from a midwife. He had used all his dexterity to dissect this foetus in the presence of his 'table-companions'. He was delighted to inform Worm about what he had observed during his dissection, not least because such dissections were rare and impossible to conduct in public, and because he was aware of Ole Worm's keen interest in anatomy. Moth provided a detailed description of his findings. He had made a special effort to identify the suprarenal gland, which other anatomical authors labelled glands for black bile. When Moth discovered the glands in the foetus, he had invited the famous Leiden anatomist, Adrian van Valkenburg, to attend the dissection, so he could observe them in 'their natural setting'. Moth had done this because Van Valkenburg had hitherto been unable to identify these glands in both his private and public dissections. As a result Van Valkenburg had proved extremely appreciative. Ole Worm was impressed and delighted that Moth continued to demonstrate his diligence and dedication and praised his achievements in dissecting the foetus. Moth, however, had dedicated at least half of his lengthy letter to Worm from March 1634 on the benefits his studies had reaped from 'the divine art of memory'. Moth claimed that his art of memory had not only benefited his medical studies but had also astonished highly learned and talented men. Bearing in mind how popular the art of memory had become among followers of Paracelsus and the Hermetic tradition in the late sixteenth and early seventeenth centuries it is noteworthy that Worm refrained from making any comments. Instead, he took the opportunity to explain why he had drawn Moth's attention towards the new method of healing hernias. Worm's experience of the terrible mutilation caused by quacks who tried to deal with hernias had inspired him to intervene. He was convinced that a capable and well-trained surgeon could do away with the mistakes made by ignorant barbers. Worm had no doubt that a surgeon who could practice this eminent art would be very successful and would benefit financially.[92]

Writing to Henrik Fuiren in May 1634 Ole Worm emphasised that he should pay attention to what his teachers taught him, and especially what they told him to observe, even if it differed from the teachings of the ancients.

---

91 *Ibid.*, no. 509.
92 *Ibid.*, nos. 512 and 521; for the art of memory, see F. Yates, *The Art of Memory*, London 1966.

In such instances, according to Worm, the present age constantly made progress and Fuiren would benefit. Worm praised Henrik for never missing any private or public occasion for educating himself. Henrik reported back to his uncle in August that he had joined a private teaching seminar in Leiden run by Johannes Walaeus. Here Walaeus explored the basic rules of medicine and solved disputed points raised by the students. Henrik also attended the lectures of Adolph Vorstius, Otto Heurnius, and Marcus Boxhorn. According to Fuiren, Boxhorn explained Ovid's *Metamorphoses* so excellently that even the professors who attended his lectures never left without having improved their knowledge. Worm praised the diligence of his nephew, especially his attendance at Boxhorn's lectures, emphasising how important it was for all students to be able to express themselves beautifully. Even so, Worm felt it necessary to remind Henrik not to forget the study of the important subjects of chemistry and pharmacy.[93]

Later in 1635 Henrik's younger brother Thomas Fuiren arrived in Franeker in the Netherlands. Like his brother, Thomas wanted to study medicine and Franeker had not been his desired destination. However, the fresh outbreak of war between Spain and the Dutch Republic which had resulted in an invasion of Spanish forces over the summer of 1635 had clearly forced him and others, 'banished by the war', as Worm put it, to seek sanctuary in Franeker. According to Worm the University of Franeker was far from an ideal place to study medicine, but he advised Thomas Fuiren that if the study of medicine could not be pursued publicly then it had to be done privately. Thomas should draw on the support of others who were in a similar situation to him, assisting each other in dissecting animals and holding disputations. Henrik Fuiren would appear to have temporarily left Leiden for the safety of Franeker and Thomas could also benefit from what he had been taught in Leiden. As always Worm was keen for his students to acquire practical, hands-on experience and he told Thomas to make the acquaintance of an apothecary or an experienced physician in order to learn the basics of chemistry, adding that he had no doubt that Thomas would prove a diligent student.[94]

A year later another Worm student Niels Bertelsen Wichmand arrived in Franeker after having survived a shipwreck. Worm still concerned about the war in the Netherlands recommended him to stay in Franeker for some time and take the opportunity to become acquainted with the town's physicians, while focussing on anatomy. Worm also warned him against travelling in France because of the disturbances there. England, on the other hand, was a possibility, and La Rochelle if he could catch a boat for that destination. After his recent shipwreck another journey by sea may not

93 *Ibid.*, nos. 520 and 606.
94 *Ibid.*, no. 577; see also J. I. Israel, *The Dutch Republic and the Hispanic World, 1606–1661*, Oxford 1982, 250–54.

have appealed to Wichmand.[95] Wichmand, however, undertook another dramatic sea journey in March 1638 to Amsterdam where he had to act as a surgeon in an emergency. Shortly afterwards he travelled to London where he stayed for a month before settling near Notre Dame in Paris. He had yet to observe how one could cut for hernia using the golden puncture. He had also made the acquaintance of skilful surgeons, but was held back because of his inability to speak French. Wichmand had visited La Charité Hospital in the company of the physician Antoine Ruffin, where they had a place where they cut for the stone inside and outside the bladder; not to mention visits to the Notre Dame Hospital and the Jardin Royal des Plantes. Worm was delighted with his industry and encouraged him to continue his interests in surgery and his visits to the hospitals. Wichmand was grateful to his mentor in Copenhagen. He informed Worm that he visited the hospitals every day and had witnessed many surgical interventions and attended the physician, Cappono's assessment of all diseases. He had become on friendly terms with Cappono and the royal surgeon La Frére. Unfortunately the latter did not understand Latin, but he could cure hernias without surgical intervention and knew secret remedies against venereal disease. Wichmand had managed to acquire some French, and had he not suffered from a fever for a couple of months he would have made greater progress.[96]

By the beginning of 1638 Henrik Fuiren had moved to Paris where he had hoped to benefit from the teachings of the famous French anatomist, Jean Riolan, who unfortunately by then had departed Paris in the company of the Queen Mother, Maria de Medici, whom he served as personal physician. Even so, Fuiren spent a year in Paris. He followed his uncle's advice and studied chemistry being fortunate to find an able teacher in the Scotsman, William Davidson, a Paracelsian iatrochemist who later became the first professor of chemistry at the Jardin des Plantes in Paris. He had then focussed on anatomy having realised that the Parisian physicians were excellent anatomists. Henrik Fuiren claimed to have witnessed no less than seven dissections, both public and private, that winter. Later he had sought instruction in botany from the well-known Guy de la Brosse, founder of the Jardin Royal des Plantes. That, however, had been a great disappointment because La Brosse had proved both unfriendly and unhelpful.[97]

Henrik Fuiren did not have a strong constitution and appears to have suffered from a number of ailments while in Paris. Ole Worm was concerned and considered the climate in Paris unhealthy and unfavourable for Fuiren's constitution. He therefore suggested that he transferred himself to a healthier place such as Montpellier. Admittedly, Worm had heard little about the University of Montpellier for a number of years, but if it was anything close

95 *Ibid.*, nos. 612 and 683.
96 *Ibid.*, nos. 721, 747, 765, and 772.
97 *Ibid.*, nos. 695 and 729.

to what it had been, then it was one of the best places to study medicine. It matched the best universities in terms of the teaching of anatomy, botany, practical medicine, not to mention the high standard of its disputations; furthermore, its healthy climate and reasonable living costs had over the years proved attractive to many medical students. Worm praised Henrik Fuiren for his anatomical observations and wanted to know who was considered the leading anatomists now that Riolan had died. Never one to miss an opportunity Worm instructed Henrik to find lodgings with a well-known practitioner, be it a physician, a surgeon or an apothecary in order to benefit from their hands-on experiences.[98]

By January 1639 Henrik Fuiren had resolved to continue his studies in Padua and to visit Montpellier en route. Worm approved of his plan, providing detailed travel advice and promising to write to his friend, the physician Johan Rhode who resided in Padua, asking him to assist Henrik Fuiren when he arrived in the city. Fuiren reached Padua at the start of June after having left Paris on 15 April. On the way he had stopped over in Lyon where he had enjoyed the company of Dr. Henri Gras, an experienced medical practitioner to whom he had been recommended by his former tutor, Poul Moth. Henrik Fuiren took the opportunity to visit the Universities of Valence and Orange on his way to Montpellier where he arrived on 6 May. He was so delighted with Montpellier that he informed Ole Worm that he regretted the time he had spent in Paris, because it would have been better spent in Montpellier, 'with greater purpose for his studies and at less expense'. Having arrived in Genoa from Marseilles Fuiren visited the University of Pisa, Florence, and Bologna before arriving in Padua on 9 June.[99]

Henrik Fuiren had arrived in Padua just when the university broke up for its summer recess. The new term started on 3 November when all the university professors began lecturing. Fifteen lecture courses were on offer, according to Fuiren, who had decide to focus exclusively on courses relevant to medicine. He provided his uncle and mentor with details of those he regularly attended: He began his day by attending the class of Johannes Vesling, who explained the properties of plants. Then he joined Johannes Domenico Sala for his interpretation of Hippocrates' Aphorisms. He also managed to attend the lectures of Johan Baptista Soncino on abdominal diseases, in the slot before lunch. After lunch he listened to Benedict Sylvaticus' lectures on fevers, which he rated very highly. Fuiren also took part in Soncino's private lectures on female diseases, and had been invited to attend Soncino's consultations in the mornings. However, Henrik preferred to join the anatomist, Pietro Marchetti, in his consultations and had by late November witnessed his surgical interventions on several occasions.[100]

98 *Ibid.*, no. 753; see also Grell, 'Like the Bees', 184–85.
99 *Ibid.*, nos. 766, 767, and 796.
100 *Ibid.*, no. 816.

Ole Worm was delighted with his nephew's undertakings in Padua. He only felt the need to remind him of one thing, namely, that he should do his utmost to follow the successful practitioners in Padua because no other place would offer him a better opportunity. Worm emphasised,

> In order to be able to treat the sick correctly in coordination with the general theoretical rules, it is necessary to have seen a great many individual cases. The sick are not cured through deliberations and considerations, but through the right use of the greatest number of observations. During your stay in Padua I therefore advice you to devote yourself entirely to this task under the guidance of practitioners, not only surgeons, but also other physicians, even at hospitals; believe me you will not regret it. It is possible to appropriate to oneself with the eyes so many things which cannot be described by the pen.[101]

By June 1640 Henrik Fuiren had managed to get lodgings with Johan Rhode in Padua and was benefiting from daily conversations with his host about medical matter. He thanked Worm for all his advice and assistance with his studies. The following spring Worm asked Fuiren for a detailed plan for his future studies in Italy. Henrik had by then spent seven years on his perigrinatio academica and it is likely that Worm thought it was about time he brought it to a conclusion. Henrik responded rather defensibly that it was not for his personal pleasure he remained in Padua, but only to make further progress in his study of medicine. He apparently needed to make up the time he had wasted in Paris, and he felt that he could not return home 'uninformed and unskilled in his field'. There was no better place, according to him, where he could acquire the necessary medical skills than Padua. Here it was possible for him to accompany practising physicians visiting their patients. Worm knew better than him the value of the experience of having seen a wide variety of patients for the trainee physician. This was enough to satisfy his uncle in Copenhagen who claimed he was delighted with his progress.[102] However, Henrik Fuiren did not focus exclusively on his medical education, but found time for travelling in Italy. During the autumn of 1641 he undertook a lengthy journey to Rome and Naples returning back to Padua via Siena.[103] Back in Padua in 1642 Fuiren spent much of his time in the company of Johannes Domenico Sala visiting the sick, and having served as Consiliarius for the German nation (1641–42) at the University of Padua he was now busy transferring this responsibilities to his successor and cousin, Thomas Bartholin. By the end of 1642 Henrik Fuiren was finally contemplating a return to Copenhagen. He planned to send his belongings via Amsterdam the following spring. He himself might be somewhat delayed by the need to

101 *Ibid.*, no. 824.
102 *Ibid.*, nos. 950 and 957.
103 Helk, *Danske-Norske Studierejser*, 217.

treat patients. Apparently patients arrived in considerable numbers in Padua during spring, which was considered a particularly fortuitous time to receive treatment and consult the resident physicians and surgeons.[104]

Evidently Fuiren was not in a rush to get home and his departure was delayed for another two years, only leaving Padua to go to Basle in order to obtain his MD on the way back to Copenhagen. He arrived in Basle in either late June or early July 1645 and was awarded his MD a little over three months later. Henrik Fuiren was granted his MD after having lectured for three days on dropsy. His published MD lecture, *Praelectiones Basilenses*, included a letter from his cousin, Thomas Bartholin, praising his achievements. Even then, Fuiren showed no urgency in returning to Denmark spending a further year in Paris and Leiden before arriving back in Copenhagen in the autumn of 1646 after a peregrinatio academica of thirteen years.[105]

No student was closer to Ole Worm than his nephew, Thomas Bartholin, for whom he acted in loco parentis, after his father, Caspar Bartholin's death in 1629, when Thomas was only twelve years old. Thomas matriculated at Leiden University in July 1637 after having studied at the University of Copenhagen for a couple of years. Apart from medicine Bartholin took an interest in philosophy and theology. Worm had not directed him towards medicine, but 'given him free range in terms of his studies'. However, by the summer of 1638 Bartholin had decided to concentrate on medicine despite his mother's opposition. However, he informed Worm that he did not intend to focus exclusively on medicine, but also wanted to study philology and philosophy which he considered important aids to medicine. He had consulted Johannes Walaeus, who had proved polite and helpful, about what medical authors he should read.[106] Bearing in mind the popularity of Johannes Walaeus among Worm's students in Leiden the choice of advisor was hardly surprising. Evidently, this first contact between Bartholin and Walaeus was a success and laid the foundations for the close friendship between the two men which blossomed rapidly.

Meanwhile, Thomas Bartholin, keenly awaiting his uncle's response, attended what would appear to have been his first dissection at the St. Caecilia hospital in Leiden, where the medical students twice a week assembled around the professor in practical medicine to undertake 'examinations of the nature, causes, and healing of diseases. The dissection had been undertaken to find the cause of death, but they had been unable to determine the cause. Worm approved his nephew's plans and agreed that the study of philology and philosophy was useful not only for medicine but also other 'sciences'. He also endorsed Thomas taking the advice of Walaeus whom

104 *Breve fra og til Ole Worm*, nos. 1064 and 1094.
105 Grell, 'Like the Bees', 188–89.
106 *Breve fra og til Ole Worm*, no. 739.

he rated highly. However, Worm gave Thomas what was his stock advice, namely, that he should make the acquaintance of one of the most distinguished apothecaries in Leiden, as well as a surgeon, and if possible find lodging with one of them. They would provide him with the hands on experience of subjects essential to the dedicated practitioner. Worm advised Thomas not to be introduced into 'the temple of chemistry' until he went to France, in order for him not to be overwhelmed.[107]

By December 1638 Thomas Bartholin had attended a public dissection of a criminal undertaken by Otto Heurnius. He also gave his uncle detailed information about the teaching of medical students undertaken at the St. Caecilia hospital. Here the professors of practical medicine instructed the students in how to perform detailed investigations into diseases and drugs. Every week four medical students were selected to attend the patients daily and make sure they received the remedies they had been prescribed jointly by professors and students. Thomas Bartholin also informed his uncle that an anatomical theatre had been constructed in the St. Caecilia hospital. This had most likely happened a couple of years before his arrival, in 1636, when the University of Leiden had begun dissections in the hospital. Here the corpses of those who had died in the hospital were opened up by a surgeon in the presence of the physicians. Thomas had recently been present at two dissections which he described in detail to Worm. Furthermore, Thomas was among a group of students being taught privately about the basic medical principles by Johannes Walaeus.[108] Worm appreciated his nephew's undertaking and expressed a wish to be informed about what he labelled other unusual things. He also encouraged Thomas to continue his philological studies. By January 1639 Worm decided that Thomas ought to be awarded the royal bursary for a medical student, by then worth 200 Thalers. This was quickly achieved and much appreciated by Thomas, who during the winter months in Leiden was present at public dissections while together with fellow student he undertook dissections of a couple of dogs in his search for the lactic veins.[109]

It is noteworthy that Worm's students in Leiden learned their anatomy and dissections from small semi-private dissections undertaken either at the St. Caecilia hospital or privately on their own initiative, like Poul Moth on the foetus, and not through the large public anatomical dissections. The sizable audiences who attended these public anatomies would have made it virtually impossible for students to get close enough to see the necessary details of anatomical structures and improve their knowledge through observation.[110]

---

107 *Ibid.*, nos. 746 and 748. For dissections at the St. Caecilia hospital in Leiden, see T. Huisman, *The Finger of God. Anatomical Practice in 17th Century Leiden,* Leiden 2009.

108 *Ibid.*, no. 758.

109 *Ibid.*, nos. 762, 768, and 773.

110 This has been pointed out by Michael Stolberg in the case of Padua, see M. Stohlberg, 'Learning Anatomy in Late 16th Century Padua', *History of Science*, 2018, 381–402.

By 1640 Thomas Bartholin had been encouraged by a number of book-sellers to publish a revised and updated edition of his father's anatomy book because of its popularity. They wanted a larger and more beautiful for-mat provided with illustrations. Johannes Walaeus appears to have been a driving force in this enterprise from the start. Thomas had the manuscript ready for publication by early April including all the updates of recent med-ical discoveries, not to mention Walaeus's letter accepting the circulation of the blood, all ready to be published if the illustrations could get ready. Thomas Bartholin did not have to wait long for the illustrations and the work; *Caspar Bartholin's Anatomicæ institutions corporis humani. Novis recentiorum opinionibus et observationibus ... figurisque auctæ a Thomas Bartholin* was published in Leiden in 1641. Worm was delighted and con-gratulated him on his achievement. If the original work had enhanced his father's reputation Thomas could only be delighted in what the revised and updated edition did for him. By 1641 he was no longer just a medical stu-dent with a famous father, he himself had acquired fame, and medical men across Europe were keen to make his acquaintance.

However, before the book had been published Thomas was seeking Ole Worm's permission to leave for France. Bartholin's health was failing. The thick and moist air in Leiden did not agree with him. He had suffered from consti-pation for years and was convinced that both his stomach and liver had been damaged through consumption caused by harm to the lungs from the outflow of juices in the head. He hoped that the signs of consumption which he regu-larly saw proof of by spitting blood, had mislead him. He had been advised by local physicians and his former tutor, Dr. Poul Moth, to go to France where he would benefit from the milder air, spas, and a general change to his situation. Worm was deeply concerned about Thomas's fragile health. He warned him against studying late at night, wasting his health thereby robbing his father-land of his splendid talents. Worm reminded him of his father, Caspar Bartho-lin, who had exhausted himself to such a degree during his youth through his draining studies, that he had proved unable to serve his country to the extent he would have wanted.[111] Worm discussed his plans for France with his grand-father, Thomas Fincke, and others. They did not appear to have embraced Thomas's plan with much enthusiasm, but Worm supported it. Expressing con-cern for Thomas's health, Worm advised him to travel to Montpellier before winter set in. Montpellier had a wealth of excellent physicians and was much cheaper than Paris, and Worm pointed out that Henrik Fuiren after having arrived in Montpellier had regretted his long stay in Paris.[112]

Disregarding Worm's advice Thomas Bartholin arrived in Paris three months later. He informed his uncle that he had befriended two profes-sors of medicine, René Moreau and Gui Patin, who had proved helpful.

111 *Ibid.*, nos. 832, 837, 842, and 844.
112 *Ibid.*, no. 845

Bartholin added that 'these together with others who match their politeness soften the boredom of this place'. Like his cousin, Henrik Fuiren, Thomas struggled with the language – clearly French as opposed to Dutch constituted a language barrier for most Danish, medical students.[113] Thomas was focussing on philosophy relevant to medicine and Worm applauded this, pointing out that anyone who had been trained in such sophistry would stand out at disputations and in all other situations. Bartholin enjoyed Paris with its variety of opinions, as he put it, but found the city very expensive both in terms of living costs and education. By the end of 1640 he had decided to leave for Montpellier by the end of winter. It is noteworthy that in the eight months Thomas Bartholin spent in Paris little of his time appears to have been spent on medicine. He had been present at a public dissection in December 1640, but had been disgusted by 'a pitiful show'.[114] Furthermore he did not appear to have taken any interest in iatrochemistry which was of such interest to his uncle in Copenhagen.

Sometime in April 1641 Thomas left Paris and travelled via Orléans and Lyon to Montpellier. Here his plans for a quiet time dedicated to the study of medicine ran into trouble, and he felt obliged to leave the city in a hurry within a few months of his arrival, due to what he described as 'the unfortunate controversies'. It would appear that Thomas had given a public disputation arguing for the new understanding of the lactic veins and the circulation of the blood, rather severely criticising the more traditional views of the local professor of medicine. This had caused 'the stubborn supporters of Galen', as Bartholin put it, not only to dislike him but also to fear him, because it had been a public event. As a result Thomas Bartholin no longer felt safe in Montpellier and had left for Italy, where he arrived in late October 1641. Worm was shocked about events in Montpellier. He found it unrecognisable from the place he had visited, and a place which talented students in future would avoid as being too dangerous.[115]

Meanwhile, Thomas set about making an impression in Padua. He befriended Johannes Vesling, the leading professor of medicine, with whom he undertook anatomical dissections, claiming Vesling had become his patron. By then he had already asked Worm to help him obtain the royal bursary which was about to become vacant. Worm had no doubt that he could secure his nephew at least another two years funding.[116] By May 1642, however, Ole Worm had become somewhat concerned about his nephew's progress and direction. Thomas had told his uncle that the difficult position of his fatherland prevented him from returning in the immediate future. One wonders whether rumours of the potential of a forthcoming conflict

---

113 *Ibid.*, no. 862; for Paris and René Moraeu and Gui Patin, see L Brockliss and C. Jones, *The Medical World of Early Modern France*, Oxford 1997.
114 *Ibid.*, nos. 874, 875, 881, and 883.
115 *Ibid.*, nos. 929, 978, and 995.
116 *Ibid.*, no. 1005; for the Royal bursary see nos. 978 and 1030.

between Sweden and Denmark was already circulating well over a year before the Torstenson War began in 1643. Simultaneously, Thomas also expressed uncertainty about where his studies were taking him. Worm dismissed what he termed Thomas's 'illusions', everything was quiet and peaceful in Denmark. Worm told him to remain focussed on his studies, informing him that his new edition of his father's anatomy book had enhanced his reputation. If he returned, Worm had no doubt that a rewarding position would be found for him. Even if Thomas Bartholin was grateful to his uncle for having drawn him to the chancellor's attention his response was not helpful. He stated that he was not sure in what direction he would take his studies. He declared that if he lost his financial support he might dedicate himself to medicine because it could provide him with an acceptable income. Meanwhile, he was spending days accompanying Johannes Domenico Sala visiting his patients and treating them for a variety of diseases. Worm was alarmed and wrote him a forceful letter, stating that what concerned the purpose and outcome of his studies he and others had advised medicine, which so far had been Thomas's intention and which had been the condition of both his bursaries. He warned Thomas not to let himself be enticed away from medicine, so that his backers in Copenhagen would lose the hope they held in him. Worm considered it acceptable for him to study philology and philosophy in his spare time, adding that 'for the rest God will take care'. If Thomas abandoned medicine he might, of course, be liable to claims for damages.

Worm informed him that he had suggested to his grandfather, Thomas Fincke, who no longer could manage his public teaching, that Thomas become employed as his deputy, when he had finished his studies and returned. Having acquired such a position at the university, through the back door so to speak, it would be difficult to exclude him.[117]

From then on Ole Worm was focussed on getting Thomas Bartholin to finish his studies and return home. In August 1642 he congratulated Thomas on having been elected Consiliarius for the German nation at Padua in succession to his cousin Henrik Fuiren. Worm had no doubt that this would help promote his career back home. A couple of months later he encouraged Thomas to write to the chancellor and the recently appointed royal physician Jacob Fabricius, pretending to want to discuss certain issues with the latter thereby drawing attention to himself. He added, that for the person who wanted promotion it was necessary to find patrons and to ingratiate himself, which was best done through a letter, which 'remained unaffected by confusion'. Worm was convinced that Thomas's elegant style would please his recipients. Again, Worm warned him against anyone seeking to divert him from his intended undertaking. Instead, Thomas should continue his medical studies with his customary energy, and only when

---

117 *Ibid.*, nos. 1044 and 1050.

tired 'seek sanctuary in the pleasure-garden of philosophy'. This advice was wasted on Thomas Bartholin who was by then busy planning a journey to Rome, Naples, and Bologna in order to meet learned men in these places. Accordingly, he told Worm that he would postpone such letters to a convenient later date.[118]

Half a year later, in August 1643, Thomas Bartholin, still remained in Padua, responding to Worm's encouragements to return home. He argued that he lacked maturity in both years and learning to take on a professorship, adding that he preferred a quiet life rather than 'public trouble', which he feared his constitution would struggle to cope with. Worm, however, was not prepared to let matters rest. He claimed that a professorship in Copenhagen would not be a burden or result in a troublesome public life. Worm was convinced that a more quiet position could not be found. Nothing was easier and more enjoyable than to lecture three or four times a week which could be done by any novice. Thomas would only exceptionally be called on to take on disputations as long as he functioned as his grandfather's deputy. The position would probably leave him more time for his own studies that he enjoyed at the moment. Bartholin should also consider that he was in the process of spending his inheritance, that the opportunity might disappear, and that his health might deteriorate. Worm was worried that Thomas was being badly advised and wanted him to reconsider.[119]

Thomas Bartholin finally left Padua for Naples towards the end of September or beginning of October 1643, eventually travelling to Rome in the beginning of November. He had been kindly received by the leading physicians in Naples, his father's friend Marius Schipanus, and the great surgeon Marcus Aurelius Severinus, who had invited him to stay with him if he returned. In Rome he was benefitting from the hospitality of the influential nobleman Cassiano dal Pozzo. Thomas Bartholin spent the first three months of 1644 in Naples enjoying the hospitality of Severinus. He informed Worm that he had travelled there for health reasons and wanted to delay his return to Denmark. Worm told him to disregard the Swedish invasion of Denmark and return home sooner rather than later. He pointed out that Thomas's grandfather, Thomas Fincke, was getting very old and infirm and could pass away any day. If that happened 'the plans of his friends' might come to nothing and a similar opportunity to find him a university position might never occur again. Meanwhile, the University of Messina had offered Thomas Bartholin a position at a considerable salary. Bartholin arrived there at the beginning of April 1644, to thank the Council for their offer, and presumably to take a look at the place. Only the physician and botanist, Pietro Castelli, impressed him. Even so, Worm was only told in May by Henrik Fuiren that Thomas had turned down the

118 *Ibid.*, nos. 1069, 1088, and 1097.
119 *Ibid.*, nos. 1154 and 1164.

offer. According to Worm Thomas had rightly declined the professorship because he was obliged to his fatherland having enjoyed the royal bursary.[120] It would appear that Worm lost contact with his favourite nephew for some months when Thomas travelled via Syracuse to Malta, then back to Naples for another three months stay with Marcus Aurelius Severinus, only to arrive back in Padua by late October 1644.[121] Worm expressed his concern for Thomas Bartholin's health, warning him not to wear himself out with all his publications, and encouraging him to return home. Thomas responded by informing Worm that he would not return until next spring to Worm's disappointment.[122]

However, travelling with his cousin Henrik Fuiren, Thomas did not leave Padua until June 1645, heading for Basle where the two of them arrived in October to acquire their MDs. Meanwhile, Ole Worm was busy trying to secure a professorship for Thomas in Copenhagen. By October he wanted Thomas to apply for the vacant professorship in philology and return as quickly as possible. Worm was sure that no one had yet been found for this position and had discussed it with the chancellor, promising him that Thomas would be back by spring 1646. Thomas did not share his mentor's sense of urgency and writing to him in November from Orléans, he told Worm that he and his cousin planned to spend the winter in Paris to enjoy the warmer climate before they returned home the following spring. Worm was far from happy with this response, pointing out that he had received no answer from Thomas about the vacant professorship in philology. He suspected that his nephew was not telling him what he was up to in Paris. Rather amusingly, Worm pointed out that so many people were getting married in Copenhagen that if Thomas did not return soon, there would be no one left for him to marry. He was desperately casting around for arguments to encourage his nephew to return home. Writing from Amsterdam in February 1646 Thomas informed him that he had been told that a candidate had come forward for the professorship in philology. If that was the case Thomas had no intention of hastening back. Worm had to admit that this rumour was correct, but, meanwhile, another vacancy, this time in ethics, had materialised. He was trying to get this reserved for Thomas and the chancellor was positively inclined towards this suggestion. Thomas should in other words come home as quickly as possible. If Worm's plan failed, Thomas could always become his grandfather's deputy which would provide him with an entry into the university.[123]

Back in Leiden in April 1646 Thomas forwarded a copy of the most recent edition of his anatomy book, beautifully bound, for the chancellor.

---

120 *Ibid.*, nos. 1168,1179, 1194, 1196, 1201, and 1224.
121 See *Helk, Danske-Norske Studierejser*, 162; see also *Breve fra og til Ole Worm*, no. 1233.
122 *Breve fra og til Ole Worm*, nos. 1233, 1246, and 1256.
123 *Ibid.*, nos. 1357, 1363, 1378, 1386, and 1394.

He would have included a letter to the chancellor if he had considered it worth his while. He informed Worm that he was annoyed that the chancellor had awarded the professorship in philology to someone else, feeling unappreciated and taken advantage of. As a result he was not going to rush home, instead he was considering giving up any thoughts of public service. He was tempted to focus on private research instead. In a further letter to Ole Worm written a couple of weeks later Thomas thanked his uncle for having taken such interest in his welfare. However, he could not hide his disappointment. He was convinced that people envied him, and he wanted Worm to support a further extension of his studies abroad. He added that even if his friends wanted him to return home, astrologers suggested that he would find employment abroad. Worm pointed out to him that the professorship in ethics had been filled by someone present and available. In other words Thomas Bartholin needed to return to further his case. Worm underlined that the position of deputy to his grandfather would be reserved exclusively for him, and it would provide an opening to something better. There was no need to complain about envy because it followed virtue in the same way as the shadow accompanied the body.[124]

Thomas Bartholin finally returned to Copenhagen in October 1646, nine years after he started his perigrinatio academica. He began his academic career as a deputy to his grandfather, as guaranteed by Worm. A year later it provided the opening to something better when he succeeded Christian Sørensen Longomontanus as professor of mathematics, on the latter's death. Only three years after his return, in 1649, he finally achieved the recognition he desired, when he succeeded Simon Pauli as professor of anatomy.

8 Conclusion

Ole Worm served the University of Copenhagen as a professor for more than forty-one years, spending the first eleven years in a number of professorships in the Faculty of Philosophy before finally becoming professor of medicine in 1624. He proved himself a hard-working member of both the Faculty of Philosophy and Faculty of Medicine. Worm was trusted and appreciated by his colleagues as can be seen from his repeated elections as dean and vice chancellor. His career progressed smoothly until May 1616 when he was refused the deanship in the Faculty of Philosophy because he did not hold a degree in philosophy. To what extent the issue was his lack of a degree is unclear, but that the case was eventually resolved a couple of years later was undoubtedly due to his strong support from within the Medical Faculty, controlled by his father-in-law Thomas Fincke, and brother-in-law Caspar Bartholin.

---

124 *Ibid.*, nos. 1396, 1401, 1403, and 1417.

In 1619 Ole Worm used his inaugural address as dean to warn the graduates against the dangerous sect of Rosicrucianism. That he should have taken this opportunity to distance himself from a movement he had been deeply interested in since 1611, even if at times, he had harboured serious doubts about it, made sense in the less tolerant climate of Lutheran uniformity which was being promoted by the professor of theology Hans Poulsen Resen, in particular. This may also help explain why his brother-in-law and university vice chancellor in 1618–19, Caspar Bartholin, asked him to give a memorial lecture on 31 October 1618 as part of the centenary celebrations for the Reformation. It was clearly considered important by Ole Worm's friends and relations to emphasise and enhance his orthodox Lutheran's credentials.

Worm may have felt it necessary to clear himself of any suspicions of being religiously heterodox, but he maintained a guarded curiosity in the Rosicrucians and a strong interest in Paracelsianism and iatrochemistry throughout his life. This was strongly in evidence in his oration when he was promoted to professor of natural philosophy in April 1621 and reflected in his later scholarly interests. However, he never embraced Paracelsianism fully or uncritically. In terms of natural philosophy Worm remained firmly rooted in the Melanchthonian tradition.

In his scholarly interests Worm always emphasised the paramount importance of anatomy for medicine. Even so, he never performed dissections of humans during his tenure in Copenhagen, but only animals. The fact that no anatomical theatre was available in Copenhagen until 1644 may help to explain this. His extensive interests in anatomy was demonstrated by his fascination with Aselli's lacteals and Harvey's circulation of the blood, which he sought to observe, demonstrate, and describe throughout the 1630s and early 1640s. Similarly his fascination with iatrochemistry and Paracelsianism was based on a hands-on, experimental approach.

Worm's role as a teacher did not end when his students left the University of Copenhagen to undertake their peregrinatio academica. He continued to provide advice and assistance through his letters and local contacts. He constantly emphasised the importance of anatomy and iatrochemistry to them, but above all underlined the importance of practical experience and observation. His students were advised to take up lodgings with local practitioners, be they surgeons, physicians, or apothecaries, in order to observe, learn, and get hands-on experience. The epistolary exchange between teacher and student proved of paramount importance for both. For the student the backing of a sympathetic tutor should not be underestimated, while the tutor was kept informed about new medical undertakings at some of the leading universities of the age.

3 The Antiquarian

Surprisingly, for a man who considered himself first and foremost a physician, and whose fame eventually came to rest on his cabinet of curiosity, it was Ole Worm's antiquarian interests which established his scholarly reputation. Within the early seventeenth century republic of letters Worm's studies of the runes and his publications about the ancient, gold horn and Danish monuments provided the basis for his international repute.

1 Runes and ancient monuments

Worm's interests in the runes may well have been awakened by his friend, the minister and later dean in Scania Bertel Knudsen Aquilonius. A Latinist letter writer and poet, who sought to correspond with a variety of learned men of the age, Aquilonius had been inspired by some of the finest philologists of the age such as Gruter, Lipsius, and Scaliger. In particular, he had been attracted to Joseph Scaliger's ambition to revolutionise contemporary ideas about ancient chronology and to demonstrate that ancient history should not be limited to that of the Greeks and the Romans, but should include that of the Persians, Babylonians, Egyptians, and the Jews, insisting that the historical narratives and chronologies of each of them should be critically compared. Ole Worm may well have befriended Aquilonius in the years following his return to Copenhagen in 1613. By 1617 the friendship between the two men was well established.[1] However, they did not have to start their research into the runes from scratch.

A generation earlier, in 1586, the nobleman Caspar Markdanner, on excavating the larger of the two runic stones at Jelling in southern Jutland, had marked the event by having a transcription of the runes on the two stones reproduced on a golden tablet and hung in the church in Jelling. Five years later a picture of the golden tablet was published by Henrik Rantzau, containing the two inscriptions plus their translation, not to mention a list

---

1 Schepelern, *Museum*, 119–20; see also Ole Degn, *Christian 4.s kansler. Christen Friis til Kragerup (1581–1639) som menneske og poitiker,* Viborg 1988, 144–45.

DOI: 10.4324/9781003290940-4

of the whole runic alphabet.[2] However, it was the Swedish polymath and antiquarian Johannes Bureus who in 1590 pioneered the runic studies in Scandinavia. He published the first runological study in 1599, an illustrated single-leaf, *Runakänslanäs Lärä-span*, and a small volume in 1611, *Runa ABC Boken.*[3]

In March 1619 Ole Worm asked Aquilonius whether he was interested in 'our' runes (Gothica). Worm wanted something to be published about them, but only in the context of other similar epitaphs about the ancient heroes in Latin. Writing to Worm six months later Aquilonius applauded Worm's interests in antiquarianism, that is, runes, and claimed they fitted well with his own pursuits. He promised to publish something about them in a different context, expecting them to gain public recognition similar to that of Latin and Roman inscriptions. Due to the publications of scholars such as Lipsius, Scaliger, and Gruter, Aquilonius was convinced that a growing interest in such ancient inscriptions existed, and he was sure that the runes which were even older, would find substantial interest within the international, scholarly community. His only concern was the difficulty in finding a printer who could manage the types needed, but he thought they might be obtained in the Netherlands from the printer who had published Bonaventura Vulcanius's *De Literis et Lingua Getarum*, in 1597. Worm owned a copy of this work, which he valued highly and later acknowledged in his publications.[4] Despite the encouragement from Worm Aquilonius failed to bring his interests in the runes to fruition. When he wrote to Worm a couple of years later, in July 1621, it was to inform him that his pupil Laurentius Asserous was about to publish a work about all the Danish epitaphs, starting with two volumes on Sealand and Scania. Worm had already seen some of the epitaphs Asserous had collected and informed Aquilonius that a careful selection was needed, avoiding the vulgar and insignificant, only selecting those relating to royals and historically famous men and the very ancient, telling his friend that he had to act as supervisor and referee on this

---

2 Published in Peter Lindeberg, Commentarii rerum memorabilium in Europa ab anno octuagesimo sexton etc., Hamburg 1591; published six years later in Bonaventura Vulcanius, *De literis et lingua getarum, sive gothorum item de notis lombardicis, quibus accesserunt specimina variarum lingua, quarum indicem pagina quae praesationem sequitur ostendit*, Leiden 1597. See also K. Dekker, 'The runes in Bonaventura Vulcanius De Literis et Lingua Getarum sive Gothorum (1597): Provenance and origins', 411–49 in H. Cazes (ed.), *Bonaventura Vulcanius. Works and Networks: Bruges 1538-Leiden 1614*, Leiden 2011.
3 Johannes Bureus, *Runakenslones Leraspan*, Uppsala 1599 and *Runa ABC Boken*, Stockholm 1611. For Bureus see, Håkan Håkanson, *Vid Tidens Ände. Om stormakt-stidens vidunderliga drömvärld och en profet vid dess yttersta rand*, Halmstad 2014, especially Chapter V, Runorna och urvisdomen, 307–62.
4 *Breve fra og til Ole Worm*, nos. 54 and 66. See also E. Moltke, *Jon Skonvig og de andre runetegnere. Et bidrag til runologiens historie I Danmark og Norge*, vol. II, Copenhagen 1958, 107; for Worm's ownership of Vulcanius's book, see *Breve fra og til Ole Worm*, nos. 124 and 137.

project. Once more Worm took the opportunity to encourage his friend to publish some of the runic inscriptions, suggesting that he put them at the beginning of the volume of epitaphs, he was about to publish with Asserous. This would in Worm's opinion encourage foreign scholars to take an interest in Danish antiquarianism realising that the country contained plenty of ancient monuments, and merited research.[5]

A couple of months later Worm received a draft copy of Asserous's first volume on Danish epitaphs which he was asked to critically read and correct before publication. The volume also contained a letter from Aquilonius to Worm dealing with some of the runic inscriptions to be found in Denmark. The letter finished with a promise to the reader that if his interest had been awakened, better and much more detailed studies of the runes were to follow.[6] Worm was happy with the draft and particularly pleased with Aquilonius's letter about the runic monuments, which he was convinced would generate considerable interest and awareness. He was satisfied that the need for Gothic/runic letters presented no problem since he knew someone who could cut them while examples could be found in the royal historiographer Claus Lyschander's genealogy.[7]

The correspondence with Bertel Knudsen Aquilonius during the autumn of 1621 served to get Worm started on his own research into the runes. Claus Lyschander had described the runic stone from Tryggevælde in his genealogy of Danish kings. On reading it Worm had realised that it was full of mistakes while offering a nonsensical interpretation. He had therefore personally made a proper drawing of the Tryggevælde stone and its inscription. He expressed the wish that a learned scholar would emerge 'who could reinsert these things in their proper glory'. Worm added that the more he contemplated the efforts of the Swede, Johannes Bureus, to interpret the runes the more he admired him, stating that it was a pity that Bureus had not continued his research and published a more detailed study. He was convinced that undying fame would be given to the person who took on this research because of its great antiquity, its intricacy, and the few who had dared tackle it. He could hardly have encouraged Aquilonius further.[8]

By the end of 1621 Ole Worm most likely had realised that the project of tracking and describing all the ancient runic monuments in Denmark and Norway was beyond the reach of a single individual. He may also have concluded that the best person to be in charge of such a project would be

5 *Breve fra og til Ole Worm*, nos. 87 and 88; see also Moltke, *Skonvig*, 108.
6 Breve fra og til Ole Worm, nos. 90 and 93 and Laurentius Asserous, *Inscriptionum Selandicarum-Daniæ antigrapha. In fine adjunct Bert. Canuti De monumentis antiquis Epistola*, Copenhagen 1621. See also Moltke, *Skonvig*, 108–09.
7 Claus C. Lyschander, *Synopsis historiarum Danicarum ... Danske Kongers Slectebog*, Copenhagen 1622. For Lyschander see K. Skovgaard-Petersen, *Historiography at the Court of Christian IV (1588–1648)*, Copenhagen 2002, 118–20.
8 *Breve fra og til Ole Worm*, no. 93; see also Degn, *Christian 4.s kansler*, 108.

himself rather than Aquilonius. Furthermore, the importance of this project which had found favour with the learned chancellor, Christen Friis, who was keen on promoting historical and cultural projects which could glorify the kingdom of Denmark and Norway would have served to make Worm realise that a prominent and controlling role in the runic enterprise might prove beneficial to him. Together with the chancellor Worm helped to produce the draft of the ordinance, which Christian IV issued to the Bishops in Denmark and Norway on 11 August 1622. They were ordered to find:

> All runes inscribed on stones, whole or in pieces, or carved in wood or on belts made of metal, to take notes of their whereabouts and produce correct copies of their inscriptions which are best made by outlining the inscriptions with chalk, and the deans and ministers are instructed to apply themselves to this and inform their bishops who shall immediately send the information to the Chancellery.[9]

Shortly after the ordinance was issued Worm made sure that a royal order was issued to Bertel Aquilonius ordering him to undertake a journey through Scania, Halland, and Blekinge to find, review, and evaluate all the runic monuments. Aquilonius was clearly excited about this commission and interpreted it as if he had also been put in charge of the intended publication about the runic monuments. Writing to Worm in February 1623 he reported, that he had already undertaken the journey and nearly finished his report. He added that when he had mastered the old language and the runes he would write a book about it. Meanwhile, he asked Worm to lend him his copy of Johannes Bureus's *Runakänslanäs Läräspan* and Bonaventura Vulcanius's *De literis et lingua getarum* so that he could finish his work before he personally presented it to the chancellor.[10]

   Ole Worm became increasingly focussed on his runic studies during the spring of 1623 when he wrote to his former Icelandic student, the later bishop of Holar, Thorlak Skulason. This proved the first of the many letters Worm exchanged with Icelandic scholars about Norse history and antiquity. By then he was already familiar with the works of the learned headmaster of the Latin school in Holar, Arngrim Jonsson. He wanted Skulason, if possible, to send him a copy of Jonsson's history of Greenland, and if not available tell him where it had been printed.[11] Having read Jonsson's *Crymogæa* he also wanted to obtain a transcription of the burial inscriptions referred

---

9 The ordinance is printed in F. C. Werlauff, 'Ole Worms Fortjenster af det nordiske Oldstudium. En Undersøgelse', in *Nordisk Tidsskrift for Oldkyndighed*, vol. 1, 1832, 288ff and in J. K. Søresen and F. Jørgensen, *Præsteindberetninger til Ole Worm*, 1–2, Copenhagen 1970–74.; cited in Moltke, *Skonvig*, 106

10 *Breve fra og til Ole Worm*, no. 124.

11 This work was not published until 1688; Arngrim Jonsson, *Groenlandia edur Groenlands Saga*, Skalholt 1688

to in this book.[12] He explained that he had enjoyed himself studying the runes and made a considerable effort to understand them. He wanted to know whether any Icelander had worked on their grammar and syntax, as mentioned by Jonsson. If so Worm was keen to know about it, as he was to learn more about Icelanders, who had written about runes in 1216. If further antiquities were found Worm begged to be informed. Skulason reported back to Worm that the work on Greenland had yet to be published and that Jonsson was not willing to provide him with a manuscript copy. He was, however, able to send Worm the signs of the runic alphabet written by the leading Icelandic specialist on runes to which he added the transcription of a local, ancient monument.[13]

Meanwhile, Worm took his time responding to Aquilonius letter from February 1623. The person who had delivered Aquilonius's letter had struck Worm as someone he was not prepared to entrust with his response and the books which Aquilonius had asked to borrow. There had clearly been a fall out, and the messenger had left Copenhagen without informing Worm, but more importantly taking Aquilonius's report about the runic stones in Scania, Halland, and Blekinge with him. Worm therefore had handed his response in July to a lady he trusted. She was also bringing Aquilonius the desired work by Johannes Bureus. Worm had, however, split his copy of Bureus's work on the Swedish runes – *Runakänslanäs Lärä-span* – into several parts. This had been done when he had been called on to explain and interpret the runes to chancellor, Christen Friis. Worm included a key to the translation of the runes which he had put together, pointing out that it was incomplete because of the ignorance of his assistant, who could not copy the runes properly. Worm was unable to send Aquilonius the work by Vulcanius he had requested, because he had lent it to his brother-in-law Caspar Bartholin, who was abroad, but intended to write a book about the variety of letters found among the people of the world, including the runes. Worm also added some of his own papers with notes about the runes which he thought Aquilonius might find useful, including some comments by the Rostock philologist Nathan Chytræus which he thought Aquilonius might be unfamiliar with. Worm thought that there was other relevant material for Aquilonius to see, when they next met. Meanwhile, he encouraged his friend to make sure that he handled the notes he forwarded with care, emphasising the hard work involved in producing them, and instructing him to return them when he had finished with them. Worm rounded off his letter by underlining how much he was looking forward to reading Aquilonius's report on the runic stones in Scania, Halland, and Blekinge.[14] Aquilonius was gratified by Worm's response and praised his friend for all

12 Arngrim Jonsson, *Crymogæa sive rerum Islandicarum libri III*, Hamburg 1609, 23
13 *Breve fra og til Ole Worm*, nos. 129 and 144; for Skulason's first letter to Worm after his return to Iceland, see no. 106.
14 *Breve fra og til Ole Worm*, no. 137.

his concern and help. He was delighted with the loan of Bureus's work, but even more so with Worm's notes about it. Despite his excitement Aquilonius had to tell Worm that it had unfortunately all arrived too late, since he had already finished his report and reached broadly similar results. However, he hoped to make use of it when revising his work for publication. He included a copy of his report for Worm to read before he handed it over to the chancellor. He expected to come to Copenhagen around Michaelmas to meet Worm and ask his advice about some of the issues around the runes, which he struggled to comprehend, and for which he had found no help in Johannes Bureus's work

We can only assume that Worm was disappointed with Aquilonius's report. By then he may have finally realised that Aquilonius was not the man for the job of supervising the collection and interpretation of the runic monuments and their inscriptions, which Worm and the chancellor had encouraged the king to initiate in 1622. As a result the contacts between Worm and Aquilonius became less regular from the autumn of 1623, and little if anything was said about the runes.[15] Instead Ole Worm must have decided to take full control of the project. Apart from his growing personal interests in the runes, the importance of the project to the chancellor and King Christian IV, as a way of emphasising the important cultural roots and international significance of the kingdom of Denmark and Norway would not have been lost on Worm. When three years later Worm asked Aquilonius to return some of the books he had lent him, he pointed out that he was surprised that his friend had remained silent for so long and refrained from communicating with him, adding that he himself was unable 'to resist the storm which had taken him out into the deep sea of antiquarian research'.[16] Clearly Aquilonius was disappointed having been passed over after what he himself had considered a promising start to his research into the runes and the ancient monuments. When visiting Copenhagen in November 1628 Aquilonius left the city without taking leave of Ole Worm who expressed his incomprehension and disappointment.[17] Relations between the two men had clearly deteriorated.

Ole Worm not only appreciated Johannes Bureus's work on the runes, praising them to Aquilonius, but he also owned a copy of the single leaf *Runakänslanäs Lärä-span* and the volume *Runa ABC Boken*. The fact that Bureus had become increasingly obsessed with mysticism, Paracelsianism, and Rosicrucianism would not have unduly concerned Worm who had a long-standing, if guarded interest in Paracelsianism, and retained a similar interest in Rosicrucianism, even beyond his public rejection of the movement as a dangerous sect in May 1619.[18]

---

15 Moltke, *Skonvig*, 107–13.
16 *Brev fra og til Ole Worm*, no. 207,
17 *Ibid.*, no. 262,
18 See O. P. Grell, 'In Search of True Knowledge: Ole Worm (1588–1654) and the New Philosophy', 218–24 in Pamela H. Smith and Benjamin Schmidt (eds.), *Making Knowledge*

Johannes Bureus, who had become royal librarian in Sweden in 1610, promoted his runic research within the context of 'Gothicism', originally espoused by Archbishop Johannes Magnus, which traced the birth of Sweden to Magog, the grandson of Noah, who was supposed to have settled there eighty years after the Flood. From there Gothic high culture had spread to the rest of Europe. Bureus inspired by the Renaissance notion of Prisca theologica claimed that all classical knowledge came from the Goths who held superior knowledge of all things, having received the wisdom revealed by God to Adam at the start of time and passed on to Noah's descendants. He saw the runes as closely linked to that knowledge and the magic associated with it. He therefore claimed that the runes constituted a sacred form of writing. Bureus was convinced that the runic characters had a double meaning. Apart from being letters of the alphabet, some of them encompassed a symbolic language, similar to, but much older, than the Hebrew Cabala and the Egyptian hieroglyphs, containing true knowledge, thereby keeping it uncorrupted for future generations. These runes Bureus labelled 'adalrunor' – noble runes – which were hidden or secret, only accessible to those who comprehended their mysticism.[19]

Ole Worm was, of course, in regular contact with Chancellor Christen Friis, who took an active interest in the runic project, registering and transcribing all the ancient monuments in Denmark and Norway. Friis was personally interested in ancient, oriental languages and monuments. Worm contacted his friend, Johannes Rhode, in Padua during the autumn of 1624 on the encouragement of the chancellor, who wanted to know whether some of the Etruscan monuments around Volterra had Gothic inscriptions. Having read a book by Raphael Volterranus. Friis had discovered that a depicted Etruscan monument had, what looked like inscriptions similar to the runes. He wanted Rhode to carefully transcribe this inscription and forward it to him. For Rhode's use Worm included a list of 'our gothic alphabet', so he could discover whether they were identical. When Rhode wrote to Friis a year later he had little of value to report about Gothic/runic inscriptions to be found in Italy in general and Volterra in particular.[20]

2 First works on runes

In 1625 Worm received a royal order to personally undertake a journey through Denmark to find any runic monuments which were relevant to

in Early Modern Europe. Practices, Objects, and Texts, 1400–1800, Chicago 2007.

19 For this see the excellent work of Håkan Håkansson, *Vid Tidens Ände. Om stormaktstidens vidunderliga drömvärld och en profet vid dess yttersta rand*, Halmstad 2014, especially Chapter V, 307–62; see also Håkan Håkansson, 'Alchemy of the Ancient Goths: Johannes Bureus' Search for the Lost Wisdom of Scandinavia', *Early Science and Medicine*, 17, 2012, 500–22.

20 *Brev fra og til Ole Worm*, nos. 169, 174, and 181.

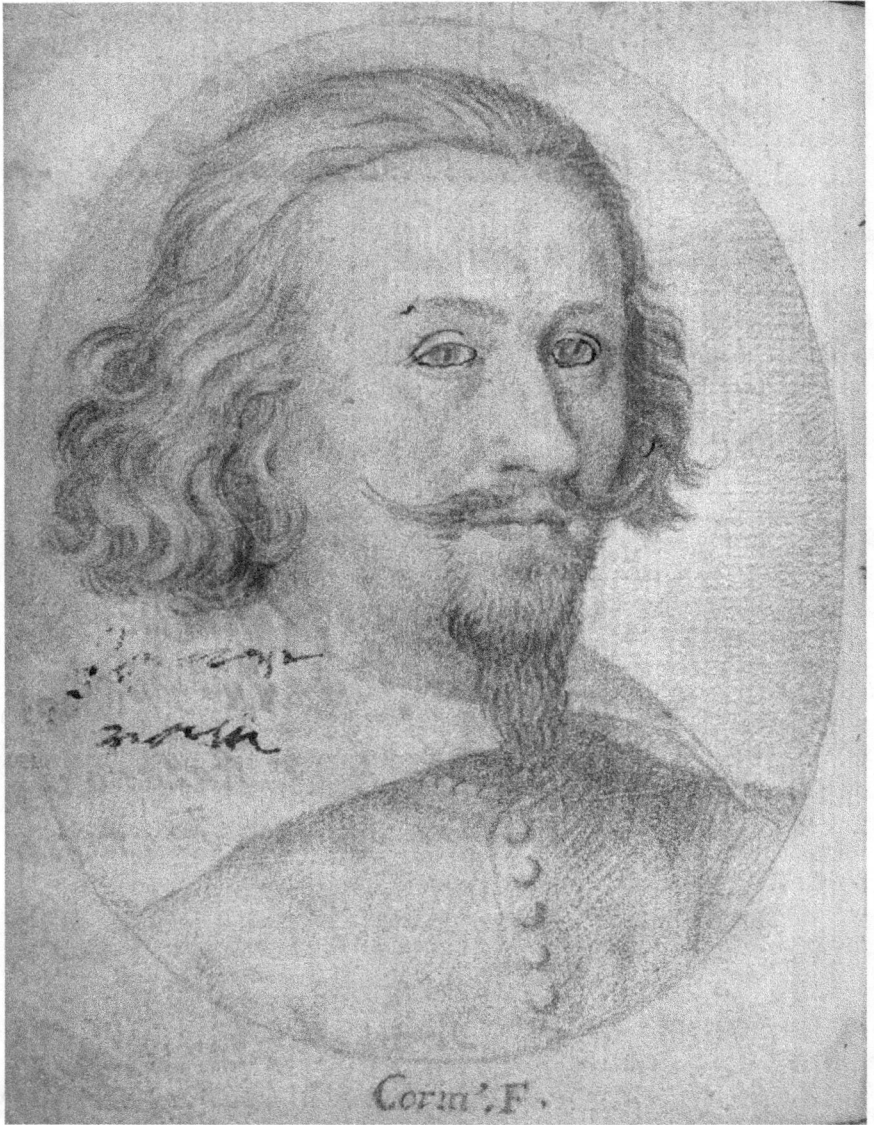

Figure 3.1 Johan Rhode (1587–1659) drawing by J. J. Corman 1632 in Johan Rhode's Album Amicorum MS Thott 573 Royal Danish Library; courtesy of the Royal Danish Library.

Danish history. By April and May the following year Ole Worm received poems from friends and assistants for his forthcoming, first work on the runes, *Fasti Danici*, about a runic calendar found on Gotland. One of his assistants, the minister Torben Hasebart, even wrote his poem in runes. He also forwarded drawings and descriptions of two ancient monuments from Halland or Blekinge for Worm's assessment. Worm was delighted with their quality and expressed the hope that others who engaged in this project would follow in his footsteps. A comment which might well refer to his disappointment with Aquilonius's efforts. Worm's friend, Steffen Hansen Stephanius was mistakenly under the impression that Worm's work on the ancient monuments was being printed in April 1626. Worm informed him that it was, in fact, *Fasti Danici* which was with the printers. The book had been delayed by the engraver who was making the depictions of the calendars. Worm added, that he hoped his work would be well received by other scholars, pointing out that only those who had themselves undertaken similar work could fully appreciate the difficulties of those who sought to bring forth matters which had remained forgotten for so long. When the first edition of *Fasti Danici* was published a few months later Worm forwarded three copies to Chancellor Christen Friis, one for the king, one for the elected-prince, and one for Friis himself. Worm added that if his work was graciously received by His Majesty then he would apply himself with even greater energy to research 'our old writing and our monuments'.[21]

Worm's research into runes and ancient monuments was to benefit tremendously from his excellent Icelandic contacts, established primarily through the students he had taught at the University of Copenhagen, many of whom had also boarded with him. Thus, it was through the intervention of his former student Thorlak Skulason, that Worm received a letter from Arngrim Jonsson in August 1626. Jonsson was mistakenly under the impression that Worm had been given responsibility for the 'study of Danish history', a position Jonsson considered similar to that of the former royal historiographer Niels Krag. Jonsson had already been contacted by the chancellor, Christen Friis, asking him to provide information about ancient Norwegian monuments on the island, but had informed the chancellor that he had nothing to add to what he had already told Niels Krag thirty years earlier. However, because the chancellor had expressed his interest in 'the old language' Jonsson had once again looked for sources and sent a number of manuscripts to the island's stadtholder, Holger Rosenkrantz. Jonsson had also sent a couple of books plus and Icelandic grammar to the chancellor, while Skulason had forwarded a runic alphabet with the Latin letters added underneath.[22]

21 For the royal order, see Moltke, *Skonvig*, 107; for the poems for *Fasti Danici*, see *Breve fra og til Ole Worm*, nos. 194, 196, and 199; for the letter to Christian Friis, see *Ibid.*, no. 201. See also Ole Worm, *Fasti Danici*, Copenhagen 1626; republished in 1633 and a new expanded edition in 1643.
22 *Breve fra og til Ole Worm*, nos. 202 and 204.

Judging from Ole Worm's correspondence, the years 1626 and 1627 proved particularly busy for registering and transcribing ancient runic monuments. Worm constantly encouraged friends and collaborators to continue to contribute to his research. Torben Hasebart was encouraged to keep up his work in Halland and Blekinge, where Worm was particularly interested in one monument. Worm evidently considered Hasebart a talented and reliable collaborator and therefore asked him to update his register of ancient monuments in Scania, Halland, and Blekinge. Never one for missing an opportunity to receive further information Worm asked his uncle Søren Olufsen to send him a detailed and precise drawing of the runic stone to be found in the garden of the Stenalt estate in Jutland. Worm wanted him to supply not only its measurements but also a full transcription of the inscription, and to tell him what local people had to say about it. He added that he planned to publish something about the runic monuments. Sending a copy of his *Fasti Danici* to the Bishop of Trondheim, Peder Schjelderup, Worm enquired whether any ancient monuments could be found in the vicinity of the town.[23]

Having been approached by the Icelandic minister Magnus Olafsson on Laufas to assist his son in receiving financial support for his studies in Copenhagen, Worm took the opportunity to ask Olafsson for help in the runic research he had been commissioned to undertake in his spare time, as he put it, since he had been informed that Olafsson was highly skilled in 'our old writing'. It would appear that Worm had by then already written the first draft of a book about the runes, *Runir, seu Danica literature Antiquissima*, which was not published until 1636.[24] He asked Thorlak Skulason who had seen the manuscript during a visit to Copenhagen to explain it in detail to Magnus Olafsson in order that he could add something to this work before it was published. Furthermore, he had been told that Olafsson owned a copy of the Edda and other books written in runes which he was keen to borrow.

More importantly for the first time in this letter to Magnus Olafsson Worm brings up the issue of the so-called 'Ram-runes', or power runes. Worm was not sure whether the 'Ram-runes', which had been used for magic, were identical with the normal runes or different. He emphasised that some ancient stone monuments could be found in Denmark which had an inscription of runes which differed from the normal. No one had so far been able to explain that to Worm who wanted Olafsson's opinion. He hoped that Olafsson's familiarity with the ancient language would prove helpful, save him time, and prevent him from making significant mistakes. Worm added that he had found that the resident Icelandic students in Copenhagen were unable to help him.

23 *Ibid.*, nos. 206 and 214 (Torben Hasebart), and nos. 209 and 210.
24 Ole Worm, *Runir, seu Danica literature Antiquissima vulga Gothica dicta luci reditta*, Amsterdam 1636.

In his response to Arngrim Jonsson written around the same time as his letter to Olafsson – late spring 1627 – Worm pointed out that he had not taken on the role of historiographer. He remained a physician who enjoyed pursuing antiquarian research when his medical work allowed him to do so. He pointed out that he received no salary for this, nor had he been tempted to take it on in the hope of reward. Worm was not exactly telling the truth here, as can be seen from his letter a couple of years later to Chancellor Friis, where he indicated that some sort of reward was needed to encourage him to keep his research going. As in his letter to Olafsson Worm sought Jonsson's opinion about the 'Ram-runes' which had been 'misused' for magic, and whether they were identical to the normal runes. Jonsson found it difficult to provide an exhaustive answer. He admitted that some people were still suspected of magic, but they would never 'reveal their mysteries to him'. However, he was convinced that the ancient magicians had used runic characters,

> especially a popular form corrupted by lines and dots, whereby the Devil had fooled them, feigning that they would become of significance when they made a bargain with him. It is not my concern to judge how Paracelsian medicine consists of rare characters. I am absolutely convinced that the runic letters originally contained nothing magic. Now the early ones have been corrupted by superstition whereby they appear to have been given the name 'Ram-runes' which means powerful runes.[25]

Olafsson proved unable to help Worm having no knowledge of the runes, but Worm was delighted with Jonsson's response. He more or less agreed with Jonsson view about the 'Ram-runes', but avoided commenting on his statement about Paracelsian medicine. Worm thanked Jonsson for confirming him in his belief that the ancient runes included a sixteenth letter, and not just the fifteen as claimed by 'a certain Swede', that is, Johannes Bureus. Appreciative of Jonsson's comments about his *Fasti Danici*, Worm send him a manuscript copy of his *Runir, seu Danica literature Antiquissima* for inspection. He was convinced that there was no one better in the whole of Scandinavia to improve and correct his text.[26]

In March 1628 Worm encouraged his student-friend in Leiden, Steffen Hansen Stephanius, to continue his historical studies. He emphasised how keen Chancellor Friis was on promoting national history, and the chancellor's appreciation of those who were dedicated to glorifying and spreading the knowledge of national history. Christen Friis had even managed to drive Worm down this route, involuntarily, and despite all his other commitments. Never one to miss an opportunity Worm forwarded some copies of his *Fasti Danici* for Stephanius to show some of the leading lights at Leiden University,

25 *Breve fra og til Ole Worm*, nos. 220 and 228.
26 *Ibid.*, nos. 229, 245, and 253

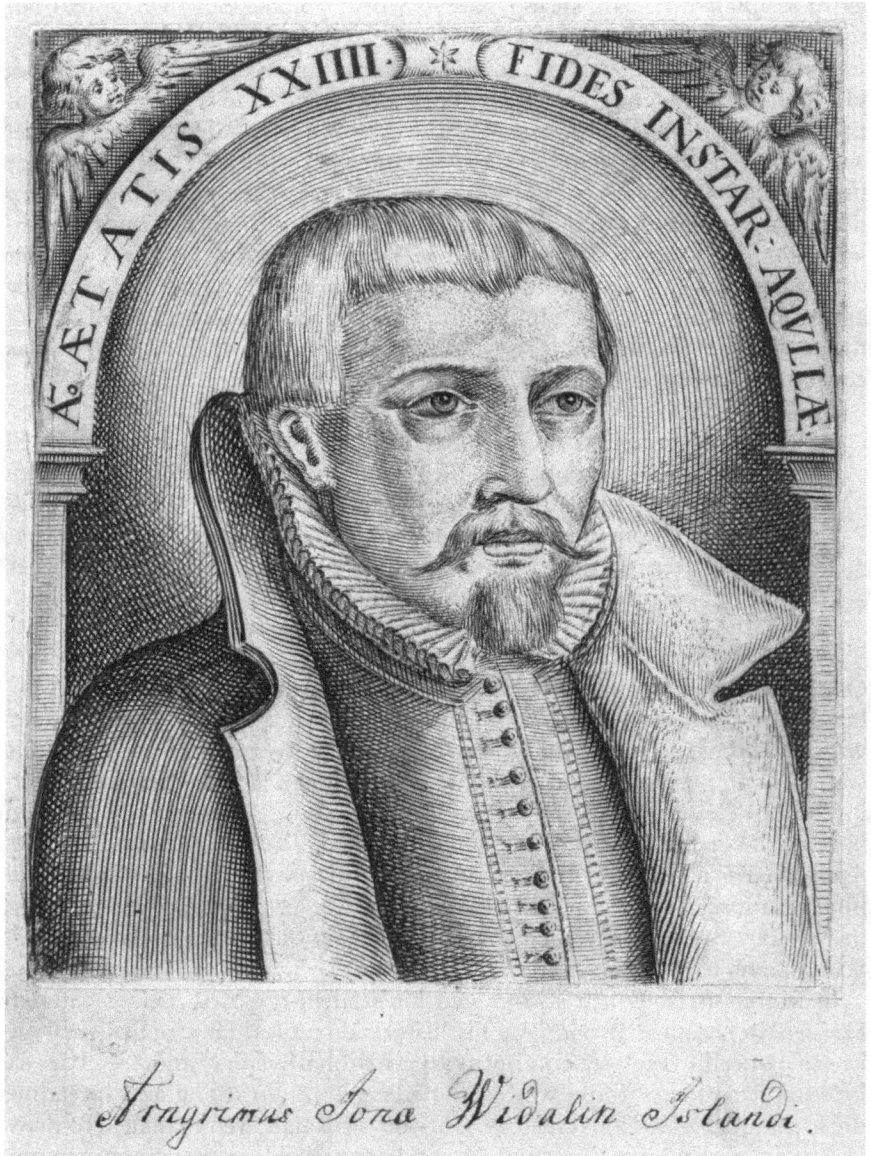

Figure 3.2 Arngrim Jonsson (1568–1648); courtesy of the Royal Danish Library.

such as the Latin scholar Daniel Heinsius and the historian Petrus Scriverius, asking him to obtain their opinion. Having just become vice chancellor of the University of Copenhagen Worm was concerned that his book about the ancient monuments would be delayed, but adding that he had already collected drawings and descriptions of a couple of hundred ancient, runic stones.[27] A bit of an exaggeration since Worm's work, *Monumenta Danica*, published in 1643 contained no more than 146 monuments.[28]

Stephanius reported back to Worm a few months later, that his *Fasti Danici* had been extremely well received in Leiden among the leading philologists, such as Heinsius and Vossius, not to mention Scriverius and Johannes Pontanus, professor in Harderwijk, who had been appointed Danish historiographer in 1618. Stephanius enclosed a collection of ancient calendars for Worm that he recently had bought on an auction in Leiden. Worm was delighted with the news, which he hoped represented the genuine opinions of these Dutch scholars rather than views filtered by Stephanius's loyalty to him. Worm then dealt with a number of issues raised by Pontanus, which he found a mixture of misconceptions and prejudice, pointing out that his book did not offer doctrines or 'articles of faith', but a number of suggestions and suppositions which were intended to result in debate. Worm was very grateful for the calendars he had received. He intended to have them drawn and added to a second edition of his *Fasti Danici*, praising Stephanius. Worm also enclosed a survey of his recently finished work on the runes for Stephanius's use and reference.[29]

When Christen Friis of Kragerup was promoted to the chancellorship in 1616 he became the driving force behind a series of national historical and antiquarian undertakings of which Ole Worm's registration and description of runic monuments came to constitute an important part. Worm's first work on the runes, *Fasti Danici* (1626), which was dedicated to Christian IV, included a reproduction and account of a runic calendar on a parchment manuscript from 1528, which Christen Friis had donated to Worm in 1622, requesting him to translate it and explain its context. According to Worm, Friis had personally discovered this runic calendar in a library in Jutland.[30] Appropriately Worm dedicated his book *Runir seu Danica literatura antiquissima*, on the origin and development of the runes, to Christen Friis.[31] Worm was convinced that the runes had been the handwriting of ancient times in a Scandinavia dominated by Denmark. He was also convinced that Icelandic as it was spoken at the start of the seventeenth century was close to Old Norse the language of the runic inscriptions. Both he and Christen Friis corresponded regularly with learned Icelanders, seeking information and obtaining ancient manuscripts. This was all undertaken in order to demonstrate the importance of Gothic or more specifically Danish culture, as having ancient and possibly biblical roots.

27 *Ibid.*, no. 232.
28 Ole Worm, *Danicorum monumentorum libri sex: espissis antiquitatum tenebris in Dania ac Norvegia extantibus ruderibus eruti*, Copenhagen 1643.
29 *Breve fra og til Ole Worm*, nos. 242 and 248.
30 See *Fasti Danici*, Copenhagen 1643 (3rd and expanded edition), 123, and Degn, *Christian 4.s kansler*, 108; see also Skovgaard-Petersen, *Historiography*, 29.
31 Ole Worm, *Runir, seu Danica literature Antiquissima vulga Gothica dicta luci reditta*, Amsterdam 1636; see also Degn, *Christian 4.s kansler*, 108

The writing of Latin, national histories for an international market was an ambition shared by many European rulers in the sixteenth and seventeenth centuries. This was also an aspiration held by Christian IV and his chancellor, Christen Friis. Throughout his reign Christian IV continuously engaged at least one royal historiographer, producing a new history of Denmark. The need to defend and amplify the cultural and political significance of Denmark grew during the early seventeenth century, as a consequence of the fierce rivalry and confrontation with Sweden for dominance of the Baltic. The fact that in 1617 the Swedish King Gustavus Adolphus had appointed the Leiden professor Daniel Heinsius as royal historiographer, and that Johannes Magnus's *Historia de omnibus Gothorum Suenumque regibus* (1554) was re-published that year, with its anti-Danish agenda and claims of Swedish cultural superiority, especially its assertion that only Swedes could lay claim to be descendants of the ancient Goths of Scandinavia, who could trace their origin back to Magog, the grandson of Noah, added urgency to the Danish government's drive to lay a counter-claim to the Gothic myths and promote its national history.[32]

Consequently, the then Danish royal historiographer Minister Claus Lyschander, was seen as not fully up to the task. In 1618 Chancellor Friis was instrumental in hiring another royal historiographer with an already established international reputation, Johannes Isaakzs Pontanus. Pontanus, who understood Danish, having been born in Elsinore in Denmark, was professor in Harderwijk in the United Provinces and had already written major historical works. In terms of international reputation he matched Daniel Heinsius, the newly appointed Swedish royal historiographer. Pontanus's remit was to produce a Latin history of Denmark from the beginning to the reign of Christian IV within six years. However, by 1624 Christen Friis and Christian IV had realised that Pontanus was not going to produce anything publishable within this time frame. They therefore hired a third royal historiographer, another Dutchman, Johannes Meursius. Meursius, who was professor at the University of Leiden and historiographer of the States General, had found life at the university challenging in the aftermath of the execution of his benefactor, Johannes van Oldenbarnevelt. Having served as tutor for the Oldenbarnevelt children he was suspected of being a Remonstrant. With his career prospects damaged he was delighted to accept the offer of a professorship at the Academy in Sorø and the position of royal historiographer to Christian IV.[33] Both Pontanus and Meursius were well paid as royal historiographers. Each of them received 500 Reichsthalers plus another 100 for assistants. Bearing this in mind it is surprising that Ole Worm received no remuneration for his antiquarian activities on behalf of the government.[34]

---

32 See Skovgaard-Petersen, *Historiography*, 26–28 and 91–95.

33 *Ibid.*, especially 37–84

34 *Ibid.*, passim, for their salaries see 27–28. The fact that Ole Worm was never appointed royal antiquarian may, of course, also explain why Worm was never remunerated, as pointed out to me by Morten Fink-Jensen.

At the start of 1629 Ole Worm was visited by the Dutch physician Johannes Narssius, who was on his way to take up a position as physician and royal historiographer to King Gustavus Adolphus of Sweden. Narssius belonged to the diaspora of Remonstrants who had left the United Provinces in the wake of the Synod of Dort in 1619. Worm had given Narssius a copy of his recently published book, *Tulshøi, seu momumentum Ströense in Scania enucleatum*, and before leaving for Sweden Narssius reciprocated by sending him a copy of what he described as 'an instruction in the runic language', namely, Johannes Bureus's *Libellus alphabetarius literis runicis cum interlinearibus sueticis editus*. Before leaving he also gave Worm a friendly warning not to define Swedish antiquities as Danish. Otherwise, he warned the two of them might have to engage in serious but friendly disagreement. Thanking Narssius Worm mentioned that he already owned a copy of Bureus's work, and took the opportunity to point out that what he ascribed to the Danes was well founded and evidenced.[35]

3 International recognition and friendship with Sir Henry Spelman

In terms of international recognition 1629 proved something of breakthrough year for Ole Worm. On his grand tour the Danish nobleman, Axel Juul, who held antiquarian interests and later donated objects to Worm's cabinet of curiosity, arrived in London in the second half of 1628. Here he took the opportunity to meet the well-known antiquarian, Sir Henry Spelman, whom he showed a copy of Worm's recent work on the Tulshøj monument. Spelman proved so excited by this work that he contacted Worm through the Danish ambassador to London, asking him to start a correspondence with him. Spelman had a number of queries about Worm's work and doubted some of his conclusions, but he emphasised that he agreed with him that Danes, Norwegians, and Goths descended from the Hebrews. In this he had been convinced by Arngrim Jonsson's *Crymogœa*. Spelman wanted to know more about the runes in particular and having heard about Worm's work on the runic alphabet he hoped to be able to obtain a copy. He also referred Worm to a number of English monuments with possible runic inscriptions.[36] Worm was obviously flattered by Spelman's

---

35 *Breve fra og til Ole Worm*, nos. 267 and 268; see also Ole Worm, *Tulshøi, seu momumentum Ströense in Scania enucleatum*, Copenhagen 1628 and Johannes Bureus, *Libellus alphabetarius literis runicis cum interlinearibus sueticis editus*, Stockholm 1624.

36 *Breve fra og til Ole Worm*, no. 271; Axel Juul took a considerable interest in Worm's research into the runes and in March 1630 gave him a small book containing characters from different languages similar to what he had seen when visiting Worm, no. 336; for Sir Henry Spelman, see *Oxford Dictionary of National Biography*; it is interesting that Spelman had obtained a copy of Arngrim Jonsson, *Crymogœa sive rerum Islandicarum libri III*, Hamburg 1609; the work on runes by Worm which Spelman wanted, was obviously *Runir, seu Danica literature Antiquissima vulga Gothica dicta luci reditta*, which was not published until 1636.

interest and praise. Having been given a copy of Spelman's *Archaeology* Worm responded by sending Spelman a copy of his *Fasti Danici*. He asked Spelman to comment on it with similar candour to what he had done about the Tulshøj monument, pointing out to him that his work only constituted an unproven attempt. Worm admitted that something might easily have escaped his attention since he had been alone in breaking new ground. If something was missing Worm hoped to be able to remedy it in his forthcoming work on the runes. Unfortunately the book's appearance had been delayed by the deplorable conditions brought about by war and the mean obstinacy of the printers. Worm was, however, delighted that Spelman agreed with him that since names of ancient, Danish heroes were identical to those used by the Hebrews, the Danes must have descended from the Hebrews.[37] Evidently Ole Worm sought to claim that Gothic history, as evidenced by ancient documents and runic monuments, was, in fact, Danish history. He was convinced that the use of the name Asser among ancient Danish heroes pointed to a link to the biblical Asher, the second son of Jacob, who founded the tribe of Asher. Furthermore, these links to the Hebrews might indicate a link to ancient, divine wisdom. There are clearly similarities between the views of Johannes Bureus and Worm here, even if Worm did refrain from making similar grand claims for a Gothic mysticism where ancient divine wisdom was linked to the runes.[38]

Ole Worm considered his runic research to be ground-breaking, a pioneering effort, and as such open to mistakes and fallacies. He was keen on comments and corrections from fellow scholars as can be seen from his correspondence with Spelman, and even more so from the correspondence with his Icelandic friends. Thus, in May 1629 Worm expressed his gratitude to Arngrim Jonsson for his detailed comments on his *Fasti Danici*. He acknowledged a number of mistakes especially towards the end of the book and promised to rectify them and a number of other issues in his forthcoming work on the runes (*Runir*), which Arngrim had recently returned to him. However, he wanted Arngrim to have kept it longer, and he therefore returned it so that he could fully benefit from Arngrim's knowledge and comments before it was published. In this Worm was not disappointed. When Arngrim Jonsson returned the manuscript in August 1630, he politely stated that he had nothing to add to Worm's 'perfect work on the runes', only to offer four pages of detailed comments.[39]

Ole Worm wrote to Chancellor Christen Friis during the autumn of 1629, asking him to find a parish in Bergen for the Norwegian minister Jon

---

37 *Ibid.*, no. 284.
38 See Håkansson, *Vid Tidens Ände*, 307–62; see also Håkansson, 'Alchemy of the Ancient Goths', 501–03.
39 *Breve fra og til Ole Worm*, no. 272; Arngrim acknowledged the arrival of the manuscript in August 1629 telling Worm he would keep it until the following year, see no. 288; he returned it in August 1630, see no. 364. Worm also instigated a translation of the Edda into Latin by the Icelandic minister Magnus Olafsson which was ready by the summer of 1629, see nos. 290 and 293.

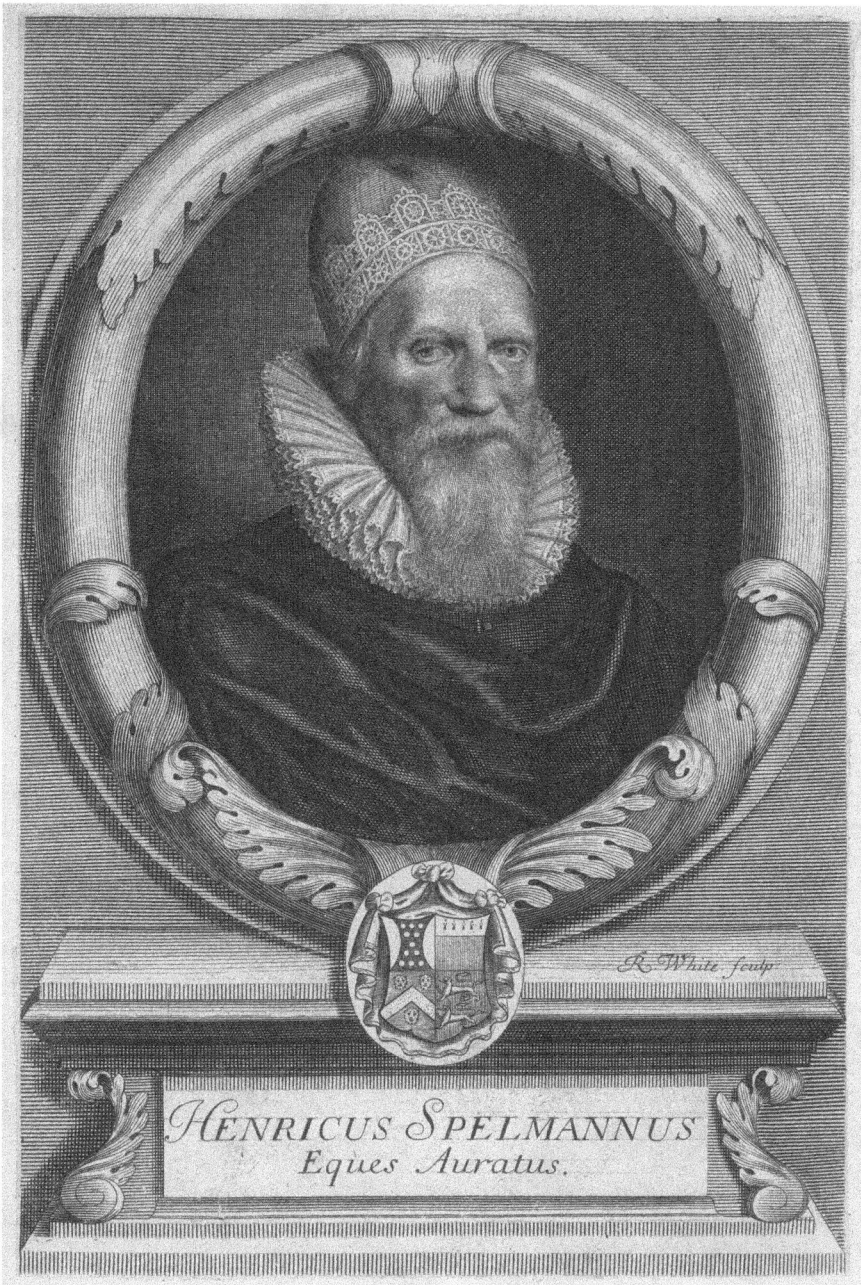

Figure 3.3 Sir Henry Spelman (1562–1641, engraving by William Faithorne, courtesy of the Royal Danish Library.

Skonvig as a reward for all his hard work helping him to track down and record the ancient monuments. Skonvig had first been employed by Worm on the recommendation of the Bishop of Bergen to undertake a survey and description of runic monuments in the bishopric in 1626. The following year Skonvig had travelled to Scania where the Bishop instructed his deans and ministers to assist him in his endeavours. Later that year Skonvig continued his work on the island of Funen, and the following year he continued his work in Jutland. By the autumn of 1629, when Worm sent his request to the chancellor for a parish to be found for Skonvig, the Norwegian was still busy finishing his survey of the bishoprics in Jutland. Most of the reports from the Danish and Norwegian bishops about ancient monuments appear to have arrived between one or two years after the 1622 ordinance was issued, but by 1629 some were still missing and may never have materialised.[40] Without Skonvig's efforts much would have been missing from Worm's final survey and description of the runic monuments. Ole Worm would not have been able to finish the project started in 1622 satisfactorily without the assistance of Skonvig who proved to be an impressive and energetic tracer of the runic monuments. In the introduction to his work on the runic monuments, *Monumenta Danica*, published in 1643, Worm stressed the importance of Jon Skonvig's help, praising his extraordinary care in recording and drawing the runic monuments.[41]

Worm's letter to the chancellor, however, did not only seek a favour for Skonvig. Worm also wanted Christen Friis to remind Christian IV about his own antiquarian efforts. The lack of any recognition or reward for his endeavours had, claimed Worm, caused him to lose interest in the ancient monuments. This clearly contradicted what he had told Sir Henry Spelman, only a few months earlier – namely, that his interests in the runic monuments was just a hobby, not motivated by greed or hope of fame, but driven solely by patriotism.[42]

Sir Henry Spelman was fascinated by the runes and had enjoyed the *Fasti Danici* which Worm had sent him. Writing to Worm in May 1630 he once again put forward his own views and questions. Spelman disagreed with Worm about the root of the word rune. He was convinced that the word did not originate from either 'ran', meaning stream, or 'run', meaning furrow, even if he admitted that many ancient words had their roots in agriculture or similar modest contexts. Instead, he was convinced that runes originated from the word 'ryne', or in Saxon 'geryne', which described something

---

40　See *Præsteindberetninger til Ole Worm*, I–II, passim.

41　For Jon Skonvig and his role in the runic project, see *Moltke, Skonvig*, 128–51, See *Danicorum Monumentorum Libri Sex e scripsis antiquitatum tenebris et in Dania ae Norvegia extentibus ruderibus eruti*, Copenhagen 1643, fol. B1v, for reference to Skonvig. For the letter to Christen Friis, see *Breve fra og til Ole Worm*, no. 315. Worm still received information about ancient monuments by 1632 while seeking further information in 1633, see nos. 434 and 468.

42　*Breve fra og til Ole Worm*, nos. 284 and 315.

mysterious or hidden. Spelman claimed they were called runes because they were both mystifying and concealed 'like the wisdom of Egyptian priests', as shown by Johannes Goropius Becanus in his *Hieroglyphica*, with a picture of an Egyptian urn.[43] These secret runes differed from the letters of other languages by their extraordinary strangeness, but also because these letters and characters (like those in Canopus in Egypt) in particular reveal themselves in their secret knowledge, namely, magic and illusion, which the Northern part of the world was distinguished and infested by. Those who deployed this writing and knowledge had to be known as runic masters and served the same function among the Danes and Goths, according to Spelman, as the Druids among the Saxons.

Worm appreciated Spelman's theory on the roots of the word rune which he thought corresponded with the facts, even if he had some reservations. He then stated what came to characterise much of his work on the runes and ancient monuments, namely, that he was not inclined to fiercely defend his own views and opinions. Instead Worm preferred to present the opinions and views of other learned people in order that the learned reader could reach the view which he found corresponded best with common sense. Worm valued Spelman's intervention for both scholarly and social reasons. That someone of the standing of Sir Henry Spelman considered research into the runes important carried weight. Accordingly Ole Worm informed Spelman that with his permission he would like to quote his letter in his forthcoming book about the runes. Worm found that it added support to his claim that rune was an ancient, original word.[44] When Worm's book on the runes was finally published in 1636 most of Spelman's letter was included in the first chapter. The books thirty chapters closely followed his intentions as stated in his letter of November 1630 to Spelman. Worm did not champion one theory, but put forward a number of opinions and views, leaving it to the reader to make up his own mind. Concerning the relationship between runes and Hebrew Worm indicated some potential links without drawing any conclusions.[45] Perhaps it is more significant whom Worm chose not to quote, rather than the many he cited. Thus, the fact that there is no reference to Johannes Bureus, who had been the first to take an interest in the runes and whose work Worm initially admired, is noteworthy. Worm would, however, have had two good reasons for not referring to Bureus. First, Bureus's claim that the runes were Swedish, having promoted them within Swedish Gothicism, would not have proved amenable to Worm's claims for the significance of the runes for Danish history. Second, Bureus's promotion of runes and 'adelrunes' within a mystic, Rosicrucian

---

43 See Johannes Goropius, *Hieroglyphica*, Antwerp 1569. Goropius was convinced that Antwerpian Brabantic was the original language spoken in Paradise. In *Hieroglyphica* he also argued that the Egyptian hieroglyphs was the written form of Brabantic.
44 *Breve fra og til Ole Worm*, nos. 346 and 389.
45 Worm, *Runir, seu Danica literature Antiquissima vulga Gothica dicta luci reditta*, Copenhagen 1636, 1 and 9–13.

setting would undoubtedly have struck Worm as a context within which he did not want his work on runes and ancient monuments to be seen.

However, before Worm's book on the runes saw publication he sought to elicit further information about the runes from his Icelandic friends. Magnus Olafsson had looked for assistance in interpreting Worm's ram-runes from a certain Jon Gudmundson, but he had fled after having been accused of being a necromancer. Olafsson was, however, able to send Worm a cipher table which the 'ancients' had used with the relevant Latin characters added. The following year, 1631, Olafsson informed Ole Worm, that Gudmundson, the most knowledgeable man about the runes in Iceland had been accused of witchcraft and was being transported to Copenhagen. The upside being that Worm might now be able to talk to him directly. However, this proved a baseless rumour, and Gudmundson remained a free man on Iceland.[46] Worm had also asked Arngrim Jonsson for his assistance in this matter. Arngrim pointed out the difficulties in finding anyone who could interpret the runes, but emphasised that people were reluctant to come forward with their knowledge about the runes because they were often suspected of sorcery, especially by the Danish stadtholders.[47]

By the autumn of 1631 Ole Worm had finished his work on the runes. He was only waiting for a dynamic printer who possessed the necessary equipment and would fulfil his ambition. Meanwhile, Worm had continued his work on the ancient monuments and had asked his friend the historian, Steffen Hansen Stephanius, to comment on the manuscript. Two years later Worm was still awaiting publication of his work on the runes and his optimism had for obvious reasons evaporated. Worm felt disappointed having been, as he put it, called away by the chancellor from his 'private medical and philosophical studies to study our ancient monuments'. He had clearly failed in recruiting a printer willing to take it on. Not surprisingly, he was pessimistic about the outcome of his work on the ancient monuments which he saw little prospect of getting published.[48] Having been informed by Sir Henry Spelman about his difficulties in getting the second volume of his *Achæologus* published due to the meanness of English booksellers and printers, Worm concluded in the autumn of 1634 that Danish printers were equally bad. Worm claimed they disliked rare and useful books and only wanted to publish those which would make money for themselves and could sell to 'the vulgar'. That was the reason why Worm's books about the runes and the ancient monuments were suppressed. Worm had little hope, as he put it, 'to penetrate the darkness unless fortune smiled upon them'.[49]

Worm worked hard to retain his contacts to Sir Henry Spelman in London instructing those of his students who travelled there to visit Spelman

---

46 *Breve fra og til Ole Worm*, nos. 369, 421, and 452.
47 *Ibid.*, no. 451.
48 *Ibid.*, nos. 435 and 489.
49 *Ibid.*, nos. 500, 510, and 536.

and convey his greetings. Thus, Peter Paulsen Winding visited Spelman on Worm's behalf in 1636 and spent no less than three hours conversing with him, informing Worm not only what Spelman was working on, but also pointed out that he had a very learned son, John.[50]

In March 1635 Worm informed his friend, Stephanius, in Sorø that he had had several visits from the Leiden-based physician and linguist Johannes Elichman, who had been extremely interested in the runes and the Gothic language. Elichman was reputed to understand sixteen languages, to speak Arabic as a native, and to be the most experienced Persian speaker in Europe. Worm was flattered by the interest Elichman took in his research and allowed him to copy more or less his whole book about the runes. He told Stephanius that he had been happy to allow Elichman to do this, because he personally doubted that the book would ever be published. Worm added that as long as his work might contribute to the knowledge of the scholarly world, he was happy for others to benefit from his efforts without acknowledgement.[51] From what we know about Worm this was undoubtedly stretching his modesty beyond the limit.

4 *Runir and Monumenta Danica*

Worm was clearly feeling increasingly pessimistic about the possibilities of having his work on the runes published during the first half of 1635. He informed his friend Johannes Cabeljau that he nearly regretted having finished his manuscripts for his books on the runes and the ancient, Danish monuments, because it had proved impossible to find a printer who would publish them. Accordingly he proclaimed that he was ready to hand the torch over to Johannes Cabeljau and 'other great names', while he discreetly remained 'in the dark'.

A few months later a congratulatory letter arrived from Stephanius in Sorø. Having looked through the recent autumn catalogue for the Leipzig book-fair, he had to his delight discovered that Worm's book on the runes had been printed in Wittenberg. As it turned out, Worm had to his great surprise made the same discovery. He found it incomprehensible, since he still had the manuscript for the book in his possession, and did not recollect having allowed anyone to copy it, except Johannes Elichman, who had borrowed it for a couple of months while in Copenhagen. Furthermore, Worm knew for certain that no printers anywhere, apart from Sweden, possessed the types for the runic letters which were needed for printing his book. He had therefore decided to investigate the case and had approached one of the Copenhagen booksellers who had recently promised him to undertake the printing of his book. When Worm had showed him the

---

50 *Ibid.*, no. 745.
51 *Ibid.*, no. 542; for Johannes Elichman, see *Nieuw Nederlandsch Biographisch Woordenboek*.

catalogue the bookseller had smiled and admitted that he had sent the title to Wittenberg in order that it would be included in the catalogue thereby giving him an idea of its commercial viability. Even so Worm was still fobbed off with empty promises by the bookseller/printer, who claimed to be unable to proceed with the printing because of a shortage of paper. Not surprisingly Worm remained glum about the book's prospect of publication. In February 1636 there must have been a glimmer of light when he told his friend Henrik Køster that his friends and the chancellor were all urging him to publish his work on the runes, but the printers proved fairly difficult. However, by then a sample of the necessary letters or characters had been carved in wood.[52]

However, by the summer of 1636 the publication prospects suddenly improved. Worm had lent the manuscripts of both his book on the runes and *Monumenta Danica* to the royal chaplain, Peder Winstrup, who was personal chaplain to the king and therefore constantly present at the court. Worm clearly hoped to draw the attention of Christian IV to his antiquarian work through the chaplain, but he now needed his manuscript for the runes returned, because he was involved in negotiations about its publication. Having failed to find a publisher in Copenhagen for Stephanius's book on Saxo due to the shortage of paper at home and abroad, Worm decided to personally pay for the publication of his book on the runes, and to buy the paper needed himself. This proved difficult and extremely costly. Worm claimed that paper prices had nearly doubled over the last couple of years, and struggled to obtain enough for the printer. Even so he hoped to see his book published shortly, but, as it turned out, at considerable financial cost to himself.[53] The difficulties in finding a publisher may explain why Ole Worm, did not use the University of Copenhagen printer, Salomon Sartor, whom he had used for his first publications about the runes, *Fasti Danici*, in 1626, and moved over to the other Copenhagen printer, Melchior Martzan for this publication.[54] His friend, Sir Henry Spelman, was among the first to receive a copy in late October 1636. Worm informed his nephew, Thomas Fuiren, in Leiden that he and his brother were to receive a copy each from the fifty transferred by Janssonius to the Leiden printer/bookseller Jacob Marci. There was also a copy for Worm's friend Johannes Elichman in Leiden and Worm emphasised that these three copies were printed on better paper than the rest of the print-run. Copies were also sent to Johan Rhode in Padua and his friends on Iceland.[55]

52　*Ibid.*, nos. 573 and 574; for the letter to Køster, see no. 579.
53　*Ibid.*, nos. 598, 599, and 603.
54　Ole Worm, *Fasti Danici: universum tempora computandi rationem antiquitus in Dania et vicinis regionibus*, Salomon Sartor, Copenhagen 1626 and Ole Worm, *Runir, seu Danica literature Antiquissima vulga Gothica dicta luci reditta*, Melchior Martzan, Copenhagen 1636.
55　*Ibid.*, nos. 614–16, and 655; Worm also forwarded a copy to his friend Stephanius, and the royal historiographer, Johannes Meursius, in Sorø, see nos. 617 and 619; see also

Having had to finance his book on the runes himself Worm also took on the job of publicising it as widely as possible. He was instrumental in having the fifty copies sent on to Jacob Marci in Leiden, and apart from personally sending copies to friends and colleagues at home and abroad, Worm also actively sought out booksellers for his book, more often than not using his students as intermediaries. One such student tried to make the London booksellers interested in Worm's book to no avail since all of them claimed there was no market in England for such a book. However, through the intervention of Sir Henry Spelman a bookseller, Philemon Stephens at the Golden Lion, was found who was prepared to take fifty copies of Worm's book in commission.[56] Books were also sent to members of the French diplomatic legation which had recently visited Copenhagen, such as François de Fleury and Johannes Tercejus, who had expressed an interest when paying a visit to Worm. Worm also made sure that a copy, sent through Stephanius, reached Charles Ogier, who had befriended him and by then had returned to Paris.[57]

In subsequent letters to friends and colleagues Ole Worm emphasised how expensive the publication of his work on the runes had been to him, and how disappointed he was with printers in general, and the Copenhagen printers in particular. They were only, according to him, interested in publishing popular, vernacular pamphlets which could be sold to the masses, despising quality works by learned men. Even so, he had to admit that times were difficult for printers due to the war disturbances in Germany which made books difficult to sell. Furthermore, paper prices had rocketed because so many paper-mills had been destroyed.[58]

It is, however, surprising that Worm was left on his own to finance and organise the publication of his book on the runes, when borne in mind that this was a project which had been encouraged and promoted centrally by both Christian IV and his chancellor, Christen Friis. It would appear that the government lacked a publication strategy, like offering subsidies, as can be seen from the publication of the two commissioned histories of Denmark. Despite the fervent interest of central government in promoting Danish antiquarianism and history from the early 1620s, and the employment of no less than two royal historiographers of international standing, Johannes Pontanus and Johannes Meursius, at considerable cost, the publication of their works were still left to the authors themselves with no financial support by the government.[59]

frontispiece of Worm, *Runir, seu Danica literature Antiquissima vulga Gothica dicta luci reditta*, Amsterdam 1636. For the copies to Rhode, Elichman, and his Icelandic friends, see nos. 630, 636, 640, 641, 648, and 652.
56 *Ibid.*, no. 650; Worm forwarded the books a year later, see nos. 718 and 719.
57 *Ibid.*, nos. 665, 667, 691, 752, 755, and 774.
58 *Ibid.*, nos. 693 and 714.
59 Skovgaard, *Historiography*, 47, 70–83.

Meanwhile, Ole Worm continued his work on the ancient Danish monuments, *Monumenta Danica*. Writing to his brother-in-law, the Bishop of Stavanger in Norway, in February 1638, he explained that he had already produced six books about them, and that the necessary information had been gathered by him and his friends. He claimed that the chancellor and learned colleagues abroad constantly urged him to publish his findings. He wanted his brother-in-law Thomas Wegner to get started on the promised collection of data from the bishopric of Stavanger which were the only missing details about the ancient monuments in Norway, in order that he could proceed to publication. Worm's letter is revealing for the way he wanted the collection of data conducted. He suggested that a young student who was reasonably capable of drawing/painting should be sent to the deans and ministers in the bishopric with a letter of recommendation. Worm then expected them to finance his travel and provide him with accommodation and food and the necessary assistance. Worm provided a list of seven subjects the student should cover when describing the ancient monuments he found. He should note: the place, county and parish; how the monument was placed, facing east, west, etc.; the size of the monument in terms of length, width, and depth. He should make a drawing of the monument, showing its appearance and structure; he should provide an interpretation; report the views of locals even if mythical; and memorable events linked to the place and other significant circumstances which might be relevant to the undertaking. Worm ended his letter with a list of examples of where ancient monuments had so far been found.[60]

So sixteen years after the royal order was issued Ole Worm was still awaiting the necessary information from at least one bishopric before his work was complete and he could write up the final version of *Monumenta Danica*. Sixteen months later Worm received copies of the runic inscriptions to be found in the bishopric of Stavanger and he promised to include Wegner's name in his book on ancient monuments. However, he was not too optimistic about its publication, having given up all hope of publishing it in the near future. Worm added that this was a bigger and financially more demanding project than he himself could sustain as a private individual.[61] Evidently the experience of having had to finance and organise the publication of his book on the runes had been stressful. Worm still received information about ancient monuments and runic inscriptions as late as December 1639. The Bishop of Lund sent him parts of stones with runic inscriptions found near Ystad and informed him that he had instructed his ministers and deans to look out for similar stones and report to him at the upcoming diocesan meeting.[62]

60 *Breve fra og til Ole Worm*, no. 700.
61 *Ibid.*, no. 781.
62 *Ibid.*, no. 820.

Worm's work on the runes – *Runir* – was generally well received at home and abroad. His nephew Thomas Bartholin, having recently arrived in Leiden, informed him that the work was highly appreciated among the Leiden professors, especially Petrus Scriverius, who was keen on acquiring Worm's portrait for his collection of famous and exceptional men, and Marcus Boxhorn, who had referred to it in a recent lecture on ancient writing and monuments. The local booksellers, however, complained about the low quality of the paper used for Worm's book which fell short of the expectations of the fastidious Dutch.[63] This was probably a fair criticism. Worm having had to finance and organise the paper himself at a time when paper prices were high may well have been constricted. That he chose to have a few copies for friends and esteemed colleagues printed on better paper would appear to confirm that view.

In August 1639 Thomas Bartholin informed Worm of the sudden death caused by a tertiary fever of his antiquarian friend, Johannes Elichman. Worm was deeply saddened by the death of a friend from whom he had expected something exceptional about 'our ancient languages'. Worm informed his nephew that a similar fate had just befallen the chancellor, Christen Friis, to the great misfortune of the University of Copenhagen. Having been told that the widow intended to auction off Elichman's library Worm advised Thomas to make a list of the Icelandic, Arabic, and Persian manuscripts in Elichman's collection, in order to find out what would be worth acquiring. He was, however, concerned that the recent death of Christen Friis may have resulted in a lack of courtiers who would encourage the king to buy.[64]

Two years after Worm had dispatched a copy of his book on the runes to his friend Johan Rhode in Padua he discovered that it had never arrived. He therefore dispatched another copy in the autumn of 1639. Worm asked Rhode to comment on his work, convinced that information relevant to his book might be found in the Vatican Library or other places in Italy. He would be grateful for any help from Rhode or his friends. Worm had noted that Athanasius Kircher and others were eagerly seeking to uncover Eastern languages and literature. Most likely Worm was referring to Kircher's *Prodomus coptus sive aegyptiacus*, which had appeared three years earlier. This was Kircher's first work on Egyptology and contained a Coptic grammar. In it Kircher suggested that there had been ancient Coptic expeditions and settlements in India, China, and other parts of Asia. Despite its shortcomings it was noticed by scholars across Europe and established Kircher as a recognised specialist

---

63 *Ibid.*, no. 702; Worm forwarded a copy of his book on the runes to Scriverius through Thomas Bartholin a few months later, see no. 739. When visiting Johannes Vossius in the spring of 1640 Thomas Bartholin presented him with a beautifully bound copy of Worm's book on the runes, see no. 842.

64 *Ibid.*, nos. 799, 810, and 818; in March 1640 Thomas Bartholin informed Worm that there were no Icelandic manuscripts in Elichman's library and that the auction would take place around Whitsun, see no. 832.

in Oriental languages and antiquities. Leading scholars of Hebrew and Arabic such as Johannes Elichman in Leiden began corresponding with him.[65] It may well have been Elichman who had drawn this work to his friend Worm's attention. Ole Worm suggested to Rhode that something similar should be done with Nordic literature and the runes, even if no assistance could be expected from others. They therefore had to do it as best they could. That their work was valued could be seen from the repeated praise it had received from certain famous Englishmen, Dutchmen, and Germans. Worm now wanted Rhode to tell him what the Italians thought of it.[66]

Johan Rhode was delighted with Worm's book on the runes. He was convinced that the Congregation for the Propagation of Faith would be able to assist Worm. Meanwhile, Rhode promised to find out whether they were familiar with Worm's book and if not proposed to forward his copy to them. He added that Nicolas-Claude Fabri de Peiresc, the famous French specialist in ancient languages, had praised Worm's book *Fasti Danici*, which Rhode had yet to see himself.[67] Worm may have been keen on gaining recognition among Italian scholars such as Athanasius Kircher, but that did not mean he was prepared to accept their scholarship uncritically, as can be seen from an exchange with his nephew, Thomas Bartholin. Bartholin, like Worm, had read Kircher's much-acclaimed *Prodomus coptus sive aegyptiacus*, while in the process of editing and expanding his father's work on the pygmees. He had already added much from new authors, but was particularly fascinated by Kircher's claims in his book that pygmees were identical with the ghosts which could be found in mines as described by Agricola and Olaus Magnus. He urgently needed his uncle's opinion. Worm approved of his nephew's intent to publish a revised version of his father's work on pygmees and offered some suggestions. However, he emphasised that he did not have to consider Kircher's 'empty opinion' which Worm explained was not based on rational argument and went against reliable observations and every probability.[68]

By the end of 1640 Worm was still waiting for news from Rhode, about a possible response from the Congregation for the Propagation of Faith to his writings on the runes. Worm, however, did not expect a positive verdict. He was convinced that the Roman scholars would consider his works no more than 'a barbarian breeze from the North', rejecting them because they were written by someone who was not a Catholic. This claim of possible confessional prejudice against his work is noticeable by being the only instance where it surfaced. Rhode eventually offered some good news in April 1641. He had given his copy of Worm's book about the runes to his close friend, Gabriel Naudé, the French librarian to Cardinal Francesco Barberini in

---

65 See Daniel Stolzenberg, *Egyptian Oedipus. Athanasius Kircher and the Secrets of Antiquity*, Chicago 2013, 94–103.
66 *Ibid.*, no. 812; see also Athanasius Kircher, *Prodomus coptus sive aegyptiacus*, Rome 1636.
67 *Ibid.*, no. 855.
68 *Ibid.*, nos. 838 and 844.

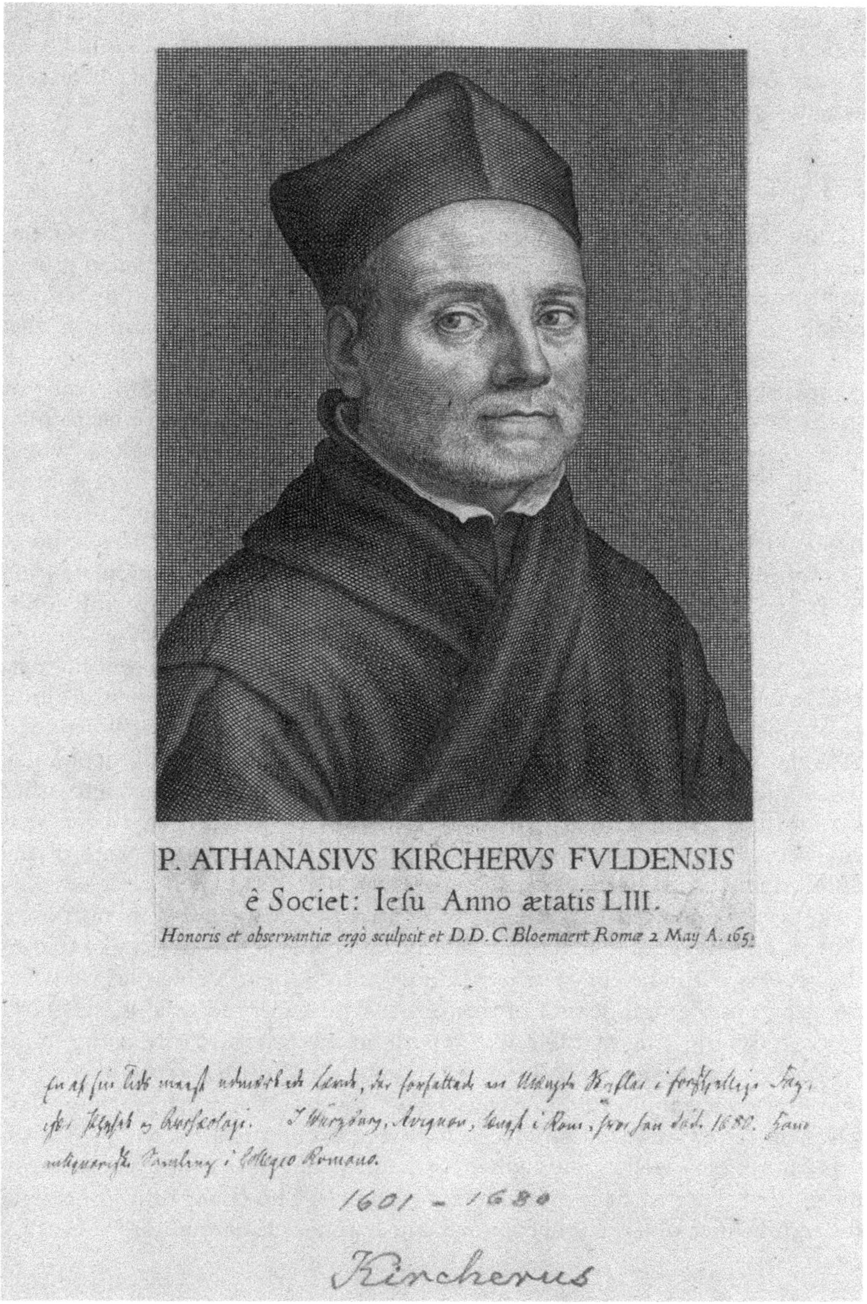

P. ATHANASIVS KIRCHERVS FVLDENSIS
ê Societ: Iesu Anno ætatis LIII.
Honoris et observantiæ ergò sculpsit et D.D. C. Bloemaert Romæ 2 May A. 165

1601 - 1680

Kircherus

Figure 3.4 Athanasius Kircher (1602–1680); courtesy of the Royal Danish Library.

Rome.[69] Naudé had then handed it over to Athanasius Kircher, in Rhode's opinion the finest linguist among the Jesuits. Kircher had found the book learned and interesting, but less useful because runes were more likely to appear on monuments than in books, whereas Naudé found it absolutely essential for the study of antiquity.[70]

5 The Gold Horn

In July 1639 an ancient, gold horn was discovered by a peasant girl at Gallehus in southern Jutland and given to King Christian IV who handed it over to his son the elected-prince, Christian. It weighed six pounds and was, according to Worm, worth at least 1200 Reichsthaler. Made of pure gold this ancient horn was decorated with runic inscriptions and animal, human, and geometric designs. Ole Worm first encountered it when visiting the court of the elected-prince in Nykøbing Falster in September 1640 in order to provide medical treatment to Prince Christian and some of his courtiers. Worm reported to his friend, Stephanius, in Sorø that among the marks of honour shown him was the gold horn discovered the previous year in Jutland. It was handed to him in the name of the prince filled with wine for him to empty. Containing well over a pint that would have presented a fair amount of wine to drink. Worm then had time to admire the horn's structure and the nobility of its material, but not surprisingly he had been particularly fascinated by the amazing combination of images and 'hieroglyphs' which decorated it. He was convinced it was ancient, but there was no trace of any inscription or of Christianity that could help determine its age or its owner. Worm had thought deeply about it and taken notes. He wanted to know if Stephanius had come across anything about such horns in his studies of Saxo and other Danish, historical authors. Worm stressed that there had been a lively discussion about what the horn might have been used for: some were of the opinion that it had been used as a cup, others that it had been a bugle, while some were convinced that the ancients had used it for religious purposes. Worm, however, did not recollect that he had come across horns like that in connection with ancient sacrifices. He urgently sought Stephanius's advice, pointing out the significance of this object which merited serious, scholarly work. It is surprising that Ole Worm with his interests and role as the country's leading antiquarian had remained unaware of the existence of such an important ancient object for nearly a year. However, the death of Chancellor Christen Friis on 1 October 1639, only a few months after the gold horn was found, may well explain why that happened. Friis's death undoubtedly meant that there was no one within government who could fully appreciate the significance of the gold horn for Danish antiquarian studies.

69 *Ibid.*, no. 886; this is the only instance where Worm expressed concern about confessional bias in non-religious matters.
70 *Ibid.*, no. 908.

Stephanius obliged Worm and responded more or less on receipt of his letter. He told Worm how privileged he considered him to have been, having held this amazing object in his hands. He had only been able to find a small number of similar objects mentioned by Saxo and other Danish historians. Stephanius, however, was convinced that the gold horn had been used as bugle, not least because it was open at the end before the elected-prince had it closed with a tap of gold. He thought that most likely it had served military purposes. Furthermore, all the horns Stephanius was aware of as having been used as cups, rested on feet or supports, of which, as far as he had heard, there were no signs. The fact that the horn had been found in a narrow and deep sitting road, also supported his view that the horn was a bugle used for communication on the battlefield. Stephanius thought that a prince or warrior was likely to have lost the bugle while fleeing along the road, only for it to be trampled down in the mud by the hooves of pursuing horses.

Ole Worm appears to have started work on a publication about the gold horn on his return to Copenhagen. He showed a first draft to Stephanius when the latter visited him in October. Worm, however, was not the first academic with interests in antiquarian matters who had been shown the horn. That honour fell to Henrik Ernst, a German academic from Helmstedt, who had been made professor of law and moral philosophy at the Academy in Sorø in 1639, after having served as tutor to Christian IV's son Valdemar Christian, Count of Schleswig and Holstein, during the latter's grand tour, 1637–39. Ernst had befriended Worm shortly after his arrival in Denmark in 1636 and had corresponded with him while travelling in Europe with Count Valdemar Christian. Worm had even asked him to keep a look out for something relevant to his research into the runes.[71] Henrik Ernst would appear to have seen the horn three to four weeks before Worm. On viewing it, Ernst had taken the opportunity to offer the elected-prince to provide him with a description of the horn including an interpretation of its illustrations and writing. The prince had then, according to Ernst, promised to send him a copy of the horn made of lead. Worm had clearly heard about Ernst's plans and had discussed them with Stephanius in Copenhagen. Back in Sorø Stephanius set about to discover what plans Ernst had about the gold horn and to discover whether or not he had put pen to paper. Having discovered that Ernst had yet to start, he encouraged Worm to speedily conclude his work on the gold horn. Worm was in Stephanius's opinion the person best suited to bring to light such an important antiquarian object, having already established his credentials in this field. By quickly publishing his work on the horn Worm would, in Stephanius's opinion, stand triumphant and earn the grace and favour of the Prince, while serving his native country and its history. Stephanius thought that it was only right and proper that such a grand object from Danish antiquity were brought

---

71 *Ibid.*, nos. 634 and 701.

to light by a Dane rather than a foreigner. He added that he was convinced that Ernst did not possess the necessary skills nor intelligence to success-fully investigate such secrets.[72]

6 The publication of *De Aureo Cornu* and the fall out with Henrik Ernst

Worm was grateful to Stephanius's for what he had discovered at the Academy in Sorø and agreed with him that he had to finish his work on the horn as fast as possible. By early December 1640 the book was already with the printers and by January 1614 Ole Worm's 72-page trea-tise, *De Aureo Cornu*, dedicated to Prince Christian, was published.[73] Among the first to receive a copy was his old friend, Henrik Køster, phy-sician to the prince. Worm asked Køster to promote it, and if necessary to explain it to any 'grumblers'. One wonders if Worm expected a nega-tive reception of his work among Henrik Ernst's contacts at the prince's court? He certainly emphasised to Køster that he had only undertaken this work on the encouragement of others. Worm expected the prince's lord chamberlain, Joachim Gersdorff, to present it to Prince Christian and wanted Køster to keep him comprehensively informed how it was received by the Prince.

Køster proved a true friend to Worm. Joachim Gersdorff was unable to join the prince when the court moved from Jutland to Antvorskov Castle on Sealand. Køster therefore took it on himself to present his own copy of Worm's treatise about the gold horn to the elected-prince. The prince read the work carefully within a couple of days, and according to Køster not a lunch or dinner passed without him praising it. Furthermore, a copy of the tract was requested for the prince's wife. Køster informed Worm that Prince Christian was delighted with the perfect drawing of the horn, but particularly relished what Worm had inferred and concluded about it from Danish history. Køster also told him that he should expect a gift from the prince of a large gilded silver-cup.[74]

Stephanius was full of praise for Worm's treatise on the horn and offered loads of helpful references and comments. Some of his colleagues at the Academy in Sorø had argued that the illustrations on the gold horn were purely decorative, which Stephanius had rebuffed with evidence. Stephanius also reported to Worm that his colleague, Henrik Ernst, disagreed with Worm's interpretation of the horn, namely, that the horn had been used as a bugle by a prince or nobleman in the reign of King Frode Fredegod,

---

72 *Ibid.*, nos. 870, 871, and 878. Ernst had befriended Worm five years earlier shortly after his arrival in Sorø, see nos. 597 and 600.

73 *Ibid.*, no. 883 and Ole Worm, *De aureo Domini Christiani Quinti, Daniæ, Norvegiæ etc. Principis, cornu dissertation*, Copenhagen 1641. The tract was printed by Melchior Martzan and published by Joachim Moltke. See also I. Ilsøe, 'Boghandleren Joachim Moltke, og hans virksomhed 1626–1664', *Fund og Fortid*, 24 (1979–80), 63–92.

74 *Ibid.*, no.894.

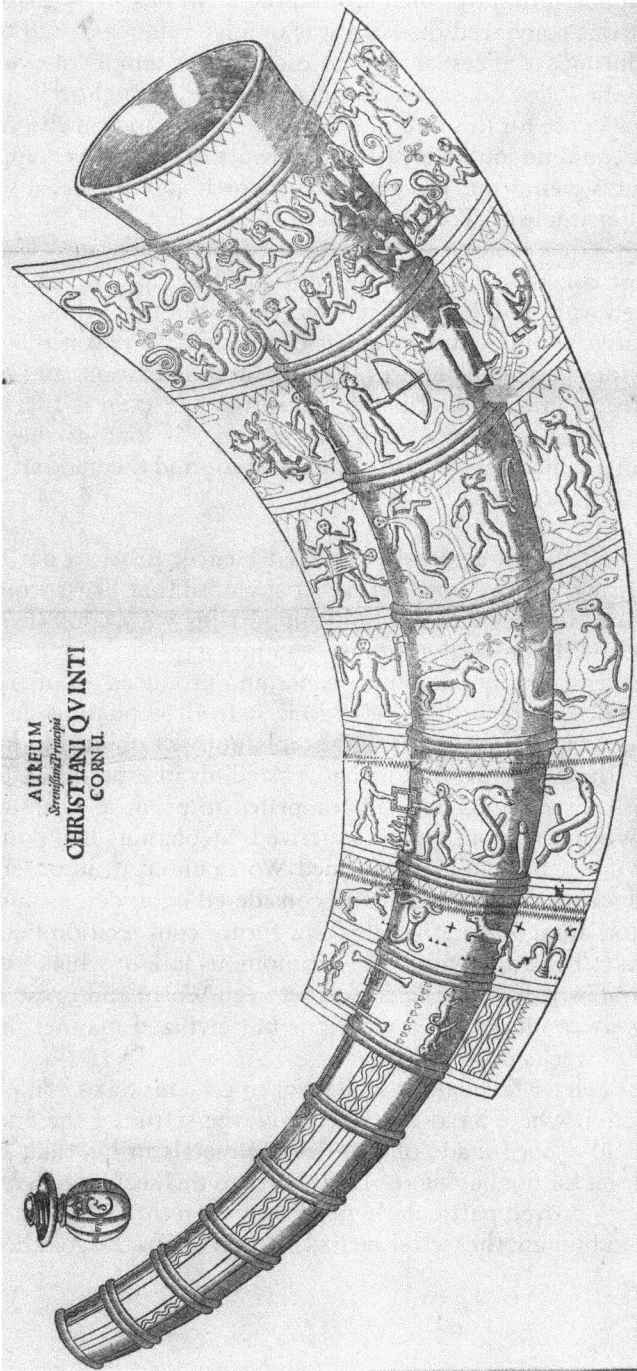

AUREUM
Serenissimi Principis
CHRISTIANI QVINTI
CORNU.

Figure 3.5 Gold horn, Ole Worm, *De Aureo Cornu* (1641); courtesy of the Royal Danish Library.

who was supposed to have ruled around the birth of Christ. Ernst, on the other hand, was convinced the horn was of a later date and had been used by priests during sacrifices, similar to those in the temple of Svantevit on Rügen near the Baltic coast. Stephanius, however, thought that Ernst had little or no evidence for this interpretation, except an ancient chronicle from Holstein he could no longer locate.[75] As always Worm proved appreciative of Stephanius's comments. His response is worth quoting, because it offers an excellent example of Worm's scholarly approach:

> I am not concerned with those who envy me, as long as my rapidly produced work will be positively received by honest scholars who love their native country. If someone is of the opinion that it is simple and easy to interpret such pictures, I ask them to take it on, and see if they can offer us another and better interpretation; even if I have broken the ice, I shall not envy them this honour, as long as they produce something which agrees with common sense and the maxims of distinguished authors.[76]

Stephanius and Worm evidently expected Henrik Ernst to put his views down in writing. Worm, however, was convinced that Ernst would struggle to find any sources which would support his view, and anyone, who was involved with national antiquity and history, who would agree with him. When Ernst finally put pen to paper and produced an interpretation of the gold horn at the beginning of March 1641 Stephanius quickly forwarded it to Worm. Not surprisingly Stephanius felt obliged to inform his colleague at the Academy, that he had posted his interpretation to Worm. Consequently, Stephanius had felt compelled to promise to show Henrik Ernst Ole Worm's response when it arrived. Stephanius had done so hesitantly, but not before he had informed Worm about it, in order that the latter could write a more careful and considered rejoinder, excluding controversial and antagonising details for a future conversation between the two of them.[77] Bearing in mind the acrimonious fallout which followed in April, it is noteworthy that the debate between Worm and Ernst about the gold horn was conducted in a vicarious but civilized manner during the first couple of weeks in March.

Three weeks later Stephanius while working on his Saxo edition discovered the section where Saxo described how the statue of the god of war, Svantevit, held a horn made of a variety of metals in his right hand. He blamed himself for not having referred Worm to this section of Saxo before. This discovery proved particularly pertinent when three days later Henrik Ernst showed him another letter he had written about the gold horn where

75 *Ibid.*, no. 903.
76 *Ibid.*, no. 904.
77 *Ibid.*, no. 905.

he specifically referred to Svantevit as proof of similar uses of the horn in religious ceremonies in Denmark before the introduction of Christianity. Ernst had no further evidence for this assumption and Stephanius rejected it as speculation. He forwarded this second letter by Ernst to Worm and asked him to analyse Ernst's point of view carefully before informing him of his opinion. As Stephanius later confirmed, this was, in fact, the letter which Ernst sent to Joachim Gersdorff, the prince's lord chamberlain. He told Worm to rely on his discretion, revealing that Ernst begrudged him his treatise about the gold horn, which had forestalled Ernst's own plans for a publication and thereby deprived him of the chance to ingratiate himself with the elected-prince.[78]

Worm was grateful to Stephanius for having shared Henrik Ernst's letter with him. He enclosed his answer in his response, encouraging him to show it to Ernst and others who might have seen Ernst's letter. Worm claimed to be surprised by Ernst's 'naivety and inability to produce a proper scholarly argument'. He was concerned that Ernst's scholarly reputation might be jeopardised. In his response Worm had therefore pretended that it was someone else who had used Ernst's name. If Ernst decided to publish his letter Worm declared his intention to publish his rejoinder immediately.[79]

Worm, in other words, was already familiar with Ernst's interpretation of the gold horn when a week later he received a letter from his friend, Henrik Køster, physician to the elected-prince, telling him that the prince had received a letter which offered a very different interpretation of the gold horn to his. This was Henrik Ernst's letter addressed to Joachim Gersdorff. Worm, unbeknown to Køster, of course, had already seen this letter, which Køster meticulously had copied out for him.[80] Worm was grateful to Køster for his loyalty. He enclosed a copy of his rejoinder already sent to Stephanius, stating,

> I find that the author firstly unfairly gibes our people and secondly tears me and my treatise to pieces in several places without adding anything new in order to fill the spindle; even so I have had to consider and assess

---

78 *Ibid.*, no. 912 and 918; for the letter Henrik Ernst sent to the lord chamberlain of the elected-prince, Joachim Gersdorff, dated 4 April 1641, see Royal Library Copenhagen, Gl. K. S. 2376b, Henrici Ernstii de Cornu Aureo ad V. III Joachimum Gerstorffium 4/4/1641.

79 Worm's response can be found in the Royal Library Copenhagen, Gl. K. S. 2376b, Notæ et Animadversiones in Epistolam cujusdam de Aureo Cornu 13/4/1641. Stephanius became concerned about his involvement in the growing confrontation between Henrik Ernst and Ole Worm. He was worried that Worm was about to publish a furious rejection of Ernst's views. It would appear that Stephanius was not supposed to have allowed Worm to see the letter addressed to Joachim Gersdorff before Gersdorff had received it. If Worm went ahead and published an attack on Ernst Stephanius was worried about his own position at the Academy in Sorø, se *Breve fra og til Ole Worm*, no. 918.

80 *Breve fra og til Ole Worm*, nos. 919 and 922.

it. Should you find my response too sharp then you have to remind yourself that the man deserves it because of his insolence. His only ambition
is to make our ancient monuments appear insignificant, and out of his
hate of all things Danish he takes every opportunity to deprive us of this
gold horn and award it to his co-nationals from Rügen.

Worm enclosed a copy of his rejoinder which he asked Køster to hand over
to Joachim Gersdorff, making sure that it reached the prince in order that
he might comprehend, as Worm put it, how Henrik Ernst was trying to
deprive the Danes of this precious treasure based on spurious and fake arguments.[81] It was, in other words, an attack on Danish patriotic history. It
was, however, not the content of Henrik Ernst's letter which angered Worm,
but the way he had made it public by sending it to Joachim Gersdorff, the
lord chamberlain of the court of the elected-prince. He emphasised that
had Ernst truly been his friend, he would have shown him his letter before
sending it. He had forced Worm to respond forcefully in order to defend
his scholarly reputation. Meanwhile, Stephanius had found himself in the
firing line at the Academy in Sorø for his involvement in the case. He had
felt obliged to let Ernst see his copy of Worm's riposte and asked Worm to
keep their correspondence out of the public sphere, emphasising that Ernst
was extremely angry. Finally, in early May Ernst contacted Worm and acknowledged that he was the author of the different interpretation of the gold
horn with its criticism of Worm's treatise. Worm responded by underlining
to Ernst how strongly he felt about the matter, claiming that Ernst had com-
mitted an injustice, not only against him but also against the Danish people.
He had been deeply disappointed by such behaviour from someone he had
considered a friend. He rejected Ernst's claim that he had only made his
views known in a private letter, pointing out that a letter which was known
in transcript by many courtiers at the prince's court could not be considered
private. Worm deemed it an attempt to smear his reputation. As a friend Ernst should have shown Worm his letter before sending it to Gersdorff. Worm
was also angered by Ernst's legal threats of a case for defamation against
him, which he summarily dismissed, pointing out that he was willing to
contemplate a 'friendly' debate, free from insults, about the issues.[82] Worm's
response only added to Ernst's ire. He proved unable to let matters rest
and wrote another letter on 17 May 1641 to Joachim Gersdorff complaining about his treatment by Worm. He also personally complained to the
chancellor, Christen Thomesen Sehested, on a visit to Copenhagen. Due to
his excellent contacts both at the elected-prince's court and within government Worm was able to nullify these complaints. On Ernst's departure from

---

81 *Ibid.*, nos. 923 and 925.
82 *Ibid.*, nos. 928 and 924; for Henrik Ernst's letter to Ole Worm, see The Royal Library, Copenhagen, Ny k. S. 4 Nr. 807, Henrici Ernstii Epistola accusatorial ad Olaum
Wormium 8/5/1641.

Copenhagen Worm was invited to dine with Christen Thomesen Sehested, who told him about Ernst's complaints. Worm not only informed the chancellor about the reasons for his robust response but also gave him a copy of his riposte to read.[83] Ernst, however, refused to let the matter rest and by the end of September Ole Worm had been informed that Henrik Ernst had distributed a written attack on him. Meanwhile, Ernst had also written a letter to the Bishop of Sealand threatening action against colleagues, presumably among others Stephanius, and the University of Copenhagen. Bearing in mind that no one at the Academy in Sorø had any knowledge of yet another letter by Ernst the rumour which had reached Worm from Nykøbing Falster most likely referred to the second letter Ernst had sent to Joachim Gersdorff on 17 May 1641.[84] Joachim Gersdorff left the court of the elected-prince by the end of 1641 and appears to have been a patron of Henrik Ernst. According to Henrik Køster no one at the court took any interest in Ernst after Gersdorff's departure. When Ole Worm attended a party in Sorø in January 1642, to which Ernst had also been invited, the latter stayed away and no one referred to their quarrel.[85] This proved the end of the matter with Worm successfully seeing off his younger rival.

Henrik Ernst was always going to be at a disadvantage in his confrontation with Worm. He was a much younger man, only recently appointed to a professorship at the Academy in Sorø, whereas Worm had been well connected with the Academy for decades, not least through his brother-in-law, and close friend, Stephanius. Furthermore, Worm was an eminent professor of medicine within the University of Copenhagen with excellent contacts within university and government. He had been particularly close to the late chancellor, Christen Friis, and it was on his encouragement that he had begun his antiquarian work, for which he was already recognised before the gold horn was discovered. Worm also regularly attended the court of the elected-prince in Nykøbing Falster providing medical treatment and advice, and he was a close friend of the prince's personal physician Henrik Køster. Ernst, having seen the gold horn in Nykøbing Falster before Worm and clearly been encouraged to write something about it, was obviously deeply disappointed when he was beaten to it by Worm, who had been kept well informed of Ernst's intentions and progress by his friends. Worm's work on the gold horn was produced within weeks. As such it had its shortcomings and omissions, as Worm recognised. However, Ernst's attempt to place the horn in a Germanic setting based on the evidence of Saxo about the horn of Svantevit did little to help him in a context where the horn was viewed and interpreted as an item of national and patriotic pride, adding

---

83 *Ibid.*, nos. 931, 933 and 941; for Henrik Ernst's second letter to Joachim Gersdorff, see The Royal Library, Copenhagen, Ny k. S. 4 Nr. 807, Henrici Ernstii Epistola ad Joach. Gersdorffium 17/5/1641
84 *Ibid.*, nos. 975, 976, and 979.
85 *Ibid.*, nos. 991 and 997.

lustre to the Kingdom of Denmark and Norway. That Ernst had a scholarly point, as belatedly recognised by Stephanius and Worm, mattered little in this context. Ernst was portrayed as a German interloper who wanted to diminish all things Danish. At play was not only scholarly reputation but personal standing and public recognition, especially by the royal household and leading government figures. Ernst bitterness against Worm and his repeated attacks on him eventually fell on deaf ears. Ernst had bitten off more than he could chew and the fact that Worm felt obliged to discuss and reject his views on the gold horn in the second and expanded edition of his work on the gold horn included in *Monumenta Danica* published in 1643 did nothing to improve his situation. For Worm the issue had never been about scholarly views, but about friendship and loyalty. Worm considered Henrik Ernst's letters to Joachim Gersdorff to be a stab in the back, an attempt to undermine his reputation, by someone he had considered a friend.[86]

7 The significance of *De Aureo Cornu* for Ole Worm's international reputation

Worm's publication about the gold horn quickly attracted interest from scholars abroad, resulting in some surprising interventions such as that from Königsberg where a local Paracelsian claimed that the ancient runic masters and scalds had, in fact, been chemists and the gold horn contained the instructions for making the philosopher's stone. This caused Worm to acknowledge that he had, indeed, given birth to 'an apple of discord'.[87]

Meanwhile, Worm was busy distributing his work on the gold horn to friends and colleagues, stressing that it had been executed on the order of the elected-prince. Friends reported that leading government figures such as the chancellor, Christen Thomesen Sehested, had proved highly appreciative of his publication.[88] When he sent a copy together with other works, such as his *Fasti Danici*, to Johan Rhode in Padua, Worm expressed his desire to have his tract about the gold horn brought to the attention of Athanasius Kircher, so he could benefit from the latter's expertise in the hieroglyphs and receive Kircher's assessment of his interpretation of the gold horn. Worm hoped that subsequently he might be mentioned in Kircher's forthcoming work about the hieroglyphs. The fact that Kircher already had proved rather unenthusiastic about his work on the runes clearly had done

86 Ole Worm, *Danicorum monumentorum libri sex: e spissis antiquitatum tenebris et in Danica ac Norvegia extantibus ruderibus eruti*, Copenhagen 1643 (De aureo Domini Christiani Quinti, Daniæ, Norvegiæ etc. Principis, cornu dissertation) Libro V, 344–434.

87 *Ibid.*, nos. 913 and 917.

88 *Ibid.*, nos. 896 and 897; Worm had also donated a copy of his treatise to the Stadtholder of Copenhagen, Corfitz Ulfeldt, Christian IV's son-in-law, see no. 898; Worm's friend and brother-in-law, Stephanius, received a copy with a request to read it carefully and suggest corrections, no. 899.

little to discourage Worm. Kircher was recognised as the linguistic scholar
of the age and an acknowledgement by him was worth its weight in gold.
Worm added that if Rhode and his learned, Italian friends approved of it,
it would serve as an encouragement for him to accelerate the publication of
his work on the ancient monuments.[89]

Ole Worm's nephews and Johan Rhode in Padua played a prominent part
in promoting his antiquarian works in Italy. Worm had sent the drawing
of the gold horn he had had made for his tract, *De Aureo Cornu*, to his
nephew Henrik Fuiren, in July 1641. It reached him a couple of months
later while in Rome, where he had shown it to local antiquarians. Eventually he donated it to Gabriel Naudé, so it might embellish Cardinal Barberini's Library. In this 'splendid library', open to all scholars, he had also
discovered a copy of Worm's *Fasti Danici*. Consequently Fuiren had obtained his cousin, Thomas Bartholin's copy of Worm's work on the runes
and donated it to the Barberini Library 'to add to the fame of Worm'. He
also intended to donate his copy of *De Aureo Cornu* to this Library when
he received it from the Netherlands. He was convinced that Naudé would
have no problem in obtaining Kircher's opinion of Worm's works.

Thomas Bartholin informed Worm that his work on the gold horn had
been donated to Cardinal Barberini's Library and that the Bolognese physician and natural philosopher Fortunio Liceti was contemplating a new
interpretation of the hieroglyphs in a publication about rings. Bartholin
also mentioned that he had recently seen a Turkish horn in the Archduke's
collection in Florence which was not dissimilar to the Danish gold horn.[90]

By December 1641 Ole Worm had finished his work on ancient, Danish-
Norwegian monuments, *Monumenta Danica*, and dispatched it to the
printer. Impatiently awaiting the responses from his nephews Worm dispatched letters to both Johan Rhode and Thomas Bartholin in Padua. He
told Rhode that the printing of *Monumenta Danica* was steaming ahead
and that he had decided to enclose a revised and expanded version of
De Aureo Cornu, in this work. He added that he would cherish nothing
more than being able to add the much hoped for comments by Athanasius
Kircher. Thomas Bartholin was instructed to find out what Henrik Fuiren
had achieved during his trip to Rome. Worm hoped Fuiren had been able
personally to show Kircher his drawing of the gold horn and to have obtained his opinion. If so it would serve to promote his *Monumenta Danica*
where he was including a revised edition of the by then sold out first edition
of *De Aureo Cornu*.[91]

89 *Ibid.*, no. 901.
90 *Ibid.*, nos. 957, 985, and 978. For Liceti's publication see, F. Liceti, *De annulis An-
tiquorum eorumque usu & cumulatione cum cadaver*, Udine 1645. See also the letter to
Henrik Køster where Worm explains that he is including a revised edition of *De Aureo
Cornu* where he has dealt with what he describes as Henrik Ernst's 'insignificant objections', no. 992.
91 *Ibid.*, nos. 989 and 990.

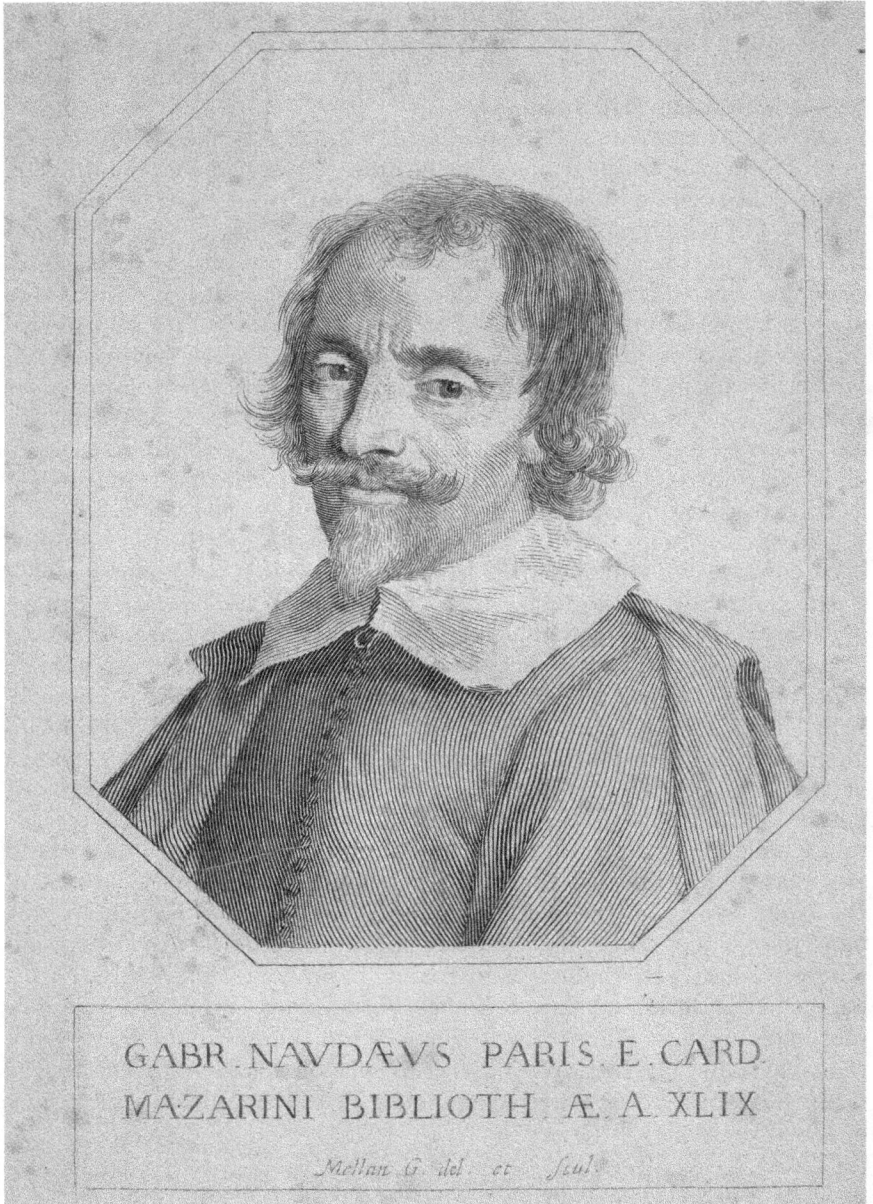

Figure 3.6 Gabriel Naudé (1600–1653) by Claude Mellan ca. 1660, courtesy of the Royal Danish Library.

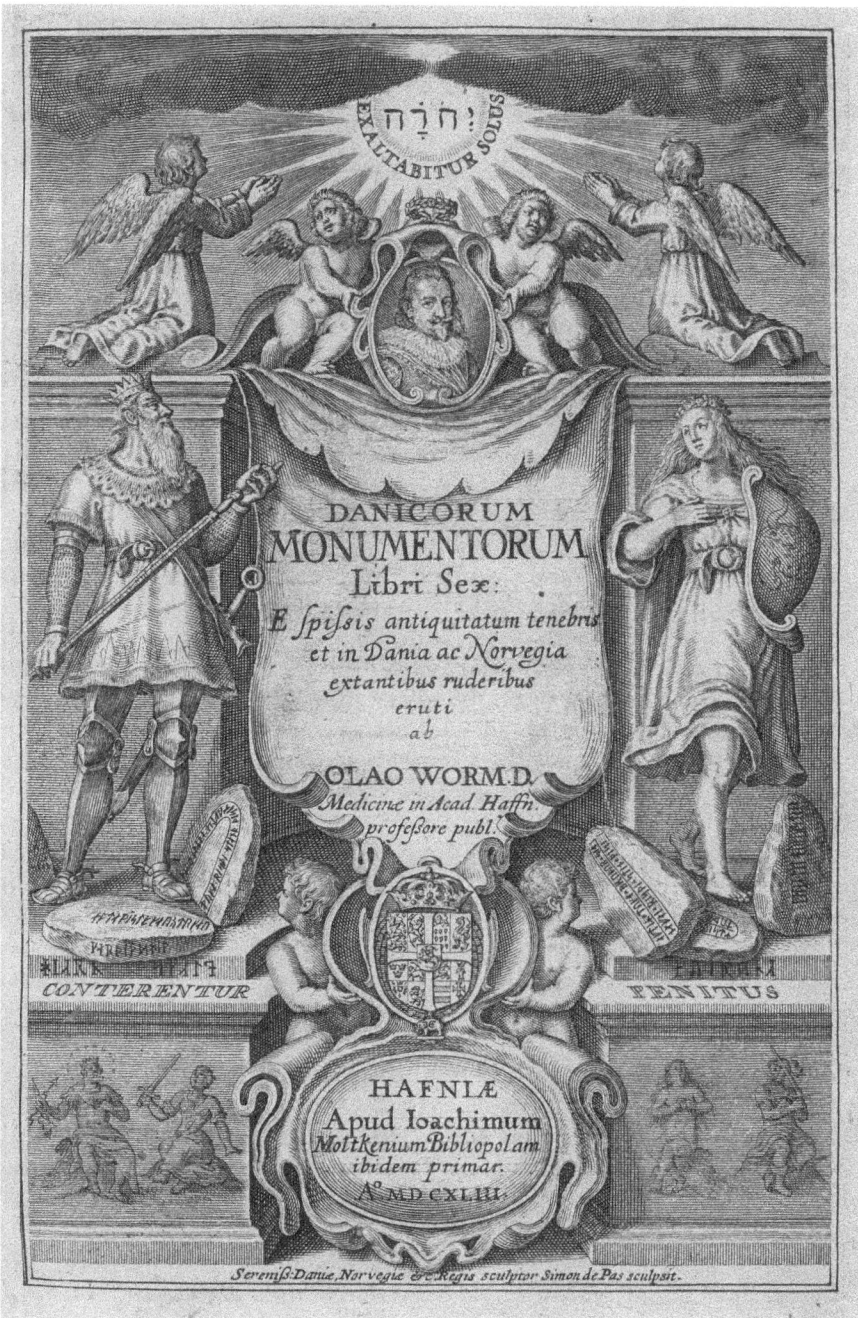

Figure 3.7 Frontispiece from Ole Worm, *Monumenta Danica* (1643); courtesy of the Royal Danish Library.

Not surprisingly Worm proved extremely grateful to Henrik Fuiren for his efforts on his behalf. He was clearly determined to achieve some sort of verdict about his work from Naudé and Kircher whose expertise on the hieroglyphs, he valued highly. Worm added that if either of them or others had found anything wanting in his treatise Fuiren should let him know immediately so he could amend it in the forthcoming edition. A month later Thomas Bartholin assured his uncle that Johan Rhode daily expected to receive Athanasius Kircher's assessment of the 'hieroglyphs' on the gold horn. Apparently it had been delayed by Naudé's trip to France, but Bartholin could inform his uncle that Liceti would include something about the gold horn in his forthcoming book on rings with an illustration of the horn. He suggested that Worm paused the printing of the relevant volume of *Monumenta Danica*, to make it possible to include the views of Liceti and Kircher.[92]

By March 1642 Worm's treatise about the gold horn was generating scholarly interest in both Germany, France, and Italy. This caused quite a stir at the court of the elected-prince in Nykøbing Falster, which in turn delighted Worm.[93] Meanwhile, Worm's nephews remained active on his behalf in Italy. Thomas Bartholin had managed to elicit a response about the gold horn from Fortunio Liceti while still awaiting an answer to his letter to Kircher in Rome. Liceti expressed his admiration for Worm's work, but offered a slightly different interpretation. Even so, Worm felt gratified enough to include Liceti's statement at the end of his revised edition of *De Aureo Cornu*, politely criticising Liceti's interpretation. Bartholin also made sure that a copy was sent to the Biblioteca Ambrosiana in Milan. Thomas Fuiren had discovered that Worm's tract on the gold horn was for sale with the booksellers in Venice. Fuiren had taken the opportunity to acquire a copy which he had sent to Cassiano dal Pozzo in Rome. Dal Pozzo was the influential secretary to Cardinal Barberini and a collector with considerable antiquarian interest. He had been very interested in the drawing of the gold horn, which Fuiren had shown him when in Rome, and the copy of Worm's treatise was a mark of gratitude for the generosity Dal Pozzo's had shown him and Thomas Bartholin during their stay in Rome. Dal Pozzo expressed his gratitude to Fuiren for having sent him 'the learned and erudite work by Worm'.

Emphasising the importance of obtaining Kircher's opinion Johan Rhode suggested that Worm delayed his publication of *Monumenta Danica* until it had been obtained.[94] Bearing in mind that Worm had been complaining to Stephanius that the printer was only making slow progress with *Monumenta Danica* he did not find it difficult to follow

92 *Ibid.*, no. 1005, Bartholin also offered to write to both Kircher and Liceti if Rhode failed to obtain an answer.
93 *Ibid.*, nos. 1008 and 1009.
94 *Ibid.*, nos. 1012, 1014, 1015, and 1041; for Dal Pozzo's response see no. 1026.

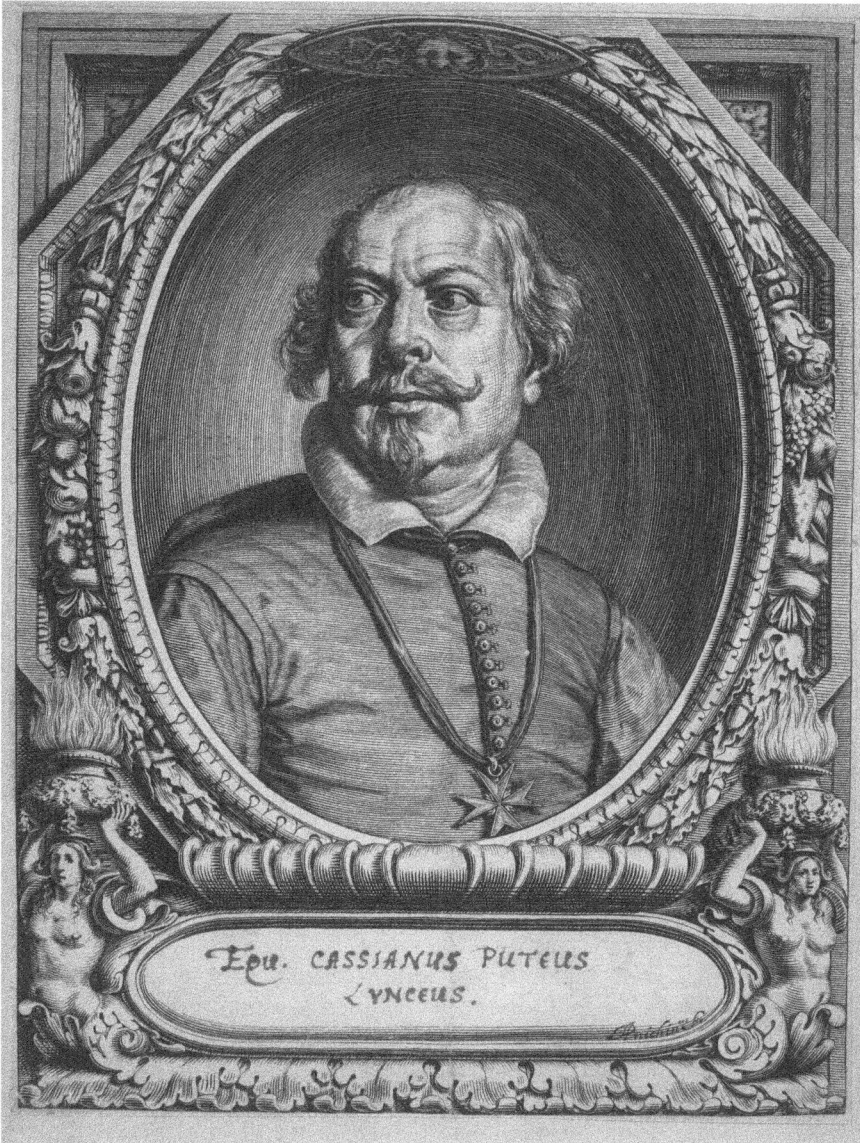

Figure 3.8 Cassiano dal Pozzo (1588–1657); courtesy of the Royal Danish Library.

Rhode's advice. He promised to delay finishing his revised edition of *De Aureo Cornu* until Kircher's opinion had been obtained. That did not stop Worm impatiently awaiting this document. As the leading European expert on the Egyptian hieroglyphs Kircher's view on the illustrations or 'hieroglyphs' on the gold horn was considered essential by Worm. Writing to Johan Rhode in April 1642 Worm expressed his gratitude to Fortunio Liceti for not disagreeing strongly with his assumptions at the end of *De Aureo Cornu*. He concluded that Liceti was a modest and educated man, and that he respected his views despite disagreeing with him. A very different response from what Worm had received from some of his home-grown critics, as he put it. Clearly the confrontation with Henrik Ernst still rankled with him.[95]

Writing to his nephews in April he told them that he was delighted to have received Liceti's opinion in time for it to be included in Book Four of his *Monumenta Danica* and that he planned to include something about a Trojan coin belonging to Johan Rhode and the Florentine horn drawn to his attention by Thomas Bartholin. Concerning the images or hieroglyphs on the gold horn Worm emphasised that they differed substantially from the Egyptian hieroglyphs. He was not surprised that other scholars such as Liceti might reach a different conclusion and would accept them as long as they were based on rational assumptions. He was happy to discuss such matters openly, pointing out that everyone made mistakes. However, he keenly awaited Kircher's opinion, because he had the greatest confidence in the latter's discernment in these matters.

Worm claimed that the gold horn needed to be discussed in the context of the other Danish monuments and therefore merited inclusion in *Monumenta Danica*, and in particular should be seen together with other ancient monuments found in the diocese of Ribe in southern Jutland. He explained to Thomas Bartholin that no one could deny it was the finest of all the monuments', but that 'a certain German', meaning Henrik Ernst, who had become his antagonist, 'had tried to wring it from the Danes' through a letter to his friends claiming that the horn was identical to that held by the idol, Svantevit, on Rügen, as described by Saxo. Though Worm had already repudiated his view he wanted to emphasise the horn's significance for the Danes and to liberate it from Ernst's stigma, which he intended to do moderately and without referring directly to him.[96]

Finally in June 1642 Johan Rhode obtained Athanasius Kircher's opinion of Worm's work on the gold horn. He claimed it was full of as much candour as well as deserved praise. Rhode enclosed a full transcription because he realised that there were those in Denmark who were prepared to challenge Worm's interpretation of the gold horn. Despite thanking Rhode for the 'friendly and beautiful statement by the learned Kircher' Worm did not include it in his revised edition of *De Aureo Cornu*. Apparently the printer had nearly finished printing the second edition so Worm was unable to add the statement in the relevant place. Instead, he decided to print Rhode's

95 *Ibid.*, no. 1027.
96 *Ibid.*, nos. 1029, 1030, and 1034

letter in full at the end of his work.[97] Perhaps Athanasius Kircher's had shown too much candour for Worm's liking and accordingly he decided not to include the long awaited opinion of the famous Jesuit scholar.

The revised version of *De Aureo Cornu* was ready by the end of May and was checked by Stephanius for any shortcomings or mistakes before being sent to the printer. Apart from corrections and changes it had grown from its original seventy-two pages to nearly a hundred pages. Worm was unhappy about the lack of urgency on the part of the printers in getting his work on the ancient monuments printed. Finally, towards the end of November 1642 Worm was able to send one of the first copies of *Monumenta Danica*, hot off the press since its year of publication was given as 1643, to Stephanius who had provided him with invaluable support throughout.[98]

Ole Worm had, at considerable cost, been forced to finance the publication of his second work on the runes. As we have seen Worm complained repeatedly about the considerable expenses he had to sustain for a task which he had been encouraged to undertake by the government. That all changed with the publication of his treatise on the gold horn in 1641. Clearly the Copenhagen printer, Joachim Moltke, considered this a publication of considerable public appeal and was prepared to bear the costs. It clearly paid off, since *De Aureo Cornu* sold out in less than a year. It was on Moltke's suggestion that Worm included a revised edition of *De Aureo Cornu* in his work on ancient monuments published two years later in 1643. *Monumenta Danica*, a large illustrated volume of 526 pages, also appears to have paid off for Moltke. It sold out within a few years, necessitating another edition in 1651 with an Additamenta of 40 pages, including a letter from Worm's friend, the French diplomat and scholar, Isaac La Peyrère, adding further information about the Gothic/runic lettering on a pyramid in France.[99]

Monumenta Danica was dedicated to Chancellor Christen Thomesen Sehested and the nobleman Just Høeg. In the preface Worm praised Sehested's predecessor, Christen Friis, for having encouraged and assisted him in his research into the runes and ancient monuments. Worm also acknowledged his

---

97 *Ibid.*, nos. 1049 and 1059; Johan Rhode's letter is printed in Ole Worm, *Danicorum monumentorum libri sex: e spissis antiquitatum tenebris et in Danica ac Norvegia extantibus ruderibus eruti*, Copenhagen 1643 (De aureo Domini Christiani Quinti, Daniæ, Norvegiæ etc. Principis, cornu dissertation) Libro V, 431–32. Bearing in mind that Kircher readily acknowledged material and information received for his hieroglyphic studies from among others Johan Rhode, and included the Danes, Thomas Bang and Thomas Bartholin, among the Northern European scholars who had influenced him, it is significant that Kircher did not make any reference to Ole Worm, see Stolzenberg, *Egyptian Oedipus*, 126–27.

98 *Ibid.*, nos. 1045, 1084, and 1091. Worm also sent a copy to his friend Johannes de Laet, in Leiden who wanted to discuss the runes with him when he had read the book, no. 1112.

99 *Ibid.*, no. 1335; for Isaac la Peyrère and his friendship with Worm, see below chapter 6.

debt to the works of Bonaventura Vulcanius, Sir Henry Spelman, the Dutch historian Peter Scriverius, and the two Danish royal historiographers Meursius and Pontanus. Finally he recognised the help he had received from Bertil Knudsen Aquilonius and Jon Skonvig in collecting the necessary information about the ancient monuments.[100] Evidently the printer Joachim Moltke considered Worm's works on the runes and ancient monuments extremely marketable by 1643. It was on his suggestion that Ole Worm produced a second and expanded edition of his *Fasti Danici* that year. As always he asked Stephanius to read through and check his work before publication.[101]

Meanwhile, Ole Worm's work on the gold horn continued to inspire scholars abroad. In a letter from Wittenberg Worm was informed that a volume, written by the minister Paul Eggers, dedicated to him and the elected-prince, had been published in Lüneburg the previous year. A couple of months later Worm borrowed a copy of Eggers' work from Henrik Køster, who informed him that it was disliked by the elected-prince who found it toadyish. The letter also informed Worm that August Buchner, the professor of poetry and rhetoric at Wittenberg University, admired his work and wanted to know more about his disagreement with Henrik Ernst.[102] A few months later August Buchner contacted Worm directly expressing his admiration and interest. In his response Worm admitted that his clash with Ernst in connection with the gold horn had differed from his normal moderation. He therefore did not want to publish it, especially since he had addressed the matter briefly in the new edition of his work on the gold horn which had been added to *Monumenta Danica*. Worm invited Bucher to comment on his work or correct mistakes, adding that someone who broke new ground could not expect to be right in all instances.

He then explained that the reason he had been so stern towards Ernst, was that the latter had pretended to be his friend until Worm on the request of the prince had published his treatise on the gold horn. Ernst had then envied him the favour and honour which his work generated, and without his knowledge circulated a letter at the court of the prince, seeking to find favour with the prince through the ruin of Worm's reputation. Worm had been alerted through his friends and taken action. However, he had no ambition to damage Ernst's reputation further now that he had regretted his action.[103] Worm, of course, refrained from mentioning that Ernst had been encouraged by the prince to produce something about the gold horn before Worm saw the horn and quickly produced his treatise. This at least might have gone some way to explain Ernst disappointment, if not to justify his subsequent action.

---

100 Ole Worm, *Danicorum monumentorum libri sex: e spissis antiquitatum tenebris et in Danica ac Norvegia extantibus ruderibus eruti*, Copenhagen 1643.
101 *Breve fra og til Ole Worm*, no. 1107.
102 *Ibid.*, nos. 1100, 1115, and 1120.
103 *Ibid.*, no. 1143

Worm kept August Buchner informed about new developments concerning the gold horn. In January 1644 he informed him that the minister in Roskilde, Enevold Nielsen Randulf, had written a pamphlet about the gold horn with some reasonable ideas taken from the Bible. Despite disagreeing with Worm on some points he had shown him his manuscript and told him that he felt unable to publish anything on the matter if Worm objected. Worm had praised his honesty which differed so profoundly from Ernst and had encouraged him to carry on with a pious enterprise which aimed at honouring God end encourage a better life. The pamphlet, in which Randulf argued that the gold horn was made by a Christian king and that its images gave instruction for the improvement of life and encouragement to contemplation, was published a couple of months later. Worm had expressed his opinion and reservations in a letter to Randulf which was printed at the end of the pamphlet. Worm informed his nephew Thomas Bartholin in Naples about Randulf's pamphlet, but pointed out that 'publications by our theologians cannot be sent securely to you'.[104]

Worm's nephews continued to promote his works in Italy. In January 1644 Thomas Bartholin informed his uncle that he was having his new observations about the unicorn printed in Padua and that he had added the views of the scholarly community about Worm's tract, *De Aureo Cornu*, at the end of the volume.[105] Worm was impatiently awaiting Liceti's book on rings which had a chapter on the Danish gold horn. In March 1644 he asked Henrik Fuiren to send him the book if it had appeared, and if that proved too difficult to have the relevant chapter copied for him. A couple of month later, in May, Fuiren informed him that he was unable to help him with Liceti's book which was still being printed in Udine. Henrik Fuiren, however, was able to inform him that another Italian, Angelico Aprosio Vintimiglia, a bibliophile Augustinian monk in Venice, had published a book dedicated to Thomas Bartholin, but with individual chapters dedicated to individuals, where the eleventh chapter was dedicated to Worm for his work on the gold horn. Fuiren had copied the introduction of this chapter for Worm to see before he received a copy of the book. A month later Henrik Fuiren obtained a copy of Liceti's book on rings, lacking introduction and conclusion which still had to be printed, and sent it to Worm, having abandoned his intention of copying the relevant chapter which, in his opinion was too long-winded.[106] Worm was so delighted by the dedication of Vintimiglia that he sent a copy of the latter's pamphlet to Stephanius

104 *Ibid.*, nos. 1184, 1192, 1193, 1194, and 1224.
105 *Ibid.*, no. 1179; see Thomas Bartholin, *De unicornu observations novæ. Accesserunt de aureo cornu Olai Wormii eruditorum judicia*, Padua 1645.
106 *Ibid.*, nos. 1181, 1201, 1208, and 1228; see also A. A. Vintimiglia, *La Sferza Poetica di Sapricio Saprici, lo scantonato accademico eteroclito. Per riposta alla prima censura dell'Adone del cavaliere Marino, fatta dal cavalier Tomaso Stigliani*, Venice 1643, and Fortunio Liceti, *De anulis antiquis*, Udine 1645.

in Sorø. Stephanius was so impressed with Vintimiglia's praise that he recommended Worm to have it printed and given to the elected-prince, so it
might be hung on a wall in the room where the gold horn was exhibited.[107]

Worm also received a letter in the summer of 1644 from the famous
surgeon, Marcus Aurelius Severinus, whom Thomas Bartholin was visiting
in Naples. Severinus applauded Worm's antiquarian works, especially his
treatise on the gold horn.[108]

Johan Rhode also worked tirelessly to promote Ole Worm's antiquarian
works among his learned Italian friends. In May 1644 he sent the copy of
Monumenta Danica which Henrik Fuiren had bought in Venice to Cassiano dal Pozzo in Rome hoping to elicit a positive assessment from this
influential man. Worm was delighted and impatiently awaiting Dal Pozzo's
appraisal, because as he stated 'the eyes of strangers form a clearer opinion
of such things than our own'.[109]

Meanwhile, August Buchner from Wittenberg heaped praise on Ole
Worm, pointing out that it was not only Denmark and the countries along
the Baltic coast but also the 'learned Germany, the clever Italy, and the
eloquent France' who admired Worm and placed him among those who
have achieved immortality through the study of antiquities and fine arts.[110]

Ole Worm's *De Aureo Cornu* also inspired a poem by the Bishop of
Lund, the former royal chaplain, Peder Winstrup. He interpreted the 'hieroglyphs and pictures on the horn as portraying the 'disturbances in our
deeply ravaged country', referring to the so-called Torstenson War with
Sweden which resulted in huge territorial losses for Denmark. Winstrup
wanted Worm to read his Latin poem before publication and discover if
any factual corrections were needed. Worm suggested a couple of minor
corrections and found that the 'heroic verse in several respects was not bad'.
Writing to Stephanius in November 1644 Worm informed him that Peder
Winstrup's poem about the gold horn was being printed in Copenhagen,
adding that he was delighted that the learned still found this topic worth
spending their precious time on.[111] In the same letter Worm recommended
the French ambassador, Gaspard Coignet de la Thuillerie, to Stephanius,
as a learned man, recommended by their mutual friend, Johan Rhode. De
la Thuillerie was a regular visitor of Worm's and admired his antiquarian
works and his cabinet of curiosity. The acquaintance with De la Thuillerie

107 *Ibid.*, nos. 1226, 1241, 1330, and 1356.
108 *Ibid.*, nos. 1223 and 1232.
109 *Ibid.*, nos. 1200 and 1222.
110 *Ibid.*, no. 1202.
111 *Ibid.*, nos. 1235, 1236, 1241, and 1257; for Winstrup's poem see *Cornicen Danicus seu
carmen de aureo Christiani, Daniæ, Norvegiæ etc. electi principis, cornu*, Copenhagen
1644; for the simultaneously published version in Danish, see *Den Danske Hornblæser,
Det er en dict om den Stormechtigste & Højborne Herres Christians Danmarckis/
Norges etc. Udualde Prindses Guld Horn*, Copenhagen 1644.

encouraged Worm to finally directly contact Gabriel Naudé, by then based in Paris as librarian to Cardinal Mazarin. Worm, who had assisted De la Thuillerie in finding books and manuscripts for Naudé, informed Naudé that manuscripts written in runes were rare

> Because foreigners who Christianised Denmark had no knowledge of this writing. In order not to be doubly troubled by trying to learn this writing and teach the people, they sought to abolish it by linking it to witchcraft and convincing the faithful that books written in runes could not be used without suspicion of ungodliness. They therefore condemned them to the fire and replaced them with their own. Accordingly manuscripts in this writing were extremely rare.[112]

The friendship between Ole Worm and De la Thuillerie brought Worm into contact with a number of prominent French scholars such as his secretary, Isaac La Peyrère, who shared his antiquarian interests.

More than anything, however, it was Ole Worm's work on the gold horn and the horn itself which continued to fascinate scholars abroad. In September 1645 Worm informed his friend Henrik Køster that De la Thuillerie was dying to see the gold horn and was likely to apply to the elected-prince to see it. Worm added that De la Thuillerie was an exceptional man and a great protector of natural philosophers.[113] In December 1645 Worm was informed that the well-known Helmstedt physician and professor, Herman Conring, wanted to correspond with him, especially about the gold horn which he apparently had something interesting to say about. Worm responded positively and contacted Conring, providing a useful resumé of the writings which had appeared in the wake of his publication of *De Aureo Cornu* in 1641. Conring was delighted and responded immediately. He had enjoyed reading Worm's tract about the gold horn and admired his learning. Unfortunately he had only been able to read through it once, because only a single copy had reached Helmstedt from Frankfurt which had quickly been claimed for the Welfern Court. Conring was unimpressed by the wild guesses of Paul Eggers, but was expecting something much better from Liceti. When Conring had read *De Aureo Cornu* he had been reminded about something Egyptian rather than Danish or German. He was convinced that the gold horn was ancient, cast at a time when gold could not be found in Germany, but when Egypt had plenty of gold from the goldmines in neighbouring mountains. Likewise, Conring was persuaded that the images on the horn corresponded closely with the Egyptian hieroglyphs, as could be seen from the different tablets which were imported from Egypt, as opposed to the ancient monuments

112 *Ibid.*, nos. 1262, 1292, and 1344.
113 *Ibid.*, no. 1351.

found in Germany which had nothing like it. However, Conring left it to Worm, who was best placed to decide whether letters used by the ancient Cimbers, Teutons, or Goths were, in fact, similar to the Egyptian hieroglyphs. Worm was delighted with the praise from Herman Conring and his rejection of Worm's detractors. Worm promised to send him a copy of his revised version of *De Aureo Cornu* which he had included in book five of *Monumenta Danica*. He found it difficult to believe that the horn had been made from Egyptian gold, not least because Saxo stated that there was plenty of gold in Denmark at the time of the birth of Christ. Neither was Worm able to detect any resemblance between the Egyptian hieroglyphs and the runes, in terms of either figures or arrangement, when comparing them. He was convinced that the runes were specific for 'our people', as can be seen from the Danish monuments, a view he pointed out that he shared with many scholars.[114]

By 1644 Worm was the recognised expert on runes and ancient monuments in northern Europe. Scholars working on different aspects of ancient languages and antiquities made contact with him. In August 1646 a Franciscan monk, at the Irish College in Louvain, Augustin Æganus, sent Worm an ancient alphabet of the Irish language which he wanted him to compare with the runes. He was convinced that the ancient people of the north had been much closer to each other in earlier times and wanted to know whether Worm had come across any Irish antiquities in his research. It would appear that Æganus was convinced that ancient Irish writings could be found in Danish archives and that the runes might prove to be of Irish origin. Worm, not surprisingly, was convinced that Æganus would be disappointed in his search, but even so he circulated the letter among his friends in case they had come across anything Irish.[115]

Ole Worm's works on the runes and ancient monuments would appear to have been widely available across Europe. They were sold in Germany, were stocked by booksellers in Venice, sold in London after some local encouragement, but appeared to have struggled to find a market in the Netherlands. When sold there, as with Worm's book on the runes, complaints had been made about the low quality of the paper. In the summer of 1647 Worm's nephew, Erasmus Bartholin, informed him that *Monumenta Danica* was not on sale in Amsterdam. Worm was not surprised because 'these people are so petty-minded that they will not exchange goods with our compatriots'. As an example of how unfair the Dutch were Worm informed Erasmus that he had been told by the Copenhagen printer/bookseller, Joachim Moltke that the books he had forwarded to Elzevir had been returned as if they were unsaleable.[116]

114 *Ibid.*, nos. 1390 and 1409.
115 *Ibid.*, nos. 1442, 1471, 1473, and 1480.
116 *Ibid.*, no. 1523.

Worm continued his research into the runes and the ancient monuments until the last few years of his life when his museum history became his preoccupation. The optimism of the early 1640s was, however, starting to evaporate by 1648. Worm even stated, that what he had written about the Danish monuments were of little significance, and that his age and failing health prevented him from continuing his research. Even so, he was working on an enlarged edition of his book on the runes, adding a glossary of old, now-forgotten, and poetic words. Worm wanted a folio edition of this to match his other publications in folio, but the printers were not keen. He had also produced additions to his *Monumenta Danica*, but because of the lethargy of the printers he doubted that they would ever see the light of day. At the same time he was, of course, increasingly focussed on his museum history.[117] A year later Worm expressed similar sentiments in a letter to his friend Isaac la Peyrére in Paris. Despite the success of his recent publications, *De Aureo Cornu* and *Monumenta Danica*, Worm was once again despairing about the printers. He was particularly angry with Joachim Moltke, whom he accused of being in the publishing business purely for himself and refusing to print his ancient monuments, on which Moltke had already made thousands, or to recognise any other God than profit.[118] However, Ole Worm eventually prevailed and had both an expanded, folio edition of his book on the runes and a revised edition of his *Additamenta of Monumenta Danica* published in 1651.[119]

8 Conclusion

For more than thirty years Ole Worm spent much of his time on research into the runes and ancient monuments, when not teaching medicine at the University or looking after his many patients. The encouragement to take on this research undoubtedly came from the then Chancellor, Christen Friis. Initially Worm might not have intended to take on the lead role in the government's scheme, launched in 1622, for collecting all data and information about the ancient monuments in Denmark and Norway. He appears to have earmarked his friend, the minister, Bertel Knudsen Aquilonius, who shared his antiquarian interests, as the right man to be in charge of this project. Two things are likely to have changed his mind. First, Worm

---

117 *Ibid.*, no. 1576; Worm consulted his Icelandic friends for the expanded edition of *Runir, seu Danica literature Antiquissima vulga Gothica dicta luci reditta*, which appeared in 1651, see nos. 1584, 1585, and 1590.

118 *Ibid.*, no. 1659; for the letter to La Peyrére, see no. 1634.

119 *Ibid.*, no. 1698, in August 1650 Worm informed Johan Rhode that the folio edition of his book on the runes was being printed; see also Ole Worm, *Runir, seu Danica literature Antiquissima vulga Gothica dicta luci reditta*, Copenhagen 1651 and Ole Worm, *Danicorum monumentorum libri sex: e spissis antiquitatum tenebris et in Danica ac Norvegia extantibus ruderibus eruti*, Copenhagen 1651.

quickly developed doubts about Aquilonius's ability to master the task and deal competently with the runic inscriptions. Second, Worm realised how important this antiquarian enterprise might turn out to be, being part of Christian IV and Chancellor Christen Friis's plans for promoting a patriotic cultural and historical understanding of the kingdom of Denmark and Norway. While Worm's personal interests in this antiquarian project grew so did his realisation of its potential advantage to him as a loyal servant of the Crown with the benefits that entailed.

It proved a difficult task, not surprising when borne in mind that this was a new and relatively unexplored field of research. Even so, Ole Worm was privileged by having access to a group of Icelandic scholars who could assist him. Worm, however, was disappointed by the lack of governmental support and reward for his efforts. He also struggled to get some his works published. *Fasti Danici*, published by the University of Copenhagen printer, Salomon Santor in 1626 appears to have proceeded to publication without any problems. Despite the work selling well and being reprinted in 1633, and again in a revised edition in 1643, Worm struggled to find a publisher for his subsequent book on the runes and eventually had to finance its publication himself after a long delay and at considerable financial cost. Despite some recognition by leading international scholars, such as Sir Henry Spelman, appreciation was only slowly forthcoming at home.

This all changed with the discovery of the ancient gold horn in Southern Jutland and Worm's rapidly produced tract, *De Aureo Cornu*, in 1641. This work more than any other established Ole Worm's reputation as an important antiquarian scholar. Worm undoubtedly benefitted from the fact that the gold horn was an extremely unusual and valuable object, decorated with curious images and letters. *De Aureo Cornu* sold out within months and helped facilitate the publication of Ole Worm's work on the ancient monuments, *Monumenta Danica*, which appeared in 1643 with a revised and expanded version of *De Aureo Cornu*. The gold horn fascinated other antiquarians and theologians who wrote tracts about it. *De Aureo Cornu* drew Worm to the attention of other leading antiquarian scholars across Europe, from Sir Henry Spelman in London, Johannes de Laet in Leiden, Herman Conring in Helmsted, Gabriel Naudé, Cassiano dal Pozzo, and Athanasius Kircher in Rome, and Fortunio Liceti in Bologna to mention some of the most prominent. At the same time the international success of Worm's publications guaranteed a growing reputation at home within both the court and university.

4 The Collector

1 Botanist and gardener

Ole Worm started life as a collector by gathering plants for his garden. He shared this interests in botany and gardening with a considerable number of early modern physicians. Undoubtedly the time he had spent at the University of Basle in 1607–08 and his friendship with one of his teachers, the physician and botanist, Caspar Bauhin, came to shape his subsequent interests in collecting plants, and objects of significance for natural history and medicine.[1]

Worm, who had returned to Copenhagen in July 1613 to take up the professorship in pedagogy, was promoted to the chair in Greek two years later. By then he had been able to establish his own garden where he could actively pursue his interests in botany. In February 1616 Worm wrote to one of his friends from his student days while studying abroad, the physician Christian Claccius in Kassel, asking him to send seeds and bulbs for his garden.[2] A year later Worm received seeds from another student friend, Niels Christensen Foss, whom he subsequently asked to approach one of his former teachers while visiting Strassburg, Dr Johannes Salzmann, and ask him for a leaf of either of two plants he remembered the latter grew in his garden, Opuntia and Ficus Indica.[3]

During the summer of 1615 Worm struggled for six weeks with a nasty tertiary fever and subsequently found it difficult to regain his physical strength in the autumn. By early March the following year he had taken up residence convalescing on the island of Amager close to Copenhagen with his two brothers-in-law, the physicians Caspar Bartholin and Jørgen Fuiren. While there the three of them used the occasion to exercise their shared interest in botany, clearly inspired and fascinated by the varied

---

1 See Schepelern, *Museum*, 57–62.
2 *Breve fra og til Ole Worm*, no. 18. Worm requested a catalogue of the plants in the medical garden in Giessen from his brother-in-law Jacob Fincke in a letter dated the same day, see no. 17. See also Hovesen, *Lægen Ole Worm*, 140.
3 *Breve fra og til Ole Worm*, no. 25.

DOI: 10.4324/9781003290940-5

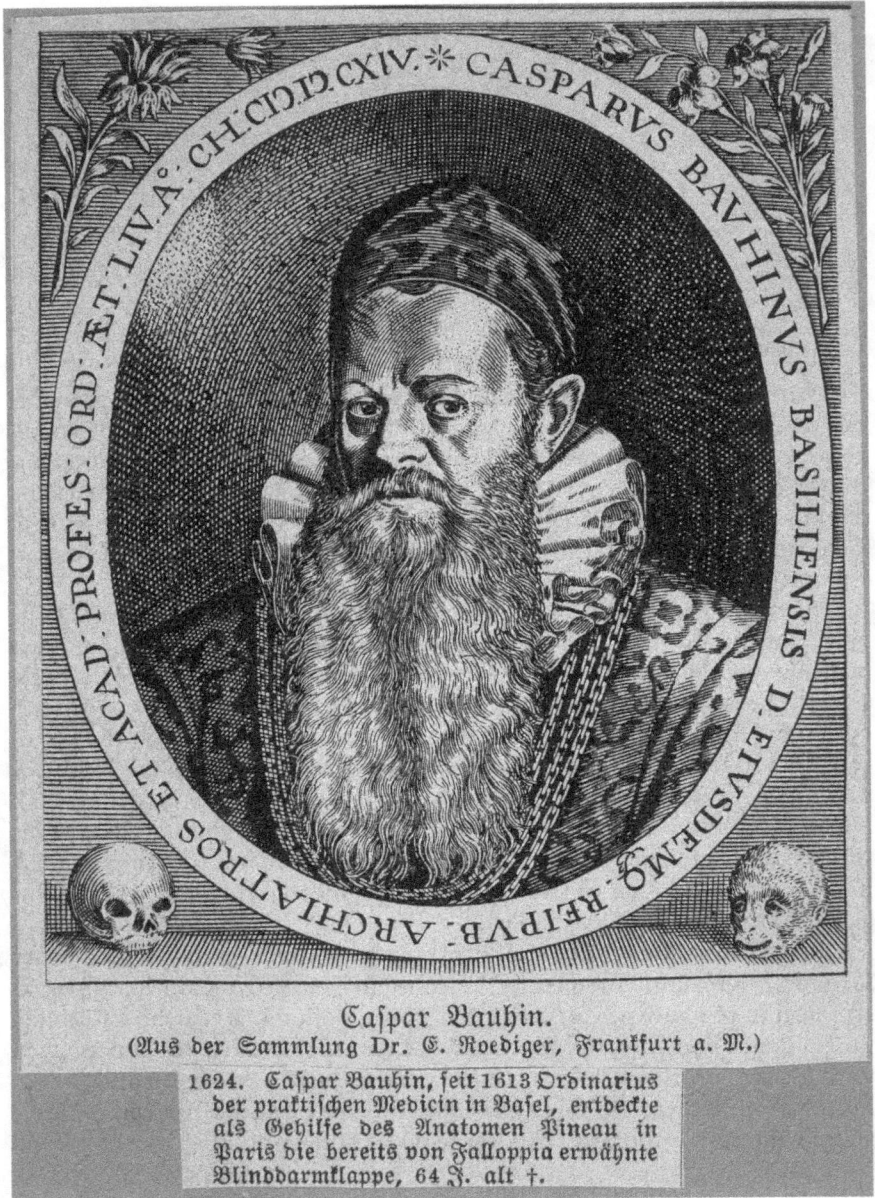

Caspar Bauhin.
(Aus der Sammlung Dr. E. Roediger, Frankfurt a. M.)

1624. Caspar Bauhin, seit 1613 Ordinarius
der praktischen Medicin in Basel, entdeckte
als Gehilfe des Anatomen Pineau in
Paris die bereits von Falloppia erwähnte
Blinddarmklappe, 64 J. alt †.

Figure 4.1 Caspar Bauhin (1560–1624); courtesy of the Royal Danish Library.

and unusual fauna on Amager. This also provided Worm with an opportunity to renew his correspondence with his former teacher in Basle, Caspar Bauhin, informing him of their findings and supplying him with samples.[4]

A regular exchange of letters between Worm and his former mentor in Basle followed over the next three years, sharing their interest in botany while Worm supplied Bauhin with samples of plants he had found on Amager. Among them was a type of Cochlearia which Worm had never seen described. Bauhin proved grateful and asked Worm to send him further samples of the plants he found on Amager. In May 1618 he asked Worm to have the two Cochlearia he had discovered drawn as they occurred naturally, promising to publish them with Worm's name attached in his forthcoming work, *Catalogus Plantarum*, Frankfurt 1620.[5]

Worm's last letter to Caspar Bauhin from August 1620 contained a detailed description of the bulbs of the Jerusalem's Artichoke, samples of which he forwarded. Worm emphasised that they had recently been brought back from America, pointing out that they were supposed to aid love-making. He added that they were edible, but should be blended with wine, butter, and pepper before being eaten, otherwise they might cause serious flatulence, as Worm himself had experienced at first hand. Worm's interest in botany, however, appears to have diminished when his correspondence with Caspar Bauhin came to an end a few years before Bauhin's death.[6]

However, a decade later, in 1630, Worm revived his interest in botany when, after the death of his brother-in-law Caspar Bartholin, he took over the latter's house. The house possessed a large well-kept garden bordering the university's botanical garden for which Worm now became responsible. Hardly had Worm moved in before he asked his student Jacob Svabe in Leiden to supply him with seeds for his garden from the famous botanical garden in Leiden. Svabe sent him a variety of seeds from what he considered the rarest plants in the hortus botanicus in Leiden. Svabe also sent the printed catalogue of the garden, adding that he would like to receive a list from Worm of the seeds he particularly wanted.[7] Worm readily made use of the opportunity and sent him a list of what he wanted most urgently. He added that he owned a rare and beautiful plant, arachidna, which he had been sent from Portugal, and which was not listed among the plants in the botanical garden in Leiden. Worm offered to send seeds of this plant to the garden if they would be welcomed.[8] Ole Worm was clearly proud of his new garden and happy to show it to visitors. His friend Niels Christensen Foss, who had become provincial physician for Scania, visited it and

---

4 *Ibid.*, nos. 20 and 24; see also Hovesen, *Ole Worm*, 141.
5 *Ibid.*, nos. 24, 34, 42, 46, 51, 58, 62 and 77.
6 *Ibid.*, no.77.
7 *Breve fra og til Ole Worm*, nos. 388 and 396.
8 *Ibid.*, no. 423.

subsequently reminded Worm of 'promised cuttings from his luxuriantly flowering red roses, not to mention seeds from his exotic plants now the planting season had arrived. They were quickly dispatched by Worm, who added that Foss should not expect too much of the seeds from the exotic plants which did not thrive in 'our climate'.[9]

In March 1633, Worm responded positively when asked by the professor in medicine and botany at the Academy in Sorø, Joachim Burser, to supply him with seeds ready to be sown. Unfortunately, he had only little to send Burser because of the disappointing flora of his 'modest' garden that year, and because his friends had brought him few new plants, which merited Burser's interest. He therefore was only able to send him some rather insignificant seeds which he promised to supplement when his garden had a better year. However, Worm considered it a good omen for the coming year that Burser had become the first of his friends to want to donate something to his garden.[10] Worm was clearly spending much time and energy on his new garden and on botany in the early 1630s and in September 1633 he informed his friend Johannes Cabeljau in Bremen that he had just finished a textbook about the Danish flora.[11] Surprisingly Worm never published this work, nor has it survived among his manuscripts.

A couple of years later another of Worm's students, his nephew Henrik Fuiren, provided him with plants and seeds from the hortus botanicus in Leiden. Some of them thrived in Worm's garden, while others such as the Indian fig, tarentine myrtle, and sinilap aggera, proved unable to cope with the inclement Danish weather. Worm was also keen on acquiring the collected works of the famous Leiden botanist, Carolus Clusius, and eventually sent money to Henrik Fuiren so he could obtain them for him in Leiden.[12]

Worm had probably befriended the physician and botanist Otto Sperling when the latter arrived in Denmark in the early 1620s and had sought Worm's patronage. In the summer of 1622 Ole Worm approached the Bishop of Bergen on Sperling's behalf, asking him to assist and support Otto Sperling whom he considered 'a clever and diligent young man'. He explained that Sperling intended to produce a catalogue of all natural objects to be found in Norway, especially plants, and needed a letter of safe-conduct to be able to successfully undertake his task.[13] By 1634 Sperling had settled permanently in Denmark and the contacts between the two men intensified. In February 1636 Sperling lent Worm his copy of Franciscus Calzolari's *Musæum naturalis et moralis philosophiæ* (Verona

---

9 *Ibid.*, nos. 423, 424, and 425. For early modern gardens see A. Cunningham, 'The Culture of Gardens', 38–56 in N. Jardine et al. (eds.), *Cultures of Natural History*, Cambridge 1996, especially 47–52.
10 *Ibid.*, nos. 462 and 466.
11 *Ibid.*, no. 489 and Hovesen, *Ole Worm*, 142.
12 *Ibid.*, nos. 561 and 596
13 *Ibid.*, no. 107.

1622) the famous botanist and pharmacist from Verona, promising him seeds from his garden within weeks. Worm reciprocated by sending Sperling some of the more interesting seeds in his possession, among them Cretica, which he had received from their mutual friend in Italy, Johan Rhode. Worm was convinced that Sperling would easily be able to identify what he was missing in his garden from what Worm had sent him, and hopefully provide him with a supply that would delight him, naming Sperling 'Flora's true son'.[14]

Shared medical and botanical interests meant that Joachim Burser and Worm stayed in regular contact during the 1630s. Burser thanked Worm for seeds for his garden in April 1637 and mentioned that the chancellor, Christen Friis, wanted him to be responsible for the creation of a new garden at Friis's estate at Lindholm, supervising the planting. Worm responded by sending him more plants from his garden, pointing out that recently he had sent the Chancellor a considerable supply of small violets for his estate at Lindholm. Furthermore, Worm had just received some seeds from the gardener at Frederiksborg Castle, which had been found among the belongings of the late royal physician Henning Arnisæus, of which Worm now forwarded half to Burser.[15] Later that year Worm received plants and seeds from Leiden from another Fuiren nephew, Thomas. Worm claimed that these had made such a change to his garden that it now could hold its own when compared with other gardens.[16]

Where Worm's students on occasion had been able to provide him with new and exotic plants from the university botanical garden during their studies in Leiden, the arrival of his nephew, Thomas Bartholin, in February 1638, for whom he stood in loco parentis, improved his access to new and rare plants significantly. In his first letter from Leiden Thomas informed Worm that the professor of botany, Adolphus Vorstius had yet to open the hortus botanicus to the public, but he promised to send his uncle any seeds, plants, and bulbs which Worm's 'well-cultivated' garden might be missing. A few months later Thomas send Worm the latest edition of the catalogue of the botanical garden in Leiden, asking him to specify what plants he wanted. Bartholin, however, added that no plants had arrived from India that year, while he himself keenly attended Vorstius's lectures on botany.[17] Worm immediately made use of the catalogue and selected some plants he would like sent for the following spring either as seeds or bulbs, as long as Thomas could obtain them without too much trouble or inconvenience. He took the opportunity to warn his young nephew against being cheated by the gardener who might provide him with old

---

14 *Ibid.*, nos. 580–83; see also Schepelern, *Museum*, 227–28.
15 *Ibid.*, nos. 643–45.
16 *Ibid.*, no. 649.
17 *Ibid.*, nos. 702 and 716.

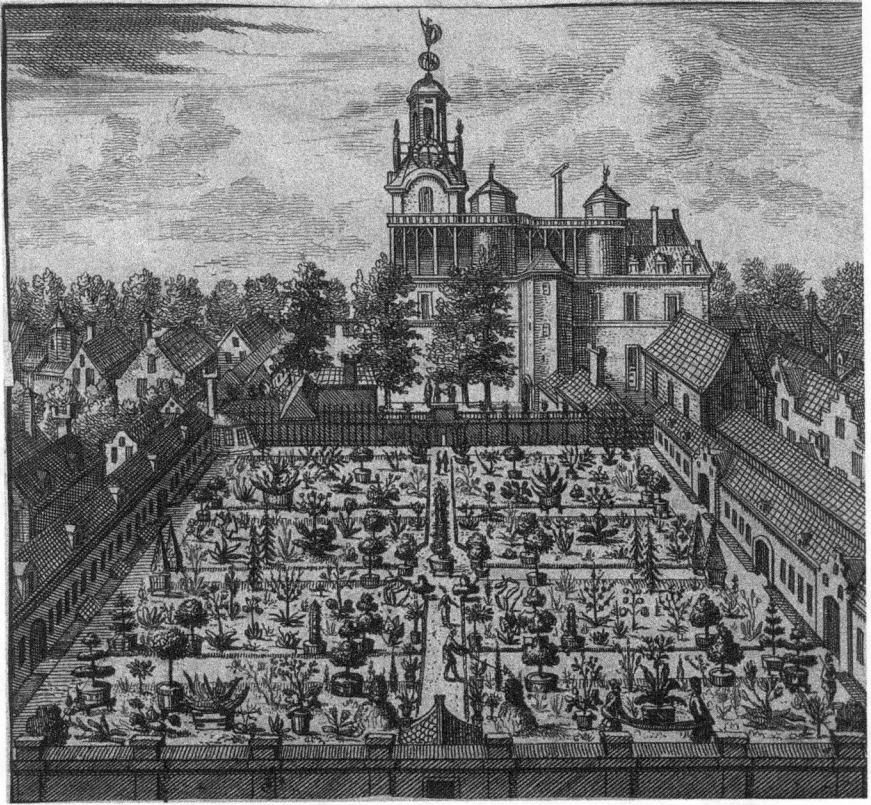

Figure 4.2 Leiden, Botanical Garden 1610; courtesy of Wellcome Collection.

and diseased stock rather than new and fresh.[18] By September Thomas Bartholin had gathered so many seeds for Worm that the package proved too heavy to send with a fellow student, who was returning to Denmark by road; instead the container had to wait until Christmas 1638 before it could be dispatched.[19]

However, Worm did not rely exclusively on Thomas Bartholin for contributions to his garden. In July 1638 he received seeds of herba vivens (sempervivum) from Henrik Fuiren, then studying in Paris, which the latter had obtained the previous year while in Leiden.[20] Worm thanked him warmly for the seeds he had received, especially of the mimosa, and hoped that his

18 *Ibid.*, no. 722.
19 *Ibid.*, nos. 746 and 758.
20 *Ibid.*, no.729.

garden would be able to produce a crop from this fine plant. He added that he was glad that Henrik still took an interest in his garden as well as his museum.[21]

Despite all the support he received for his garden from interested friends and students Worm was unhappy about the state of it by 1639. Writing to his friend and later brother-in-law Steffen Hansen Stephanius, professor at the Academy in Sorø, Worm complained that its poor condition now forced him to beg others for support, informing him that Stephanius's colleague at the Academy, Joachim Burser had recently send him a variety of seeds and bulbs. A few months later Ole Worm contacted Stephanius again and asked to be supplied with more seeds for his garden, especially amaranthus purpureus, to make good the losses it had suffered during the cold winter. Worm added that he felt that he could not ask Stephanius for seeds of rarer plants.[22] To judge from the extant correspondence Worm's interest in gardening was on the wane after the disappointments of 1638–39. Apart from some seeds received in June 1639 from his student Hans Leyel in Leiden his garden does not feature in the correspondence until a couple of years later when he received seeds of herba viva from his friend and colleague, Henrik Køster, in Nykøbing Falster. From Worm's comments we can assume that he had failed to grow the identical seeds he had received the previous year from Henrik Fuiren. Nevertheless Worm planted some of them while donating others to Otto Sperling, even if simultaneously expressing his misgivings.[23] His pessimism proved justified and a couple of months later he informed Køster that both he and Sperling had been unable to get the seeds to grow, adding that most of them had been rotten while others had been unable to sprout due to their age. Worm wanted Køster to let him know if the gardener to the elected-prince had fared any better with his seeds.[24]

Half a year later, in March 1642, Thomas Bartholin, now in Padua, forwarded some 'rare' seeds to Worm on behalf of Henrik Fuiren, who evidently had not forgotten Worm's garden. In August that year Henrik forwarded the freshly printed catalogue of the botanical garden in Padua to his uncle and mentor. Worm thanked him warmly, expressing his admiration for the wealth and rarity of the plants in the garden, but also his surprise that he was unable to find herba viva or mimosa in the catalogue. Worm pointed out that he had been able to grow one of these plants in his garden from seeds he had received, even if he was unsure whether it was the right plant. Among the other plants he had successfully grown was Laplab and

---

21 *Ibid.*, no. 753. Writing to another student in Paris a couple of months later Worm wrote that he was anxiously waiting to see if the Danish climate would allow it to the flower that summer, see *ibid.*, no. 765.
22 *Ibid.*, nos. 770 and 778.
23 *Ibid.*, no.792, 941, and 946.
24 *Ibid.*, no. 960.

Bebiora which he could not find in the catalogue either. Unfortunately the latter had been consumed by ants which were also attacking his mimosa. Worm concluded that the Danish soil and climate did not prevent such exotic plants from growing even if they might prevent them from flowering and producing seeds.[25] This positive message encouraged Henrik Fuiren to intensify his collection of exotic seeds in Padua, even if he had some doubts about collecting bulbs which he thought might struggle to cope with the long journey, unless Worm could inform him of a way to preserve them. Worm was delighted and asked him in particular to supply him with Dens caninus, Granadilla, and Mimosa. He informed Fuiren that Otto Sperling had just published a catalogue of the royal garden in Copenhagen. He would have sent him a copy if it had been possible and Henrik Fuiren would have been surprised that so many exotic plants could be grown in Denmark; unfortunately most of them only generated leaves and shoots and never flowered or produced seeds. Worm recommended that Fuiren sent the bulbs he collected wrapped in moss placed in a wooden box which should be enough to preserve them. In a postscript he informed Henrik that he had received a drawing from Peder Charisius of an Italian plant which grew on Mount Zibio, known locally as Fumana. Worm was keen to know whether Henrik Fuiren knew anything about it or could obtain seeds from the plant in order that Worm and his colleagues might better understand it.[26]

By 1644 Worm's interest in his own garden, and gardening in general, appears to have declined rapidly. Clearly his cabinet of curiosity and his antiquarian interests were now taking precedence. Still, in a letter to his brother-in-law Henrik Motzfeld, from January that year he corrected him by pointing out that the garden belonging to the Copenhagen mayor, Hans Nielsen, had never been as splendid as Henrik believed. Worm admitted that it was full of flowering bulbs, but contained nothing unusual or rare of any significance, and furthermore after he had become mayor Nielsen had lost interest in it. It was therefore not worth a visit. The royal garden, on the other hand, was worth seeing having acquired a variety of rare and unusual plants under Sperling's care and supervision, as was evident from his catalogue.[27] Apart from a couple of requests from Stephanius in Sorø for seeds, bulbs, and roots of flowering plants, among them lilac, from Worm's garden during 1647, Worm would appear to have taken little interests in gardening. When, in September, he sent a copy of Sperling's *Hortus*

---

25 *Ibid.*, nos. 1064 and 1075.
26 *Ibid.*, nos. 1094 and 1106. For Peder Charisius's letter see no. 1096; based on this letter Hovesen thinks Worm received the plant from Charisius, Hovesen, *Ole Worm*, 143. Sperling who had been appointed superintendent of the royal garden at Rosenborg Castle in 1638 published his catalogue in 1642, see O. Sperling, *Hortus Christianæus seu Catalogus plantarum, quibus Ser. Principis Christiani IV ... viridarium Hafniense Anno. 1642*, Copenhagen 1642
27 *Breve fra og til Ole Worm*, no. 1183.

Christianæus, to Johann Friedrich Slezer in Hamburg he informed him that he should no longer expect to find many of the plants mentioned in the catalogue in the royal garden. Not only had Sperling lost his directorship of the garden, but due to the disturbances of war the grants for its maintenance had been discontinued. Worm, however, told Slezer that he would be delighted if he could supply him with copies of the two catalogues of rare plants he had shown him while in Copenhagen and inform him how these plants could be obtained.[28]

Worm may have lost interest in his garden, but that did not mean that he lost his interest in botany. Thus, he encouraged his son Willum, newly arrived in Leiden, to pay great attention to the study of botany. As always Worm valued a practical and hands on approach, telling Willum to befriend the gardener by tipping him in order that he might benefit from his personal insight and obtain plants.[29] He also continued to collect rare plants for his cabinet of curiosity, and botany eventually played a prominent part in the history of his museum, *Museum Wormianum*, which was published shortly after his death. Its thirty-five richly illustrated chapters covering more than a hundred pages constitute a significant part of the work. Worm was primarily concerned with the medical use of these plants and only dealt with rare plants which were difficult to obtain.[30]

2 From collector to creator of a cabinet of curiosity

When did Ole Worm begin to collect natural and manufactured objects? Most likely already while he was on his peregrinatio academica. Among Worm's teachers at the University of Basle were Felix Platter who wrote in Worm's album amicorum in April 1608. Undoubtedly Worm would have been impressed by Platter's large collection of natural and artificial objects much of which he had inherited from Conrad Gesner.[31] During Worm's subsequent time at the University of Padua from November 1608 until spring 1609 he may have visited Verona and seen the late Francesco Calzolari's museum. But bearing in mind that Worm never explicitly stated that he had visited the museum this remains speculation. The modest first catalogue of Calzolari's collection from 1584 was no more than a short unillustrated text advertising the breath of the pharmacopeia Calzolari had amassed. It was more of a sales catalogue than a publication to entice visitors. The second catalogue commissioned by his grandson and published in 1622 proved a totally different kettle of fish – ten times longer, illustrated,

28 *Ibid.*, nos. 1489, 1542; for the letter to Johann Friedrich Slezer, see no. 1535.
29 *Ibid.*, no. 1770.
30 Schepelern, *Museum*, 249; see also Ole Worm, *Museum Wormianum*, Book 2.
31 See Schepelern, *Museum*, 60. For the significance of Felix Platter, See Brian W. Ogilvie, *The Science of Describing. Natural History in Renaissance Europe*, University of Chicago Press 2006, 41–42.

and more of a natural history of the objects in the collection.[32] Not surprisingly it served to raise the reputation of the museum and attract visitors. The timing of Worm's arrival in northern Italy may simply have been wrong for him to have prioritised a visit to Calzolari's museum in Verona.[33]

Likewise Worm does not appear to have visited Ulisse Aldrovandi's famous botanical garden and museum in Bologna when he spent a couple of days in the city in the second week of May 1609. Could the reason be that Aldrovandi's museum remained closed to the public after his death in 1605? The fact that the Senate of Bologna who took over the responsibility for Aldrovandi's museum after his death did not appoint a custodian until 1610 would seem to support such an interpretation. This is further supported by the fact that the museum had been closed for some time when Worm's student Hans Andersen Skovgaard visited Bologna in the autumn of 1627, coinciding with a delay in the appointment of a new custodian.[34] Skovgaard had only been able to see Aldrovandi's museum through the intervention of 'an influential gentleman' because it had remained closed for three years. He reported it was full of the most marvellous objects, but not to be compared with Imperato's in Naples.[35] Furthermore, it is worth remembering that by the time Worm was travelling in Northern Italy very few of Aldrovandi's works on natural history had yet been published, making a visit less imperative.[36]

Worm's journey to Rome and Naples in the spring of 1609 may well have been influenced by his ambition to see Ferrante Imperato's museum in Naples, and Worm managed to get Imperato's signature in his album amicorum during his visit.[37] Worm would undoubtedly have been well informed about Imperato's cabinet of curiosity from Imperato's book about his collection published in 1599. As opposed to Calzolari's catalogue Imperato's work was an abbreviated, illustrated, natural history based on the objects displayed in his museum; it was also the first work to show what a cabinet of curiosity looked like.[38]

32 See Schepelern, *Museum*, 65; for Calzeolari's museum see Paula Findlen, *Possessing Nature. Museums, Collecting, and Scientific Culture in Early Modern Italy*, University of California Press, Los Angeles 1996, 37–38.

33 Worm never claimed to have visited Calzeolari's museum and when referring to objects in it used the term as can be seen rather than seen by me which confirms this, see Schepelern, *Museum*, 91, note 73.

34 Findlen, *Possessing Nature*, 24–25, especially note 25.

35 *Breve fra og til Ole Worm*, no. 233. Skovgaard also visited Giovanni Pona's museum in Verona.

36 Findlen, *Possessing Nature*, 24–27 and Schepelern, *Museum*, 222.

37 Schepelern, *Museum*, 65–66.

38 Findlen, *Possessing Nature*, 38–39. See also L. Daston and K. Park, *Wonders and the Order of Nature, 1150–1750*, Zone Books, New York 2001, 153. Schepelern thinks that Worm may have visited Calzeolari's museum in Vorona on his journey to Padua, but admits that there is no evidence for this. Similarly, Schepelern implies that Worm visited Ulisse Aldrovandi famous botanical garden and museum during his stay in Bologna,

Worm was evidently keen on visiting famous museums on his peregrinatio academica. In 1610 he visited Enkhuizen in the Dutch Republic and saw Bernhard Paludanus's cabinet of curiosity which was particularly famous for its many exotic objects from the Far East and the New World. Not only did Worm sign Paludanus's album amicorum, but Paludanus reciprocated by signing Worm's. Furthermore Worm was given two objects by Paludanus, which he eventually included in his own collection, a perfumed tube, calamus aromaticus, and a coffee bean.[39]

Paludanus had started his collection and cabinet of curiosity when in 1586 he became city physician in Enkhuizen, then a major centre for overseas trade in the Dutch Republic. Ten years later he helped co-author Jan van Linschoten's travelbook to the East Indies, which added further to his fame. Linschoten's *Itinerario* was later repeatedly consulted by Worm when writing his magnum opus, *Museum Wormianum*, where he cited it five times.[40] In 1603–04 Paludanus had sold his cabinet of curiosity to Duke Friedrich of Württemberg, but within a few years he had put together an even more impressive collection full of objects from Africa, Asia, and the New World. This was the collection Worm saw in 1610 and which some time after Paludanus's death in 1633 was sold to the Duke of Schleswig and Gottorp.[41]

On the second part of his peregrinatio academica Ole Worm spent five to six weeks in Kassel during the autumn of 1611, where he had the opportunity to see the famous cabinet of curiosity belonging to Duke Moritz, the Learned, of Hesse-Kassel. Even if the museum primarily contained works of art, coins, and valuable natural objects such as horns of 'unicorns' and rhinos in costly and elaborate fixings, it also contained a section on natural objects. The fact that Worm was able to spend a considerable time inspecting the collection would undoubtedly have served to inspire him to start collecting himself.[42]

---

even if he acknowledges that Worm never referred to it. These tentative suggestions have been upgraded to certainty by later historians, see Jens Erik Kristensen, 'Det kuriøse og det klassificerence blik – naturens indsamling og forordning fra Renæssancens samlere til det modern naturhistoriske museum med *Museum Wormianum* som udganspunkt', *Den Jyske Historiker*, 64, 1993, 31–41, especially 35; and Camilla Mordhorst, *Genstandsfortællinger. Fra Museum Wormianum til de moderne museer*, Museum Tusculanum, Copenhagen 2009, 34

39 Worm, *Museum Wormianum*, 144 and 189; see also Schepelern, *Museum*, 70–71 and 145.

40 Jan van Linschoten, *Itinerario: voyage ofte schipvaert van Jan Huygen van Linschoten near Oost ofte Portugaels Indien, 1579–1592*, Amsterdam 1596; see also Schepelern, *Museum*, 226.

41 H. J. Cook, *Matters of Exchange. Commerce, Medicine, and Science in the Dutch Golden Age*, London 2007, 115–16, 124–30.

42 Schepelern, *Museum*, 76–77.

In 1639 responding to an inquiry from his Icelandic friend Arngrim Jonsson, Worm explained that he was still working on a catalogue of the objects in his cabinet of curiosity, and had yet to finish it. From his answer it is clear that he considered his collection an ongoing enterprise which he had started on his peregrinatio academica:

> I collected different objects on my travels abroad and I gradually receive a variety of items from India and other far-away places, such as samples of soil, stones, metals, plants, fish, birds, and terrestrial animals, which I carefully preserve with the intention that together with a short account of their history I am able to let my audience touch the objects with their hands and examine them, in order to personally determine to what extent what has been stated corresponds with the objects, thereby acquiring a more exact knowledge about them.[43]

For Worm the link between description, observation, and handling was paramount to which more often than not could be added the consultation of prominent scholarly works.[44]

Ole Worm may have collected a few objects while a student, but more than a decade passed after his return to Copenhagen before he began to collect natural objects in earnest. During the summer or autumn of 1623 he wrote to his student Hans Andersen Skovgaard, then in Wittenberg, that he had begun to collect natural objects, 'especially the rarer objects from the animal and mineral kingdoms and objects from the sea'. Worm requested Skovgaard to bear this in mind on his journey, if he came across such things. He was aware that there were mountain works and mines close to Wittenberg and he asked Skovgaard to send him small samples of minerals and metals labelled with their names, if he could obtain them. He promised to keep them for 'mutual benefit'. Another letter from around that time asks the headmaster at the Latin school in Viborg to assist Worm in getting rarities from the local physician for his newly established collection.[45] By then he had already received the cranium of the giant bird Semenda from one of the participants in the recent Danish expedition to East India, Ove Gjedde.[46] Evidently Worm was collecting natural objects in earnest by the autumn of 1623 and he was looking at a variety of ways for enhancing his collection. Thus, he tried to obtain some of the mineral samples such as the 'Norwegian magnet-stone' which the nobleman Anders Bille had brought back from Norway a few year earlier when commissioned by Christian IV to discover what minerals could be extracted in Norway. Worm had no

43 *Breve fra og til Ole Worm*, no.787.
44 For the significance of this approach see Brian W. Ogilvie, *The Science of Describing. Natural History in Renaissance Europe*, Chicago University Press 2006.
45 *Breve fra og til Ole Worm*, nos. 142–43.
46 Worm, *Museum Wormianum*, 309

doubt that such objects would enrich his 'treasure chamber'.[47] This is the first indication that Worm was moving from an occasional collector to becoming a creator of a cabinet of curiosity.

In a letter to his friend Johan Rhode in Padua written around the same time Worm informed him that:

> I have started a collection of peculiar natural objects, especially the rarer ones; towards this I have received contributions from several of my friends. Since you live in a region where many of these occur daily, I ask you to remember me. I ask you to send me everything that is available be they from among the animals of the land, sea, and air, or made of stones and metals.

Apart from specifically asking for a whole, dried, poisonous snake and some conchs from Venice Worm emphasised:

> You should on my behalf consider what suits this aim. It is not precious objects I want, but objects which are rare here, but common where you are and which can be acquired for nearly nothing.[48]

Such *rariora*, however, were not exclusively to be found abroad, but were also available locally. Of particular relevance were objects which broke with traditional categories and challenged established views and concepts. This explains why Worm included common animals such as owls, crayfish, and bees in his collection. The crayfish were included for their specific use in drugs, the owls for their exceptional vision, and the bees for the way they built their hives.[49] Rare objects should in other words have unusual and surprising qualities, often bordering on the marvellous and incomprehensible. By collecting them and studying and describing them they could be made comprehensible.[50] They were, indeed, examples of some of God's most beautiful and surprising creations as emphasised in recent scholarship. But they were more than that. They offered exceptional examples of how God had created the natural world and as such provided particular insight into the Book of Nature. The collection and detailed description of natural rarities became the physicians and natural philosophers encyclopaedia of the exceptional, a compendium which eventually would lead to a better if not full understanding of the Book of Nature. These *rariora* may well initially appear to be opaque and fragmented and therefore difficult to interpret or give meaning to, as pointed out by a number of scholars, but the

47 Schepelern, *Museum*, 146.
48 *Breve fra og til Ole Worm*, no. 147.
49 Worm, *Museum Wormianum*, 296.
50 See K. Whitaker, 'The Culture of Curiosity', 75–90 in N. Jardine et al. (eds.), *Cultures of Natural History*, Cambridge 1996.

ultimate ambition for a Lutheran natural philosophers and physician such as Ole Worm was to seek to understand and make sense of these marvellous objects, thereby coming to an understanding of the created world.[51] Where the reading and understanding of the Bible was of paramount importance to every Lutheran, so was the investigation and comprehension of the Book of Nature for a Lutheran natural philosopher like Ole Worm.

Rhode was more than happy to assist in providing Worm with the 'rarities' from Northern Italy which he was missing in his cabinet of curiosity. Johan Rhode had, in fact, already begun collecting objects for Worm. He had had two snakes, one male and one female, stuffed and preserved, and would have sent them on, but had been unwilling to trust them to sailors. He had therefore placed them in a chest with other items and sent them over land rather than by sea.[52]

By then Ole Worm must have felt that his cabinet of curiosity had become interesting enough to show it to friends. His friend Steffen Hansen Stephanius thanked him for his kindness by giving him access to his cabinet of curiosity 'full of different and even rare objects'. Worm responded by inviting Stephanius to visit him again when he was next in the capital. In particular he wanted him to inspect a considerable number of Roman and Danish coins he had recently acquired for his collection.[53]

Worm also made good use of his friends and contacts on the Faeroe Islands and Iceland in obtaining objects for his museum. In May 1625 he thanked the minister in Thorshavn, Hans Rasmussen, for remembering his collection of 'curious natural objects'. Telling him his museum had benefitted from a supply of rare mussels which the Stadtholder of the islands had sent him, Worm encouraged Rasmussen to collect different species of fish, birds, and shells for him, which he considered rare.[54] A year later Worm received a variety of stones from Thorlak Skulason, the Bishop of Holar on Iceland. Among them was an eagle-stone or aetite, which Skulason considered to be pregnant because it contained another smaller stone inside; an emerald-coloured flint stone; plus two whitish pebbles, which when ground together produced flames, but failed to generate fire when hit against steel. Worm thanked him for this contribution to his 'cabinet of natural objects'. He claimed it had served to extend it considerably, which, if not just excessive politeness, would indicate that the collection was still in its infancy. Worm took the opportunity to put Skulason right on a number of points. What he labelled as an eagle-stone was, in

51 For the view that these objects defied rational explanation, see Daston and Park, *Wonders*, 244. For the importance and significance of the Book of Nature for Protestants, see P. Harrison, *The Bible, Protestantism, and the Rise of Natural Science*, Cambridge 1998.
52 *Breve fra og til Ole Worm*, no. 174.
53 *Ibid.*, nos. 194 and 196.
54 *Ibid.*, no. 198.

fact, a type of sea-bean which was often sold as eagle-stone. It was softer than stone and could be ground into a flour. Worm already owned shells which contained these fruits. He was, however, highly appreciative of the emerald-coloured flint-stone, which was very rare. The white pebbles were also found in Denmark and Worm thought they were what Aristotle called pyrimachoi.[55]

Around this time Worm was given a skeleton to 'adorn his museum', which had originally been donated to the university by the royal physician, Henning Arsinæus.[56] Otherwise, more modest natural objects continued to dominate what Worm received for his museum at this stage. His student Christen Stougaard sent him a couple of curiosities while residing in London. Even if they were not valuable Stougaard considered them worth attention. He forwarded three fossilised mussels plus several pieces of wood, some of which had begun to fossilise, others which were half-fossilised, like stone on the outside, but like wood on the inside, and finally those which had turned into a stony mass because of the sea and its salinity. Worm promised to find a place for these objects among his rarities, even if he pointed out that the fossilised wood would quickly rot or dissolve when in contact with the air.[57]

In 1628 Worm began to collect man-made objects – artificiosa. He received a chess set from Iceland probably made from walrus tooth, and he began collecting coins. He told his friend Bertel Knudsen Aquilonius that the coin he had given him had Arabic lettering similar to some already in his collection. Worm was still hoping to find a coin inscribed with runes.[58]

By 1629 Worm's cabinet of curiosity had clearly become important enough to be shown to foreign visitors. Among the first was the Dutch physician, Johannes Narssius, recently appointed royal physician to King Gustavus Adolphus of Sweden. He had enjoyed the occasion so much that he wanted Worm to show his 'wonderful objects' to the Swedish antiquarian and polymath Johannes Bureus, who was soon to arrive in Copenhagen. Worm responded that there was nothing in his cabinet of curiosity he would not happily show Bureus.[59] If Bureus undertook the planned visit to Worm's cabinet of curiosity, he and Worm would have had plenty to discuss from runes and antiquarianism to Paracelsianism and mysticism.[60]

55 *Ibid.*, nos. 204 and 219.
56 *Ibid.*, no. 208.
57 *Ibid.*, nos. 223 and 256.
58 *Ibid.*, no. 245; see *Museum Wormianum*, 377, see also Schepelern, *Museum*, 307; the single chess-piece of the king made from walrus tooth is probably what little has survived of this set, see Mordhorst, *Genstandsfortællinger*, 31. For the coins, see *Ibid.*, nos. 250–51.
59 *Ibid.*, nos. 267–68.
60 For Johannes Bureus see Håkan Håkansson, 'Alchemy of the Ancient Goths: Johannes Bureus's Search for the Lost Wisdom of Scandinavia' in *Early Science and Medicine*, 17,

If the visit took place it did not result in any correspondence between the two men. Johannes Narssius was among the first of a growing group of foreign visitors who took the opportunity to visit Ole Worm's cabinet of curiosity when in Copenhagen. Later Worm appears to have started a visitors-book for guests to his museum, not dissimilar to Aldrovandi's book of visitors. A contemporary reported that 'many royal persons and envoys visiting Copenhagen ask to see the museum on account of its great fame and what it relates from foreign lands and they wonder and marvel at what they see'.[61]

By the autumn of 1629 Worm had begun looking for more unusual and exotic objects for his museum. Thus, he asked his friend Otto Sperling to check whether it was true that a skeleton of a giant had been discovered a couple of years earlier when foundations were dug for a new mill on the estate of Selsø. If so, Worm wanted to recover a few bones for his collection.[62] Not surprisingly nothing came of this inquiry. However, Worm was later able to include a tooth from a giant in his museum which he acquired from the Bishop of Aalborg, Christen Hansen Riber.[63]

The number of distinguished visitors to Worm's museum would appear to have increased considerably by 1634. The French diplomat Charles Ogier and another member of the embassy who attended the wedding of the elected-prince in September 1634, François de Fleury, visited Worm after having attended his lecture on Hippocrates. In his account of the trip Charles Ogier mentioned that they visited Worm at his house and that he showed them many unusual things especially books without specifically mentioning a cabinet of curiosity. Perhaps Worm's collection was too modest at this point to be considered a museum by a learned diplomat like Ogier? The Frenchmen were particularly impressed by a large relic container made of mountain crystal and filled with a variety of relics which Worm had been given by a Swedish army captain who had obtained it as booty while serving in Germany. De Fleury later asked Worm in a letter from Stockholm to donate this object to them because it was of greater value to Catholics than Protestants.[64]

Worm not only received further exotic, natural objects from Otto Sperling in 1636, such as amianthus from Cyprus, a type of asbestos with long

---

no. 5, 2012 and the same, *Vid Tidens Ände. Om stormaktstidens vidunderliga dröm-värld och en profet vid dess yttersta rand*, Halmstad 2014

61 Cited in Findlen, *Possessing Nature*, 137; see also Arthur MacGregor, 'Collectors and Collections of Rarities in the Sixteenth and Seventeenth Centuries', 80 in Arthur MacGregor, *Tradescant's Rarities: Essays on the Foundation of the Ashmolean Museum 1683*, Oxford University Press 1983.

62 *Breve fra og til Ole Worm*, no. 303; Worm was clearly getting impatient for an answer from Sperling, pointedly stating in his next letter: 'What am I to expect concerning the skeleton of the giant?' *Ibid.*, no. 314.

63 *Museum Wormianum*, 43 and Schepelern, *Museum*, 151.

64 *Ibid.*, no. 540; and Schepelern, *Museum*, 158–60

silky fibres considered incombustible, but he also borrowed Sperling's copy of Francisco Calzolari's *Musæum naturalis et moralis philosophiæ.* Thanking him, Worm apologised for his impatience in receiving the book, but excused his keenness in seeing and touching such a valuable and rare item. He begged Sperling to let him hang on to the book for a while so he could fully enjoy and explore it.[65]

From 1637 Worm benefitted in particular from objects sent to him by his nephews and his other students studying abroad. From Leiden Henrik Fuiren sent him the bristles of an American hog. Worm planned to include them among his rarities referring to Henrik Fuiren by name. He was convinced the hog was called Zachinus by the Indians, but otherwise known as Coya Metl.[66] The following year Thomas Bartholin sent him a couple of tortoises from India.[67] From Amsterdam his student Niels Bertelsen Wichmand sent him an Indian nut, three calabashes, sea apples, the tooth of the Indian animal Odonda, an Egyptian Canistra, and a rosary.[68] Another student in Leiden, Jørgen Eilersen, sent him a stunning collection of shells.[69]

By June 1639, Worm's nephew Thomas Bartholin proved a particularly valuable contributor to his cabinet of curiosity. Evidently having developed excellent contacts in Leiden Thomas Bartholin managed to obtain one of the large pods from the Brazilian Cassia tree which had been donated to the botanical garden in Leiden by Willem Piso, physician to Prince Mouritz, Governor of East India for the States General. It had been difficult for Bartholin to 'wrest' the pod from the gardener. Bartholin understood that no cleansing quality in this Cassia had been discovered, as opposed to what was generally assumed. Piso claimed that there were forests of these trees in Brazil, and when the wind made the pods clash they made such a noise that they scared passing sailors. Bartholin had discovered that the eastern variety differed from the western both in size and shape, the former was flatter the latter more round. Worm was flattered and excited by the gift of the 'American Cassia' which he promised to 'permanently exhibit among the rarer fruits in his museum with Bartholin's name attached'. He mentioned that Otto Sperling had already given him a pod, but that it was nowhere near as beautiful, nor large. However, had Worm not been told that it grew on trees, he would have been inclined to think that it was the Brazilian bean mentioned by Carolus Clusius in his *Exotica*, especially since it lacked the

---

65 *Ibid.*, nos. 580–83. If Worm had visited Calzolari's museum on his academic travels at the start of the century he would surely have referred to this in his exchange with Sperling.
66 *Ibid.*, no. 633; see also *Museum Wormianum*, 340 and Schepelern, *Museum*, 151.
67 *Ibid.*, nos. 716 and 722.
68 *Ibid.*, no. 721 and Schepelern, *Museum*, 150.
69 *Ibid.*, no. 749; another student in Leiden, Hans Leyel also sent shells for Worm's museum, no. 792.

cleansing power which Cassia was supposed to have. Firmly dedicated to observation and experiment Worm concluded that the only way to prove whether it was the Cassia or the bean was by cutting it up.[70]

Worm also received some rather odd objects for his cabinet of curiosity. His friend Henrik Køster sent him a sealed chest containing a folded napkin with a flat bread 'which the Persians eat not by using a knife but by pulling it apart lengthwise with their hands'. Presumably it was a glass case so the content could be seen – one can only wonder when this pita bread would have gone mouldy.[71] In January 1640 Worm received a whole collection of objects from the minister Laurits Christensen Bording in Ribe. Worm offered to pay him his expenses thanking him for adding to his collection. Among them were a sea horse, different from the one he already owned. A fish labelled sea hen, which Gessner named cuculus marimus and which Worm thought might be related to cataphractus, even if there were differences. It also contained Indian coins of which Worm already possessed some, an eagle stone, a small piece of Japanese paper, of which Worm already owned two sheets, and some material which looked like a spider's web. Worm thought this was rare even if he remembered that he had seen much of it 'flying in the air the previous summer', but planned to include something about its emergence in his museum history which he was working on.[72]

Once more, during the summer of 1640 while awaiting transport by boat from Vlissingen to Paris, Thomas Bartholin was in a position to send his uncle in Copenhagen some rare and valuable objects for his museum. The most precious object in the package was a bird of paradise unusually with its legs preserved. Birds of paradise had been the focus for natural historical curiosity and aesthetic desire in Europe since 1522, when five skins of the lesser bird of paradise had reached the Continent. Portuguese sailors later brought back bird of paradise skins from Indonesia. Their richly coloured plumes captivated European imaginations, as did the fact that they had no legs, because they had been removed during their preservation. This gave rise to speculation that the birds, unable to alight, remained perpetually in flight, suspended between heaven and earth. Worm was delighted with his bird of paradise, 'especially because it had legs', which most commentators denied. Worm was, however, concerned that his nephew bought him such expensive gifts.

Bartholin also included some Chinese fans made of silk paper, pointing out that fans made in normal paper was all the fashion among the ladies in the Netherlands. Among the other objects was a Brazilian root used for

---

70 *Ibid.*, nos. 780 and 795.
71 *Ibid.*, nos. 815 and 817.
72 *Ibid.*, no. 823; this is only the second time Worm referred to his work on his museum history, which was published as *Museum Wormianum* in 1655. In June 1639 he had told Arngrim Jonsson that he had yet to finish this work, see no. 787.

food and named Patart (potato) by the inhabitants; they added the bread, which Bartholin included, baked from the root Cassava (as they call it) after all the juice has been squeezed out of it because of its poisonous qualities. Bartholin was unable to label the red and black beans in the parcel, because the sailors from whom he had obtained them had no knowledge of them. However, the black nut he included was from a tree locally known as Papaya. This was a major contribution to his uncle's cabinet of curiosity and Worm was extremely appreciative. Unfortunately the messenger had broken off the head and one of the wings of the bird of paradise and damaged some of its feathers. He had also managed to break the most beautiful of the fans. The experience caused Ole Worm to complain about students as irresponsible when it came to delivering letters and items for his collection, as opposed to merchants who were far more reliable and careful.[73]

From the later Bishop of Oslo, Niels Bang, Worm received a dagger plus buckles all made in narwhale tusk in June 1641. Despite expressing his appreciation and promising to exhibit them with Niels Bang's name in his cabinet of curiosity Worm eventually forgot to do so, when referring to them in *Museum Wormianum*.[74] By now Ole Worm seems to have received a steady stream of objects from friends and colleagues, often single objects such as the lump of copper from Stephanius which was included in the collection of minerals, the 'artfully worked glass threads' from the schoolmaster in Landskrona, and a handle for a dagger made of jasper which was supposed to have belonged to Luther's brother, the physician Paul Luther. Henrik Motzfeld studying in Wittenberg had obtained the latter from Luther's grandson.[75] This was evidently as good a souvenir as a Lutheran physician could hope for, and Worm was extremely grateful. It was to be placed among the 'exceptional' objects in his cabinet of curiosity. Motzfeld had also sent some balls from a garland which had belonged to Luther's brother, Paul, which were also much appreciated. Typically for Worm, he examined his gifts meticulously. He was unable to determine whether the jasper came from the East Indies or Bohemia, but he considered it of good quality coming close to a 'heliotrope because of its drops of blood and blood vessels'. As such Worm was convinced that it might be able to cure haemorrhages. He concluded that the stone had been shaped as a handle for a dagger by a craftsman, but never fixed to a blade because no hole had been drilled in it for fixing. Worm also noted that the black ball from Paul Luther's garland had been kneaded together by perfumed materials.[76] Motzfeld provided

73 *Ibid.*, nos. 851 and 883; see also Schepelern, *Museum*, 163 and *Museum Wormianum*, 294–95. Already in 1641 Worm used one of his medical disputations to point out that the common perception that the bird of paradise had no legs was wrong using a drawing of the bird Bartholin had sent him. He reproduced the same in *Museum Wormianum*.
74 *Ibid.*, no. 949; see also Schepelern, *Museum*, 155 and 157.
75 *Ibid.*, nos. 1092, 1102, and 1100.
76 *Ibid.*, no. 1118

further items for the museum in February 1645 when he forwarded coins plus two wax portraits of Luther and Melanchthon which unfortunately were broken in transit.[77]

3 The friendship with Johannes de Laet

It was Ole Worm's antiquarian publications which led the polymath and director of the Dutch West India Company, Johannes de Laet, to write to him in March 1642 seeking information relating to his own Anglo-Saxon interests. Early on, however, Worm made sure that their exchange increasingly focussed on the collection of natural objects. He informed de Laet that he had heard that the Dutchman owned many exotic articles which had been brought back from America. These Worm would be extremely keen to examine. He explained that he himself had managed to gather 'a not insignificant collection of different objects'. Worm, who owned a copy of Johannes de Laet's *History of the New World* or description of the West Indies, had compared the description and illustration of the animal named Haut in that book with the illustration of the Ignavus (sloth) in Carolus Clusius's work, wondering whether or not the two were identical. Worm was convinced that de Laet would be able to answer this question, because he possessed such exotic objects in considerable numbers. Worm, however, despite having spent considerable time and energy in collecting natural objects had so far been unable to find such items. Implicitly there was an unstated expectation in Worm's letters that Johannes de Laet might be able to remedy this situation. To facilitate this Worm offered to supply de Laet with a catalogue of his collection when the opportunity arose.[78]

In 1642 Worm published the first of two small catalogues of his collection. They were intended for other collectors and natural philosophers as a source of information and reference, especially if they wanted to exchange or donate items. Entitled *Musæi Wormiani Catalogus Anni MDCXLII* the first catalogue listed more than a thousand objects divided into four groups similar to that of his museum history, *Museum Wormianum*, published in 1655.[79] Worm distributed a number of copies of this catalogue to friends and contacts during the summer of 1642. Johannes de Laet thanked him

---

77 *Ibid.*, nos. 1283 and 1295.

78 *Ibid.*, nos. 1019, 1031, and 1040; Jan de Laet published his *History of the New World* in 1625, *Nieuwe Wereldt Beschrijvinghe van West-Indien*, Leiden 1625; a second edition entitled *Beschrijvinghe van West-Indien door Johannes de Laet*, Leiden 1630. Worm acquired the Latin edition published in 1633 via his nephew Henrik Fuiren, then a student in Leiden, see no. 596. For Jan de Laet, see Jaap Jacobs, 'Johannes de Laet (1581–1649): Leiden Polymath,' *Lias* 25, no.2 (1998), 135–229; and Rolf H. Bremmer, 'The Correspondence of Johannes de Laet (1581–1649) as a Mirror of his Life', *Lias* 25, no. 2, 1998, 139–64.

79 Schepelern, *Museum*, 166–68; The catalogue consists of only 34 pages; for other recipients, see nos. 1056, 1058, and 1065.

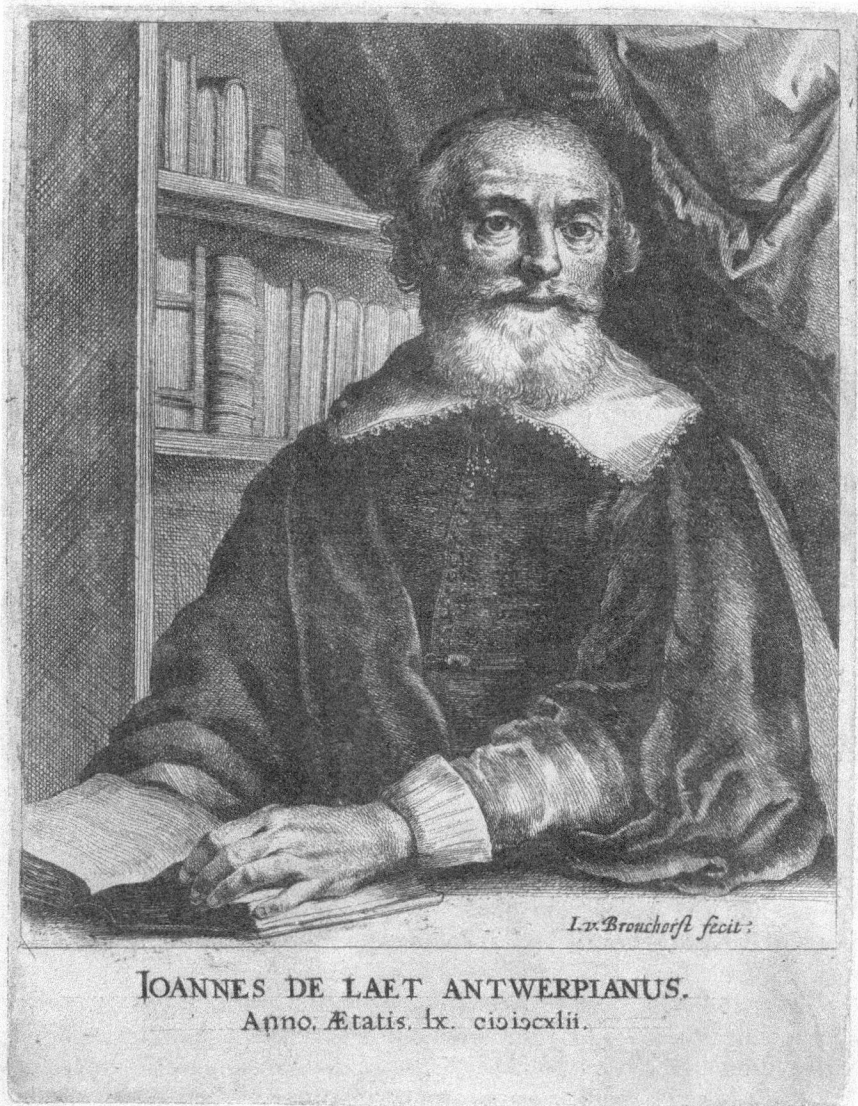

Figure 4.3 Johannes de Laet (1581–1649) by I van Bronchhorst 1642; courtesy of the Royal Danish Library.

for his copy in August, commenting that Worm had organised his museum 'quite well'. de Laet explained that he too had been collecting natural objects, but that he did not display them in an organised manner, because he did not want to be obliged to show them to unwanted visitors whom he could not refuse without insulting them. He would create a catalogue if he could find the time, indicating that this was not his top priority. One can only assume that a glut of visitors, who would have been an inconvenience in cosmopolitan Leiden, would not have been an issue in Copenhagen. However, if Worm would inform him what he was missing from each of his categories, de Laet would be keen to help him. In the meantime he sent him some smaller objects.[80] An exchange of natural objects and letters followed. Worm undoubtedly proved the winner when it came to the exchange of natural objects, for the simple reason that de Laet had virtually unrestricted access to objects arriving in the Netherlands from the New World while also proving a generous friend.[81]

In March 1643 he informed Worm that the rosary he had recently sent him was made from American balsam, and the elongated fruit was a type of oblong pepper from the same part of the world. de Laet had noted Worm's complaint that he only had very few of the natural objects described in de Laet's American history, but took the opportunity to point out that he himself did not have them all. In some cases he had relied on the description of others. A practice which was considered acceptable by natural historians of the period. However, if Worm could draw up a list of the items he wanted, de Laet promised to make an effort to obtain them. Meanwhile, he sent some objects which Worm would be able to compare with the illustrations in his book. He also included another type of Lapis Nephriticus which was highly valued in the Netherlands. Johannes de Laet had often tried the properties of a similar object on his wife. He was clearly valuing its supposed diuretic qualities as a remedy against bladder and kidney stones. The small precious stone Worm called the eye of the world de Laet identified as a type of opal, because he had conducted similar experiments with others. They tended to regain their opaqueness relatively slowly, similar to what he had observed in the stone Worm had sent him. He remembered having seen a totally different opal at a jeweller in the Netherlands which was opaque like a small piece of bone, but became transparent fairly rapidly. The jeweller had refused to sell it and had given it a name de Laet had now forgotten.[82]

In May 1643 Ole Worm expressed his profound gratitude to Johannes de Laet for the generosity he had shown him. He was only able to reciprocate with a number of modest, smaller items originating from the Faroe Islands and Norway, but he took the opportunity of informing de Laet that he had so far been unable to obtain the tiny bird, huitzitzelin or tominia (hummingbird) and the fruit known as ahovay, evidently hoping for de Laet's assistance in obtaining them. As always Johannes de Laet proved helpful.

---

80 *Breve fra og til Ole Worm*, no. 1072;
81 29 objects are listed in *Museum Wormianum* as having been donated by Jan de Laet, see Schepelern, *Museum*, 173.
82 *Breve fra og til Ole Worm*, no. 1112.

The Dutchman emphasised that so far he had never possessed more than one specimen of the tiny hummingbird. Unfortunately he had neglected to sprinkle it, and many other small birds which he had collected over the years, with hops with the result that moths had consumed all their feathers. He promised to try to obtain the ahovay fruit through friends in Brazil. Johannes de Laet also addressed Ole Worm's query whether or not the two animals, Ignavus and Haut/Haythi were one and the same, but without offering much clarification. Some years back he had seen a live specimen of the sloth called Ignavus in the Netherlands, and like everyone else had been amazed at how slowly it moved, but unfortunately it did not survive for long. De Laet confirmed Clusius's illustration of Ignavus as correct. The illustration of the Haut/Haythi in his own work de Laet had borrowed from Andreas Thevetus's *Les Singularitez de la France antarctique autrement nommée Amérique* .... Those, however, who had seen it alive had told him, that it did not look like the illustration. It moved so slowly that it hardly covered half a mile in eight days; at times it was spending five or more months in the top of a tree, which the 'barbarians' call Ambaiba, eating its leaves. Despite their likeness in character, shape, and manner their names were distinct and different, but de Laet promised to try and find the truth.[83]

By the end of 1643 the contacts between Johannes de Laet and Ole Worm would appear to have faded. The fact that de Laet had acquired Georg Marcgraf's manuscript for his *Historia Naturalis Brasiliae* on the latter's death in 1644, with a view to edit and publish it, may go some way to explain this. Marcgrave had written his manuscript in cipher and de Laet had to put in a considerable amount of work to crack the code.[84]

To reinvigorate his contacts with Johannes de Laet Ole Worm encouraged some of his students to seek him out during their time in Leiden to convey his greetings, but more importantly to remind de Laet that Worm was hoping to receive a number of objects for his cabinet of curiosity. In October 1644 Worm urged his Icelandic student Gisli Magnussen to seek out de Laet, who, he thought, might well be keen to discuss the Icelandic language with him. A couple of years later he asked Thomas Bartholin to look up de Laet before he returned home from Leiden and convey Worm's good wishes to him. Significantly, Worm also wanted Thomas to ask de Laet if there were any exotic articles he would like him to forward to Worm. The visit proved a success and Bartholin gave Johannes de Laet his own copy of the new catalogue of Worm's collection which had been printed in 1645, so he could check what was missing from Worm's museum.[85]

83 *Ibid.*, nos. 1127 and 1138; for the work used by de Laet, see Andreas Thevetus, *Les Singularitez de la France antarctique autrement nommée Amérique* ..., Paris 1558.
84 See Harold. J. Cook, *Matters of Exchange. Commerce, Medicine, and Science in the Dutch Golden Age*, New Haven 2007, 210–16.
85 *Ibid.*, no. 1408.

As a result of this visit the correspondence between de Laet and Worm picked up again. de Laet had been delighted to hear that Worm was working on his museum history which he was convinced would prove of public benefit, providing valuable information about the objects displayed. Worm responded by telling de Laet that he had, in fact, finished a description of all the objects he had collected, but there was still a lot to do before he could contemplate publication, not least because of so many generous donations of friends such as de Laet, as could be seen from his most recent catalogue, not to mention all the items Johannes de Laet had recently sent him.

The new 1645 catalogue served its purpose, because de Laet started to go through what he himself had collected over the years in order to find articles which Worm was missing. By doing so de Laet realised that he needed some sort of register for his collection which apparently was widely dispersed. He promised to send Worm a copy when it was finished.

Meanwhile, de Laet was filling a chest with items which were missing from Worm's cabinet of curiosity. These he would give to Thomas Bartholin for safe transport. The trunk contained the bones of a hand and the rib of a sea monster common along the coast of Angola, and known among the Portugese as Perxe de Moliher, meaning siren or mermaid. de Laet was expecting to receive a picture of the live creature shortly, adding that the pellets turned from the ribs of this sea monster were supposed to be a perfect remedy against haemorrhoids. He had taken the trouble of making a list for Ole Worm of the content of the chest. He would also be able to provide Worm with further information about some of the objects, but for the majority he only had a name. A number of shells were included for which no names were provided, but which could easily be identified from the works of among others Aldrovandi. Of greater significance was the inclusion in the trunk of the brain of a shark (canis carcharia or lamia). In powdered form it had proved especially useful for expelling kidney-stones, even if de Laet warned that it should be used with care.

Johannes de Laet also informed Worm that his book on jewels and stones was nearly finished. He intended to include illustrations of the many petrified shells he had received from friends in France and England. Bearing in mind the disagreement among scholars of natural history about their origin he wanted Worm's opinion. In this he was not disappointed. Worm spelled out three scenarios. First, there was the natural stone which had taken the shape of a living creature or part of another natural or artificial object. Second, there was what had previously been a plant, artificial item, or animal, which had been turned into stone. Third, there was the object which in essence remained unchanged, but have had a stony surface added. Worm was convinced that the genesis of these three categories differed. The genesis of stones, which materially were stones, but were imitating different objects, were no different from normal stones, apart from the place they had been created. When a stone-making juice fall on a place where previously a foot rested, a head, or similar, then it would reproduce its shape. However, when an item was turned into stone, Worm was convinced that a salty, stone-making, and fine spirit had penetrated the object's pores and combined with the object's inborn moisture to turn it into a stone. Because the stone-making spirits differed some stones were hard, others soft and disintegrating. The last kind, which should probably be called the crusted, struck Worm as being produced not through a solidifying spirit, but through a liquid full of tartar. When an object fell into such a liquid, often at hot springs, then the phlegm of the juice evaporated through an interior or exterior heat which left the tartar sitting on the object as one or many crusts. Worm had several examples of this in his museum.[86]

Johannes de Laet agreed with Worm's view of petrification and took the opportunity to inform his friend in Copenhagen that he had received several tongue-stones or glossopetrae from Bordeaux where they had grown. A learned friend of his claimed that these stones could alleviate the pain from inflammation and blisters in the mouth caused by unclean food or the bitterness and acidity of liquids. One of the stones should be placed in spring water whereupon it would generate bubbles in the water. When settled the water should be used for gargling two to three times a day until the pain and inflammation disappeared. de Laet had yet to undertake his own experiment because he had no access to spring water, but he intended to try with water from his well.

Worm discussed this report with Thomas Bartholin who was excited about the observations and wanted to include them in his work about tongue-stones, promising to acknowledge de Laet.[87] Worm also provided an opinion of the pebbles Johannes de Laet had received. They were two types, one black like agate or marble, the other looked like linseed, shaped like an eye, compact but hollow. According to de Laet they were able to extract grit from the eyes. When one of these pebbles were placed in the eye it moved around without causing pain and when it encountered what was damaging the eye it attracted it and enclosed it in its cavity. The one which looked like linseed had proved the most efficient. According to de Laet they both looked like highly polished marble or precious stones from a jeweller's shop.

Worm was convinced that the pebbles or stones were Lapides Bufonius, known as toadstones coming from the head of the toad, and Chelidonius, known as swallow-stones, coming from the stomach of the swallow. Worm

86 *Ibid.*, no. 1462; see also E. Hoch, 'Diagnosing Fossilization in the Nordic Renaissance: An Investigation into the Correspondence of Ole Worm (1588–1654)', 307–27 in C. J. Duffin et al. (eds.), *A History of Geology and Medicine*, Geological Special Publication no. 375, London 2013.

87 Thomas Bartholin had written *De glossopteris Melitensibus dissertatio* in 1644. He never published his unfinished manuscript on the tongue-stones which was lost when his library burnt in 1670, see Thomas Bartholin, *On the Burning of his Library and on Medical Travel*, ed. Charles D. O'Malley, Lawrence 1961.

identified the black agate similar to stones as toadstones, referring to Anselm Boethius de Boodt, but adding that Johannes de Laet himself had identified them as such in his recent work on stones. The other kind that had the colour of linseed, Worm thought, were swallow-stones, referring once again to Boethius. Having had to identify them from the drawings provided by de Laet, Worm emphasised that it was far more difficult to ascertain natural objects under such circumstances than when handled directly, so he wanted to know whether or not de Laet agreed. Worm already possessed some swallow-stones from Malta, where they were believed to be snake eyes turned into stones. This, however, could not be the case because Worm owned a spectacular lump of three or four which Thomas Bartholin had brought back for him from Malta. He was not surprised that they could extract foreign bodies when placed in the eyes, since he knew of other similar shaped stones less smooth having the same effect. Worm had achieved a similar result with the so-called crayfish eyes, which were not eyes but pebbles or stones sitting along the bellies of lobsters.[88]

In his letter from June 1646, Johannes de Laet had taken the opportunity to inform Worm that he had taken possession of George Marcgrave's description of all the animals and plants in Brazil. It was supplied with fine drawings of most of the animals and plants. De Laet was keen to have it published, but was held back by a shortage of craftsmen who could turn the drawings, of which there were nearly 500, into woodcuts. He hoped to solve the problem over time in order that he could publish at least some of the manuscript. Worm was excited about the prospect of the publication of a natural history of Brazil, which he was convinced would reveal many new rarities. By seeking to accelerate its publication Johannes de Laet, in his opinion, would be of the greatest service to all those interested in natural history.[89]

In July 1647 Johannes de Laet reported to Worm that the editing and printing of *Historia Naturalis Brasiliae* was finally progressing with some speed, even if he could not guarantee that the work would be published before the onset of winter. Three books about plants had been printed as had one about fish and one about birds, while the printing of the book about the four-legged animals had begun. This would be followed by the book on insects and the last book about the inhabitants. Four of the 500 woodcuts had finally been produced despite a shortage of qualified artists. Johannes de Laet was rightly proud of his achievement and convinced that Worm would take delight in the finished work. Worm did not have to wait long. Marcgrave's *Historia Naturalis Brasiliae*, edited by de Laet, was published in Amsterdam the following year. Worm's nephew, Erasmus

---

88 *Breve fra og til Ole Worm*, nos. 1512 and 1513; Worm referred to Anselm Boethius de Boodt, *Gemmarum et Lapidum Historia*, Hannover 1609.
89 *Ibid.*, nos. 1430 and 1462.

Bartholin received a copy from de Laet for his uncle, which he had had bound before sending it to Copenhagen.[90] Worm was ecstatic, thanking de Laet for 'a golden book extremely useful for everyone who has an interest in rare natural objects'. Always eager to augment or improve his collection Worm enquired whether anything new had arrived from America. He also took the opportunity to remind de Laet that he had promised to help him obtain the Ourisia and the Ahovay. Worm informed Johannes de Laet that some birds-nests made of what looked like fish glue had arrived in Copenhagen. They were dissolved in soup and given to those who wanted to be 'eager warriors for Venus', in other words a love potion. Worm wanted to know from which birds they originated and from where they came.

The war in Brazil between the Dutch and the Portuguese had seen the arrival of new natural objects from that part of the world dry up. De Laet had no memory of having promised to help Worm obtain the Ourisia, but he was busy trying to find the Ahovay both for himself and Worm. De Laet was able to tell Worm that the birds-nests came from the Coromandel Coast in India where they were made by 'small birds building these half-circular nests of a sticky material'. Like the swallows they attached them to inaccessible, and steep boulders, where the natives pulled them down and sold them at great profit. No agreement existed, according to de Laet, about the effect on those who ate them, even if some claimed that they worked as a love potion. They were considered a delicacy when dissolved in soup and eaten with a fork. de Laet had relied on two former governors of these provinces for his information, thereby adding further credibility to his information.

De Laet intended to write something about stone plants which grew in the sea and wanted the assistance of Ole Worm. He had been told that a wealth of them could be found along the coast of Norway and was keen to hear what Worm had observed. Finally, he enclosed a copy of the catalogue of his collection of natural objects. He emphasised that it was still a work in progress, but forwarded it to Worm for his personal use. Worm was delighted and amazed to find a number of objects unknown to him. He also realised that the Ourisia bird he was missing in his collection was listed by de Laet under the name Hvitzitvil or the tiny bird Tomineus.

Like de Laet Worm was having difficulties preserving the plumage of the birds in his museum. He had already lost some of his finest birds and was particularly concerned for his Gvara Brasiliana and his precious paradise bird with feet. He had tried hops, wormwood, and even steam from sulphur with little success.

The wood de Laet labelled Nephriticum Brasilianum had, according to Worm, none of the characteristics of the real Nephrit. It did not colour

---

90 *Ibid.*, nos. 1512, 1513, 1572, 1575, and 1577. See also G. Marcgravius, *Historiæ rerum naturalium Brasiliæ, libri VIII*, Amsterdam 1648 (edited by Johannes de Laet).

water, when plunged into it, and differed in colour from the real Nephrit, which was light and whitish, while this was heavy and black. Worm thought that it could not be labelled as a Nephrit, unless de Laet through experiment and observation had determined that it expelled stones. Worm was also very grateful for the details de Laet had provided about the birds-nests, especially since no one else could offer him any information about them. Consequently Worm wanted to include the paragraph about the nests in de Laet's letter in his forthcoming museum history. Concerning Johannes de Laet's inquiry about stone-plants Worm referred him to his own catalogue. Some stone-plants he had a number of and he was happy to share them with de Laet.

In what proved to be his last surviving letter to Worm, dated 2 November 1648, Johannes de Laet informed him that he had finally obtained the Avohay fruit for him which he enclosed with his letter. He admitted that the labelling in his draft catalogue might well be problematic since he had been short of time and unable to verify them against descriptions by reliable authors. Concerning the preservation of the plumage of birds de Laet knew of no other remedy than hops, but they had to be renewed annually. They would preserve the plumage for years, but in the long run de Laet was convinced that these things could not survive the ravages of time. He agreed with Worm's observations about the Brazilian Nephrit-wood as being different from the variety from 'New-Spain' (Mexico). It was, however, a root rather than wood and had the same quality as the Mexican variety. de Laet referred Worm to his recently published *Historia Naturalis Brasiliae*.[91] The correspondence appears to have stopped around this time. A year later Ole Worm encouraged his nephew, Erasmus Bartholin, then a student in Leiden to seek out de Laet, who had not responded to his last letter, and convey his greetings. This was a similar approach to the one taken in 1644 when contacts had faded. As always Worm was not one for missing an opportunity telling Erasmus to remind de Laet that if he had received new objects from India not to forget his friend in Copenhagen. This time, however, it proved too late because Johannes de Laet had died in The Hague before Erasmus could contact him.[92] In his museum history Worm eventually listed Johannes de Laet as having donated thirty objects to his cabinet of curiosity,

---

91 *Ibid.*, nos. 1606 and 1613
92 *Ibid.*, nos. 1667 and 1670; see also Bremmer, 'Johannes de Laet', 161. Worm was constantly trying to find a better way to preserve the birds in his collection. In May 1649 one of his students informed him that he had visited a museum in Orléans belonging to a canon named Tardificus. Among his collection were some tiny birds from India whose feathers were wonderfully well preserved by placing a 'corrosive sublimate of ground pepper or pyrethrum' between their feathers killing the maggots which might otherwise cause their destruction, see no. 1631. Again in November 1650 when complaining to Klinger that he had lost the Eurasian bittern he used to have in his collection to 'moths and worms', Worm reminded him how he had so far been unable to find a remedy to preserve the beautiful birds in his museum from bore worms in particular. Worm would

making him by far the largest donor. Only Worm's nephew, Thomas Bartholin, came close, having donated twenty objects.[93]

A postscript was provided when Ole Worm's son Willum newly arrived in Leiden in the summer of 1653 managed to buy Georg Marcgrave's herbarium which had belonged to Johannes de Laet and was described in de Laet's edition of Marcgrave's *Historia Naturalis Brasiliae*. Worm was delighted when he received the herbarium emphasising how valuable and rare it was. It arrived just in time to be included in his museum history.[94]

4 The cabinet of curiosity takes shape

Ole Worm would appear to have intensified his efforts in obtaining objects for his cabinet of curiosity in the years following the publication of his first museum catalogue in 1642. Thus, he approached his friend Henrik Køster after having heard a rumour that Køster's son, studying in Königsberg, kept some liquids in a glass which rose with the sun and sank at sunset, not to mention some other marvels. Worm was keen to know how this was done and eager to obtain such an object for his museum. Køster informed Worm that the object in question belonged to his son's host, but he could bring the artefact back for him, when he returned the following spring. He added that Worm no doubt knew that the Paduan professor, Sanctorius, had observed the temperature in a container of liquid – the so-called thermoscope.[95]

Bearing in mind how diligent Ole Worm was in distributing his museum catalogue to friends and students it is surprising that by the autumn of 1643 he had yet to supply his nephew, Thomas Bartholin, with a copy. Not least because Thomas had already shown himself keen on obtaining objects for his uncle on his peregrinatio academica. Thomas's presence in Italy clearly provided Worm with access to objects otherwise outside his reach. However, another nephew, Bertel Bartholin, provided Worm with interesting news about the hummingbirds he had recently discussed with Jan de Laet. While in Paris Bertel had obtained access to an unnamed collector's cabinet of curiosity. Among other rarities he had recently observed some tiny birds of the size he had shown in his letter. He noted that the female was slightly smaller than the male. They had reached Paris from those parts of America which had been colonised by the French who had named them Mouches de Canada after that part of America. Bertel had no idea why they were called Mouches, but assumed it might be because they were not much bigger than flies or wasps or because they ate flies. He asked his uncle

be grateful if Klinger could discover some remedy from Loesel or others which could contribute to their preservation, see no. 1705.

93 Schepelern, *Museum*, 173–74

94 *Breve fra of til Ole Worm*, nos. 1742 and 1752; see also Schepelern, *Museum*, Kat 261a, and 210 and Mordhorst, *Genstandsfortællinger*, 31.

95 *Ibid.*, nos. 1161 and 1165.

to let him know if they were of any significance, adding that they were sold in Paris for hefty prices.[96] Worm was obviously fascinated, but felt no need to seek Bertel Bartholin's assistance to obtain an expensive hummingbird from Paris. Instead he pointed out to Bertel that the picture he had sent him was of the American Ourisia or hummingbird. Among a number of works Worm referred to were those of Carolus Clusius and Jan de Laet, especially the latter who mentioned several types in his work on 'Westindia'. Worm explained that de Laet over several years had donated many exotic objects to his museum and recently promised to obtain several examples of the hummingbird for him.[97]

Meanwhile, in April 1644 Thomas Bartholin had reached Messina in Sicily on his travels. Here he obtained some corals for his uncle's museum. He had also befriended the famous botanist and physician, Pietro Castelli, who in 1635 had laid out the botanical gardens at Messina where he cultivated a variety of exotic, medicinal plants. Castelli had also established a museum where he, according to Bartholin, had assembled a variety of rare natural objects. He had gathered the skeletons of animals as diverse as the musk rat and the swordfish and he exhibited several petrified shells and an Indian palm fruit which it was impossible to break. Bartholin had given him a copy of Worm's museum catalogue which he appreciated, even if his comment that it contained 'the most common apothecary seeds' would appear to have been less than positive. Thomas clearly thought so too, adding that there could be no doubt that they were necessary for the totality and diversity of nature. On his way to Messina Thomas had found time to visit Imperato's museum in Naples where he had seen the head of a swordfish; while in Messina he had visited the collection of a nobleman which contained among other items two large horns from rhinoceros' and others which were said to be from unicorns. Thomas Bartholin, however, felt unable to determine the truth of this claim, not least because it was fairly common to put horns of gazelles on craniums of horses.[98]

Around this time Ole Worm received a somewhat strange object for his museum. It was an egg which a respectable woman was supposed to have given birth to in Norway. Already a mother of twelve children the woman had fallen ill a year before she gave birth not only to one but two eggs. Assisted by her neighbours she had first given birth to the one egg which on being broken revealed the normal white and yolk. The following day she gave birth to a second egg which she begged her helpers not to break because doing so would expose both her and her neighbours to the greatest danger. Worm had been given this egg which looked like a chicken egg, except it had now lost its normal whiteness and gone dark like eggs which

96 *Ibid.*, no. 1168 for the letter from Thomas Bartholin and no. 1177 for the letter from Bertel Bartholin.
97 *Ibid.*, no.1188.
98 *Ibid.*, no. 1196.

were rotten. That the woman's name and address was known, the event was described in detail, and a public document had been signed by three reliable witnesses, implying the credibility and truthfulness of the event. Worm, however, did not believe it could have happened naturally, but was convinced that the woman had been bewitched. Significantly, not only did he exhibit the egg, but he found the event significant enough to discuss it in detail in his museum history.[99]

If it had been possible, he might have wanted to include the elephant which had arrived in Copenhagen in January 1640. This female elephant, which had been brought to the city by a merchant, clearly impressed Worm with its size and cleverness. He claimed it could do things with its trunk which no man could do better with his hands. It jumped and danced and could challenge its adversaries with a sword, bend its knees, clean itself with a brush, dry itself with a towel, and put a hat on and take it off again. It allowed people to sit on it and it more or less did everything its master ordered it to do. It had proved an occurrence of such magnitude that the elected-prince set out for Copenhagen with his wife to see the animal.[100]

Worm proved impressively proactive in obtaining items for his cabinet of curiosity during the 1640s. He explained to Jens Dolmer, the tutor of Christian IV's son, Ulrik Christian Gyldenløve, that he had recently been given a fine Scythian bow by the Emperor's ambassador when the latter had visited his museum. He now wanted Dolmer's help in getting the young Gyldenløve's consent in obtaining some Scythian arrows and a quiver which he had been given. 1644 would appear to have been a good year for Worm's collection when it came to ancient and decorated weaponry. From his brother-in-law Steffen Hansen Stephanius he received 'a beautifully decorated Rutherian bow'.[101] Later that year Stephanius added some 'spectacular items' from Norway to Worms 'sanctuary'. He was particularly excited by a bow which was supposed to have belonged to 'Holy Olaf' which he was convinced would be a jewel for Worm's 'cupboards', as he referred to Worm's display cabinets. A number of the objects had unfortunately been broken in transfer, such as a bush of coral, the bow, which was, in fact, not a bow, but a stone shaped as such by Nature, and one of the sea urchins. Surprisingly Worm considered 'a knotty stick' to be of exceptional value among these items without explaining why.[102] Stephanius also acted on behalf of Worm, negotiating with possible contributors to his museum, especially among his colleagues at the Academy in Sorø, such as the professor of mathematics, Hans Lauremberg. Thus, Lauremberg promised to produce a list of the rare and unusual objects he owned in order that Worm

---

99 *Ibid.*, no. 1183 and *Museum Wormianum*, 311; see also Schepelern, *Museum*, 287.
100 *Ibid.*, nos. 827 and 829.
101 *Ibid.*, no. 1210; for the Rutherian bow see nos. 1211 and 1226.
102 *Ibid.*, nos. 1244–45.

could choose what he wanted for his museum.[103] In June 1647 Stephanius sent Worm a beautifully crafted chest, designed by his father, full of rare objects. He inserted a list of them, but also added other items from his own collection after having sealed the chest. Stephanius expressed the wish that Worm would incorporate them in his cabinet of curiosity as 'a modest but permanent commemoration of their friendship'. Worm was grateful and promised to include Stephanius's name in the history of his museum. He was, however, somewhat unsure about some of the objects, but promised to place them in the sections of his museum where they belonged. As always Worm offered corrections and clarifications. The stone which looked like a loaf had never been a loaf. No virgin had ever extracted a swallow-stone from a swallow. Worm already owned several such stones originating from Malta where they were plentiful and presumed to be petrified snake eyes. The fire stone (pyrites) had a different consistency from what Stephanius presented as Gold-Minera, and from which one extracted copper not gold. Another stone which showed the eye of a cow was a particular type of marble, which children tended to play with. Even so Worm felt obliged to state that it was all most welcome and interesting.[104]

Stephanius not only donated objects to Worm's museum he also offered his expertise in cataloguing his friend's growing collection of coins and medals. He apologised to Worm in December 1647 for having been slow in fulfilling his task, explaining that he was awaiting the arrival of a couple of books by Hubert Golzius on antique medals and coins before he could finish his work. It proved a greater task than Stephanius had expected, cataloguing and describing the medals and coins. He sent Worm a catalogued page describing twenty-one coins from the reign of the younger Emperor Claudius and twenty-seven from that of Emperor Posthumus. Worm told Stephanius that he should not tire himself with long descriptions, just an indication from the inscriptions from which province and Emperor they originated. He was happy to wait for more details at a convenient time. Worm realised it was a time consuming task he had given Stephanius and that there were still 152 items to be dealt with. He would be delighted if Stephanius could master twenty a month.[105]

In September 1649 Stephanius donated the Iron Age burial urn from Vejrum to Worm, which he himself had been given by the nobleman, Just Høeg. He was convinced it had belonged to a noble woman, possibly a queen, judging from the size of the urn, and the bones and jewellery it contained.[106]

---

103 *Ibid.*, no. 1410.
104 *Ibid.*, nos. 1504 and 1510.
105 *Ibid.*, nos. 1550, 1554, and 1563.
106 *Ibid.*, no. 1654; see also Schepelern, *Museum*, 332, no. 21; and *Museum Wormianum*, 349.

Ole Worm maintained his contacts with French diplomats he had initiated in 1634, and renewed in 1644, when they travelled through Copenhagen on their way to the peace negotiations between Sweden and Denmark in Brømsebro. Through the French ambassador to Denmark, Jacques Hennequin, he managed to engineer what turned out to be a very favourable exchange of coins with Archille Harlay, Marquis de Breval, in 1649. This also brought him into contact with Pierre Chanut, the French ambassador to Sweden, who helped facilitate the exchange while taking the opportunity to express his admiration for Worm's museum. Furthermore, Chanut brought Worm and his museum to the attention of other French scholars such as the writer Louis du May not to mention his master, the Duke of Württemberg, who enjoyed visiting Worm's museum.[107]

5 The importance of the Fuiren and Bartholin nephews

From the mid-1640s Worm's nephews studying abroad became increasingly important for the expansion of his cabinet of curiosity. Not only did they find new objects for him, but they also brought him into contact with other collectors. Thus, via his nephew, Thomas Bartholin, Worm came into contact with the famous physician and anatomist, Marcus Aurelius Severinus, in Naples. In June 1644 Severinus contacted Worm praising him 'as someone who had comprehended all of Nature and recognised all its hidden secrets'. He also admired Worm's cabinet of curiosity which according to him was highly regarded in all of Italy. Severinus took the opportunity to send Worm some rare objects for his museum with his nephew, Thomas, who had been his guest.[108]

Worm also remained in close contact with another nephew, Henrik Fuiren, with whom he had extended communications about rare and unusual objects. A letter from August 1644 is particularly revealing for how Ole Worm gathered information, through texts, descriptions, observations, and critical assessment of the available information. From reading Fabio Colonna Worm had gathered that the so-called glossopetrae or tonguestones were fossilised teeth from the great white shark – canis carcharias. This made sense to him, when born in mind that in Malta where they were mainly found together with other parts of fish which had been fossilised. Worm had recently been given some rarities from Malta, among them a petrified vertebra and a lump of soil filled with that type of teeth by another of his students. These objects appeared to Worm to support Colonna's view and illustrate that in those places you found a petrifying juice or

---

107 *Ibid.*, nos. 1625, 1627, 1628, 1634, 1650, and 1651; see also Schepelern, *Museum*, 191–92; for Pierre Chanut, see O. Garstein, *Rome and the Counter-Reformation in Scandinavia. The Age of Gustavus Adolphus and Queen Christina of Sweden, 1622–1656*, Leiden 1992, 502–10.

108 *Ibid.*, nos. 1223, 1232, and 1233.

rather an exhalation which could bring this about by penetrating the bones and transforming them. However, Worm questioned whether many of the stones sold as tongue-stones were, indeed, fossilised teeth of the great white shark. When he considered where glossopetrae were found he had serious doubts. Some were found in the alum mines in Lüneburg in Germany, others on the sandy areas near Deventer, and many other places untouched by the sea and the great white shark. Worm also remembered that Calzolari had tongue-stones in his museum which had been found in the area around Verona between rocks and stony soil. He did not believe these stones had ever been shark teeth.

Furthermore, the great variations in their shape caused Worm to have further doubt about their provenance. Some had pointed edges and looked like shark teeth, others were totally smooth, some were triangular or dagger shaped, some had a hunched back very different from the real teeth of the great white shark. Then there was the colour: shark teeth were white while the tongue-stones were anything from black, via red to grey. Worm was, however, prepared to concede that the colouration might have been due to the nature of the local exhalation. But more than anything else it was their size which caused Worm to question their origin. They were so big that no fish, in his opinion, would be big enough to have them in their mouths unless they were whales. Worm had been given such a tongue-stone for his museum which was five inches long, had a circumference of a foot, and weighed six and a half ounces. It would have demanded enormous jaws to contain 200 of those, which was the number of teeth in the head of the shark Worm had in his cabinet of curiosity. Worm had noted that they were placed in three rows in both upper and lower jaw with the smallest teeth closet to the throat and the largest further forward in the mouth. The biggest teeth were no more than half an inch long, all white and jagged, and flatter than those which were supposed to be petrified. Worm therefore was of the opinion that teeth of dead fish were transformed into stone in maritime areas only, especially where lots of these fish had been present together with large quantities of mud that had petrifying power. He added that Nature through its whims produced stones of similar shapes in other places in the Mediterranean, adding that similar developments could also be observed in other objects. Thus, Worm was exhibiting peculiarly shaped flint stones in his museum, one which looked like a human torso, another which looked exactly as the left foot of a human, one which looked like a bird, one like a horn, and one like a petrified unicorn. Worm concluded that 'Nature pursued its wonderful play where it makes use of petrifying juice or air'. He considered the investigation of the 'Nature of such things and their creation to be a beautiful occupation for a free-born spirit'.

Worm informed Henrik Fuiren that he had asked Bertel Bartholin, who had recently left Padua to bring back some of the luminous stones from Bologna which 'received light from the sun in daytime and returned it during the night'. Worm was afraid that Bertel would fail to obtain these stones and therefore asked Henrik to try and get hold of some. Worm was convinced that this was what Athanasius Kircher had labelled phosphor. He was certain it would prove useful in both raw and treated form, and from reading Petrus Poterius he was also convinced it could be found in Norway, presumably the silver mine in Kongsberg.[109]

Petrus Poterius, a French, Paracelsian physician, had been among the first to write about the so-called Bologna stone which had been discovered in 1602. In 1622 he published *Pharmacopoea Spagirica*, which Worm must have either owned or had access to, since he specifically referred to chapter 28 as having been dedicated to the Bononian stone, also known as the luminous stone, the sun stone, or the moon stone. Athanasius Kircher, the Jesuit scholar who by then had become the luminary of early seventeenth century learned society, had included the Bologna stone in his work on magnetism, *Magnes sive de arte magnetica*, published in 1641. Here he claimed that the stone acted similarly to a magnet, pulling in light the same way as magnets attracted pieces of iron. This work must have been available for Worm to consult at this time, even if he had to wait until the end of 1644 before he obtained his own copy from Henrik Fuiren.

A few months earlier Henrik Fuiren had informed his uncle that to the best of his knowledge Bertel Bartholin had included the luminous Bologna stone among his possessions forwarded to Amsterdam and awaiting transport to Copenhagen. He added that Bertel had also included a copy of *Litheosphorous sive de lapide Bononensis*, recently published by the Bologna professor, Fortunio Liceti, and recognised as the authoritative work on the phenomenon. At this point Henrik, however, was unaware that Kircher had written about this topic too, but he promised Worm to do his utmost to secure him an untreated sample of the stone either through Fortunio Liceti or Thomas Bartholin who was travelling home via Bologna. If that failed, Henrik was convinced that the small lump of the stone he already possessed would suffice.

Eventually, in 1645, when Bertel Bartholin finally returned to Copenhagen, Ole Worm received his long awaited samples of the Bologna stone for his cabinet of curiosity. He would undoubtedly have been delighted to obtain such a rarity seldom found in the museums of Northern Europe. A couple of years later he informed the son of his old friend Henrik Køster that he owned both a prepared and a raw sample of the Bologna stone. Unfortunately, the prepared stone had lost its ability to attract the light and Worm was convinced that such stones only retained this ability for little more than two years.[110]

---

109 *Ibid.*, no. 1227; see also Schepelern, *Museum*, 287, Schepelern has translated *canis carcharias* as blue shark rather than great white shark. Worm was referring to Fabio Colonna, *Minus cognitarum rariumque nostro cælo orientum stirpium ...*, Rome 1606.

110 *Ibid.*, nos. 1227, 1240, 1251, 1259, 1269, and 1543. For the publications about the Bologna stone, see Petrus Poterius, *Pharmacopoea Spagirica*, Bologna 1622, Athanasius

6 The influence of Athanasius Kircher and Cassiano dal Pozzo

Ole Worm was an avid admirer of the most famous polymath of the age, the Jesuit Athanasius Kircher but never managed to get into direct contact with him as opposed to his nephew, Thomas Bartholin, who conveyed Kircher's greetings to Worm while in Venice in October 1644. Rather obliquely Bartholin informed Worm that Kircher was convinced that 'the larger root bought from an Arab was that of a heliotrope'. This is the first hint that Worm and Bartholin had been discussing Kircher's sunflower clock, one of the Jesuit's most famous 'magnetic' inventions. Kircher provided detailed instructions for this in his *Magnes sive de arte magnetica*. He believed in a magnetic relationship between the sun and the vegetable kingdom as an explanation why flowers faced the sun, especially heliotropes. Kircher designed his sunflower clock by attaching a sunflower to a cork floating in a basin of water. The flower would rotate to face the sun while an indicator would tell the time on the inner side of a suspended ring. He admitted that the clock did not always work well, when the sunlight was weak or when too much wind disturbed the water in the container. He also acknowledged that his sunflower clock barely lasted one month even under the most optimal conditions Even so Kircher's invention of the sunflower clock was strongly criticised by leading scholars such as Descartes. Kircher, however, maintained a sunflower clock in his museum, which he constantly modified and showed visitors. Thomas Bartholin saw the sunflower clock when visiting Rome.[111]

Ole Worm had been inspired by Thomas's letter and tracked down a heliotrope in his garden. He dug it out with its roots in order to find out whether or not Kircher had pulled Thomas Bartholin's leg. Having cleaned and dried his heliotrope Worm had placed it on a woodchip and put it in bowl of water to find out what direction it indicated and what movement it undertook. It had proved a waste of time. Initially, the plant had followed the movements of the water a little, but after the water had settled it remained still. Worm had then carefully marked the directions in which it pointed on the side of the bowl. He returned several hours later to find absolutely no change. He then placed the heliotrope directly in the water. It floated, but with the same result. Worm therefore had serious doubts. He could not believe that Kircher had not achieved similar results long

Kircher, *Magnes sive de arte magnetica*, Rome 1641, and Fortunio Liceti, *Litheosphorous sive de lapide Bononensis*, Bologna 1640. See also Helge Kragh, 'Phosphors and Phosphorus in Early Danish Philosophy', *The Royal Danish Academy of Sciences and Letters*, 88, 2003, 16–18.

111 *Ibid.*, no. 1246; see Paula Findlen (ed.), *Athanasius Kircher: The Last Man Who Knew Everything*, London 2004, 1–48, especially 13–15 and Joscelyn Godwin, *Athanasius Kircher's Theatre of the World*, London 2009, 197–98.

ago, especially since he was normally quite concerned about all aspects of his cases and claimed not to advance anything without prior experiment. Bartholin was delighted that Worm had taken up Kircher's view of the heliotrope while seeking to discover its validity through experimentation and observation, something, Bartholin claimed, only few people were prepared to do in their day and age. However, he defended Kircher by pointing out that the Jesuit had told him that the different conditions across the globe often caused the effects to vary. Bartholin added that he left the evaluation of this statement to Worm as 'an exceptional connoisseur of natural phenomena'.[112]

Not only Kircher but another Italian scholar of great repute, Cassiano dal Pozzo, loomed large in Worm's correspondence from the early 1640s. Trained as a physician Dal Pozzo had become secretary to Cardinal Barberini in 1623 and quickly rose to become a leading figure in the intellectual life in Rome. Centrally placed in Barberini's household and as a member of the Accademia dei Lincei he became a notable character within the republic of letters with his antiquarian and natural historical interests. It was through his friend Johan Rhode in Padua and his nephews Thomas Bartholin and Henrik Fuiren, who, while in Italy, had donated some of Worm's antiquarian publications, including his work on the gold horn, to Dal Pozzo, that Worm was drawn to the latter's attention.[113] Seven years later when his student Laurits Bording was on his way to Rome, Worm encouraged him to convey his greetings to both Dal Pozzo and Kircher, but more importantly to try and obtain a copy of *Nova plantarum, animalium et mineralium Mexicanorum historia* which Worm had heard Dal Pozzo was secretly planning to publish. The work Worm had heard about was the second edition of Francisco Hernández's work, entitled *Nova plantarum, animalium et mineralium Mexicanorum historia*, edited by Nardo Antonio Recchi, which was eventually published in Rome in 1651. Bording, however, was beaten to it by another of Worm's students, Peder Scavenius, who in January 1650 could inform Worm that the publication of *Nova plantarum, animalium et mineralium Mexicanorum historia* had been paid for by the secretary to the Spanish ambassador to Rome and for some reason had been held back. Scavenius had, however, been promised that Dal Pozzo would obtain a copy for Worm when the opportunity arose. A couple of months later Laurits Bording reached Rome and visited Dal Pozzo who claimed to have done his utmost to secure a copy of *Natural History of Mexico* for Worm, but that a variety of delays and additions to the work had prevented him. A year later, in March 1651, it finally fell to another of Ole Worm's students, Willum Lange, while in Rome to obtain a copy of

---

112 *Ibid.*, nos. 1256 and 1278.
113 *Ibid.*, nos. 1005, 1014, 1026, 1048, 1064, 1095, 1168, and 1200; see also above Chapter 3.

Nova plantarum, animalium et mineralium Mexicanorum historia from
Cassiano dal Pozzo, despite the fact that the book was yet to go on sale.
Sadly, Ole Worm never received the book, which was lost in transit. Having
spent so much time and energy in obtaining a copy of this important
work it must have been a grave disappointment to Worm. He had obviously
expected more from Willum Lange, who, in his opinion, had failed to take
proper care when sending this precious book. He sent a copy of his work
on the Norwegian lemming, plus his museum catalogue to Erasmus Bartholin in Padua, with instructions to forward them to Cassiano dal Pozzo
in Rome, thanking him for the copy of *Nova plantarum, animalium et
mineralium Mexicanorum historia* while pointing out that unfortunately it
had been lost. Evidently Worm hoped that Dal Pozzo might be able to find
him another copy. In this he was disappointed.[114]

7 The stimulus of Isaac La Peyrére and other French intellectuals

From 1644 Worm's cabinet of curiosity was repeatedly visited by a number
of the French diplomats who arrived in Copenhagen on their way to take
part in the peace negotiations between Denmark and Sweden in Brømsebro.
Thus, in November that year Ole Worm informed his friend Stephanius in
Sorø that the French ambassador Gaspard Coignet de la Thuillerie often
visited his museum and had shown an interest in his antiquarian works.[115]
It was on the suggestion of the French ambassador that Ole Worm in
December 1644 wrote to the librarian of the Bibliothéque Mazarin in Paris,
Gabriel Naudé, informing him that he had been delighted to help La Thuill-
erie find books and manuscripts for Cardinal Mazarin's rapidly expanding
library. As a recognition of his help Worm was promised a medal with the
portrait of the cardinal which was being minted.[116]

Other members of the French diplomatic mission took the opportunity to
visit Worm's cabinet of curiosity such as Du Buisson and Isaac La Peyrère.
Thus, during his final visit to Worm's museum before returning to Paris Du
Buisson had asked Worm to provide him with a short explanation for how
amber came into existence, where the horn of the unicorn originated, and
how corals grew, which Worm produced in February 1646. The heterodox
millenarian Isaac La Peyrère, La Thuillerie's secretary, proved by far the
most interesting and durable of the contacts Worm made with members of
the French delegation. He became a friend and regular correspondent of
Worm, taking a particular interest in matters linked to Iceland and Greenland. In April 1645 La Peyrère had inquired whether Worm considered the

114 *Ibid.*, nos. 1648 and 1671, 1674, 1686, 1708, 1715, and 1758.
115 *Ibid.*, no. 1257.
116 *Ibid.*, nos. 1262 and 1292; see also Schepelern, *Museum*, 188, 190–92.

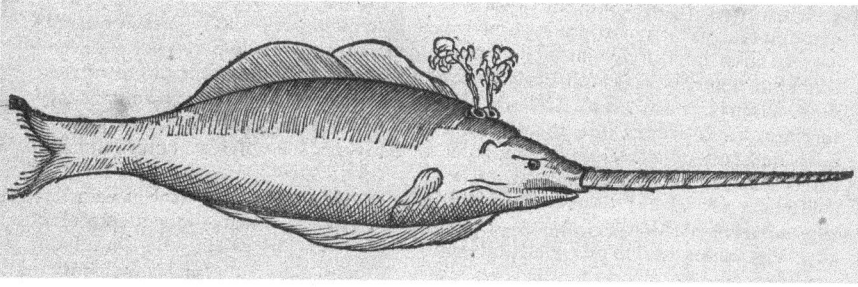

Figure 4.4 Narwhale, from Ole Worm, *Museum Wormianum* (1655); courtesy of the Royal Danish Library.

unicorn an animal living on land or a monster in the sea. Worm provided him with a detailed answer, pointing out that the bones collected by noblemen as horns of unicorns were, in fact, teeth of a whale which was common in the Greenland Sea close to the Strait of David. He kept a drawing of this whale in his museum made by an artist from the tooth/cranium belonging to the Danish chancellor Christen Friis. Worm had briefly been given the use of this head and tooth of a narwhale. He had taken the opportunity to show it to friends and students and he had written a dissertation about the nature of this animal and the purpose of the tooth. In particular he recommended La Peyrére to consult Caspar Bartholin's work about unicorns which had recently been expanded and revised by his son, Thomas, and published in Padua.[117] La Peyrére, however, was not entirely satisfied with this response and wanted to know what a live narwhale looked like and whether or not the tooth might not be a horn, causing Worm to write a comprehensive letter providing all the evidence he possessed, reaffirming his view.[118]

Before Isaac La Peyrére had taken on the role of secretary to La Thuillerie he had been in the service of the Prince of Condé. In 1643 he had anonymously published his philosemitic and millenarian work, *Du Rappel des Juifs*, without official permission, name of publisher, nor place. By then the work had already circulated in manuscript and many of his friends knew he was the author, such as Marin Mersenne and Pierre Bourdelot, physician to the Prince of Condé. It was on Bourdelot's suggestion that they both joined the French diplomatic mission to Sweden in 1644. While in Copenhagen La Peyrére had taken the opportunity to discuss not only his millenarian ideas

---

117 *Ibid.*, nos. 1300 and 1303. For Ole Worm's disputation, see *De Unicornu*, in *Institutiones Medicæ*, liber 1, sect II, Copenhagen 1638; see also Thomas Bartholin, *De Unicornu*, Padua 1645.

118 *Ibid.*, nos. 1306 and 1311.

with Ole Worm but also his so far unpublished work on the pre-Adamites. Worm inquired in his first letter to La Peyrére, after the latter had returned to France, whether or not he was having his work on the pre-Adamites published in the Netherlands as 'he intended'. If so, Worm wanted a copy not only of that but also of his already published work about the recall of Jews. Worm had clearly been so fascinated by La Peyrére's heterodox ideas that he had brought them up while providing medical assistance to the elected-prince in Nykøbing Falster. The prince, according to Worm, had been captivated by what he had been told and regretted not having made contact with La Peyrére while he was in the country.

Worm joked, knowing La Peyrére's obsession with alien people, that he had been worried that his friend had joined 'the pre-Adamites in America', but he would be delighted if La Peyrére could help him with an important inquiry. Worm had recently re-read the learned work, *Unheard of Curiosities*, by Jacques Gaffarel, and noted that a method was mentioned whereby plants could be resurrected from ash in a glass. This process, known as palingenesis, Worm had discovered had been demonstrated daily to an audience in Paris by a learned chemist, Etienne de Clave. Worm wanted to know whether La Peyrére knew this man. If so, he wanted him to obtain the ash from a plant for him. Worm would pay whatever it took, and he was convinced it would prove an 'adornment to his museum'.

Worm was right in approaching Isaac La Peyrére for this purpose. Together with Jacques Gaffarel La Peyrére had belonged to the circle of 'learned libertines' in Paris which also included such scholars as Pierre Gassendi, Marin Mersenne, and Gabriel Naudé. La Peyrére confirmed in his response that it was, indeed, true what 'our friend' Mr Gaffarel had written about the chemist Etienne de Clave. La Peyrére personally knew De Clave and had seen him in action, even if he had never seen him reproduce the flowers in a glass. He was, however, able to confirm that De Clave had undertaken several successful experiments of this nature. Etienne de Clave was no longer in Paris, having left some years earlier, but his collaborator or assistant known as Philosophus Miles, whom La Peyrére also knew, was still around. But La Peyrére was reluctant to approach him, because he had recently been imprisoned accused of making counterfeit coin. Otherwise La Peyrére was sure that Miles could recommend someone who could teach him how to resurrect flowers from ash and salt. When that happened he would immediately inform Worm 'so he could obtain not only one flower but a garden of flowers for his museum'.[119]

---

119 *Ibid.*, nos. 1421, 1463, 1470, and 1483; for Issac La Peyrére, see Richard H. Popkin, *Isaac La Peyrére (1596–1676). His Life, Work, and Influence*, Brill, Leiden 1987, 5–25, especially 6–11. For Etienne Gaffarel, see Hiro. Hirai (ed.), *Jacques Gaffarel. Between Magic and Science*, Rome 2014, especially Hiro Hirai, 'Images, Talismans and Medicine in Jacques Gaffarel's Unheard-of Curiosities', 73–84; see also J. Gaffarel, *Curiositez*

Having received La Peyrére's response and read Gaffarel's statement Worm was convinced that the resurrection of plants was possible, even if he admitted that he had harboured some doubts. Many scholars had written extensively about palingenesis, but Worm had so far remained unconvinced unless they had personally witnessed the process. So far Worm had been unable to bring it about himself having used methods recommended by friends. He referred specifically to the Leipzig professor Philipp Müller's work *Miracula chymica, et mysteria medica*, which described the whole process. Despite following it closely Worm had failed to achieve anything. What he wanted was an example from someone who had mastered the art and carried out the 'mystery'. Because of the pettiness which was typical of people who communicated such secrets to others they tended to conceal the most important details. The result was that those who followed their instructions wasted their time.[120]

In September 1647 Ole Worm contacted la Thuillerie to enquire about the Roman coins he had been promised and to ask why he had not heard from Gabriel Naudé and La Peyrére. Shortly afterwards he received a letter from La Peyrére explaining why he had been incommunicado. La Peyrére underlined that Naudé was a great admirer of Worm and was trying to make sure that he was properly rewarded for his contributions to Bibliothéque Mazarin. Furthermore, he informed Worm that he was also much admired by his friend Pierre Gassendi, who intended to write a biography of Tycho Brahe. La Peyrére also took the opportunity to send him a copy of his recently published book about Greenland where he repeatedly praised Worm.[121] A couple of months later another letter from La Peyrére arrived. In it he had inserted a note from Gabriel Naudé, and a copy of Gassendi's work on Epicur, not to mention the gift of a gold coin and an ingenuous clock enclosed in gold and inlaid with mosaics of amber from Cardinal Mazarin.

Isaac La Peyrére also informed Worm about the debate in France concerning the experiment conducted by Evangelista Torricelli five years earlier, in 1643, recording the first incidence of creating a permanent vacuum. He was very keen on obtaining Worm's opinion about this experiment, informing him that the young Danish nobleman Tønne Reedtz, who was delivering his letter, had witnessed several experiments creating permanent vacuum while in Paris, and would prove an excellent witness. La Peyrére's letter was the first Worm had heard about Toricelli's experiment. He struggled to understand what precisely the experiment was about, and he found Tønne Reedtz

inouyes, sur la sculpture talismanique des Persans, horoscope des patriarches et lecture des etoiles, Paris 1629.

120 *Ibid.*, no. 1483. See also P. Müller, *Miracula chymica, et mysteria medica*, Wittenberg 1611.

121 *Ibid.*, nos. 1538, 1540 and 1545. See aso Popkin, *Peyrére*, 10–11 and I. La Peyrére, *Relation du Groenland*, Paris 1647.

to be a less than reliable witness and unable to explain the experiment in the necessary detail. Worm thought it was similar to what happened in glass containers when the air temperature was being investigated. However, even if the liquid in them went up and down no other conclusion could be drawn than air was compressed by coldness and took up less space when it was diluted; the liquid then rose against its nature (which is heavy), fearing the empty space and filling up the greater part of the glass. From that Worm was inclined to assume the impossibility of the concept of the empty space rather than its existence. Wisely Worm decided to hold back his judgement until he had fully understood the issue. Worm left it at that, being far more interested in 'the spiritual revival of plants' and making contact to Etienne de Clave in order to obtain a sample for his museum.[122]

In April 1648 Ole Worm, as we have seen, received an inquiry from his nephew, Erasmus Bartholin, asking him if he had managed to get hold of the herb which grew in a bottle of water, as described by Athanasius Kircher, clearly mistaking it for paligenesis. Erasmus's promise that his travel companion, Joel Langlot would share the secret of paligenesis with Worm meanwhile came to nothing. Worm was, of course, not interested in Kircher's herb, but only in the 'resurrection of plants via their salts or spirit as described by Joseph du Chesne, in other words paligenesis which he had yet to see performed. He hoped that Erasmus might encounter it in Paris and report back to him.[123]

On his forthcoming visit to Paris Worm also desired Erasmus to solve another mystery, namely, how engravings printed on paper were coloured with such fine colours that they could not be seen unless exposed to sunlight. Worm had been told that the inventor lived in the city. As always well informed from the works of Athanasius Kircher Worm acknowledged that the method was described in the tenth book of his work on light and shadow (*Ars Magna Lucis et Umbrae*, 1645), but that those who had tried to follow his instructions had been disappointed. Worm had recently seen a sample belonging to Otto Sperling who had brought it back from France, but had told him that the inventor refused to share his secret.

Meanwhile, Worm doggedly pursued palingenesis: how it could be achieved and how to obtain the ashes or salts of at least one plant for his cabinet of curiosity. He therefore wrote to Joel Langlot, congratulating him on becoming personal physician to the Duke of Holstein, with the purpose of asking him to share the secret with him which Joseph du Chesne had referred to, namely, 'how plants could be awakened in a gaseous state with bright colours and all its parts from philosophical ash by the use of heat' Worm reminded him, that he had promised to send him a specimen for his museum as a recognition of 'their old friendship'. He asked Langlot to do so urgently because he was involved in an argument with a friend who

---

122 *Ibid.*, nos. 1554, 1570, 1581, 1589, and 1598; see also Schepelern, *Museum*, 190.
123 See Chapter 2.

denied the possibility of palingenesis. Worm admitted that he already possessed a number of methods of how to produce such plants, given to him by friends, but the ones he had tried had failed, possibly because he was failing to implement them correctly. Worm emphasised that he relied on the assistance of Langlot, having been unable to contact Etienne de Clave who had recently demonstrated palingenesis to a wider audience in Paris. Despite his efforts Worm received nothing from Langlot. Not until his son Willum visited Joel Langlot on Gottorp Castle in 1653 did Worm receive an account of the Gottorp physician's method for paligenesis. It differed from what Worm had so far received from others. He was, however, not particularly interested in the method, but only in the outcome. Unfortunately Joel Langlot proved unable to guarantee that his method worked.

In the autumn of 1649 Erasmus Bartholin had visited the Jesuit Alexander Barvoetius in Louvain who worked on the anatomy of insects. Erasmus reported excitedly to his uncle in Copenhagen that Barvoetius had shown him the anatomy of the eye of a fly by inserting it in a microscope thereby demonstrating what the Italian, Giambattista Odierna, had published five years earlier was true, namely, that the eye of the fly consisted of innumerable tiny parts connected like a net. Odierna's work was the first detailed account of microscopic anatomy of organic tissue based on the use of a microscope. Alexander Barvoetius must have been among the first to confirm Odierna's observations and was convinced that the eyes of all insects were similar. Surprisingly, apart from congratulating his nephew on his trip to visit scholars in Flanders Worm appears to have taken no interest in these ground breaking observations of the eye of the fly, and he passed them over in silence.[124] Perhaps this revolutionary approach to anatomy with the use of the microscope simply proved too novel for the elderly Worm.

Ole Worm certainly kept abreast of other new developments within natural history. In 1650, his student Christen Foss had sent him a copy of the English physician Walter Charleton's newly published work, *Spiritus Gorgonicus vi sua saxipara exutus*, which provided an account of the formation of stones in the body and the cure, drawing on Paracelsian and Helmontian sources. Consequently Worm was extremely keen to find out what kind of stone Charleton's Ludus was, which he claimed could be found in Antwerp. He therefore asked Erasmus Bartholin to try and obtain a sample through a friend and to send him a small piece at his convenience. Worm had always shared the opinion of 'the other Paracelsians', namely, that Ludus was a small stone secreted or cut from the human body. He encouraged Erasmus to find out more about Walter Charleton's Ludus. On his trip to England in 1647 Erasmus had not been able to have a conversation with Charleton or any of his friends. However, his travelling companion, Joel Langlot, had been given a piece of the Ludus by the son of Jan Baptist van Helmont which Erasmus had

124 *Ibid.*, nos. 1663 and 1667.

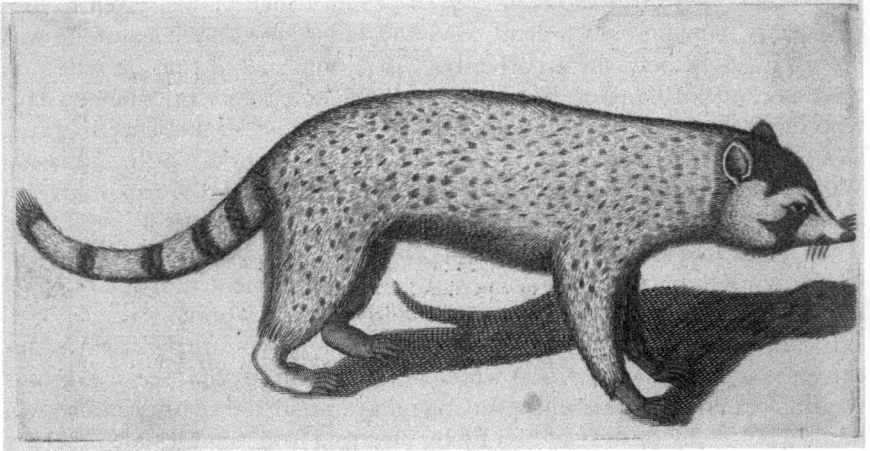

Figure 4.5 Live Coati, from Ole Worm, *Museum Wormianum* (1655); courtesy of the Royal Danish Library.

seen, adding that Charleton had obtained many things from Van Helmont. Erasmus described it as a type of flint stone coloured like clay and shaped like a cube to be found near the river Schelde.[125] Later that year he was sent a particularly fine example of antimony by Henrik Køster, the Younger, and a stone which Køster presumed was Helmont's Ludus. Worm told him he had serious doubts about the Helmontian Ludus. From the Netherlands he had already received a type of flint which shaped into small squares or dice which apparently was the reason they were called Ludus. The stone was hard and smooth, could resist iron, and had a colour close to yellow, and was sold as Helmont's Ludus. If Ludus was a type of flint then the one Køster had sent him could not be a ludus, because it was a soft stone which could be scraped with a knife and was nowhere close to flint in hardness.[126]

Christen Foss, who had sent Worm Charleton's work on stones had given him a far more spectacular present in July 1649 when from Amsterdam he sent him a live Coati, an animal described and depicted in Johannes de Laet's edition of Georg Marcgrave's *Historia Naturalis Brasiliae*. Worm managed to keep it alive for a number of years. It was still alive when his German student Georg Seger published a systematic survey of his collection in 1653. As a result Worm was able to provide interesting details about its behaviour in his museum history. He even had it drawn by an artist because the illustration in *Historia Naturalis Brasiliae* failed to do it justice.[127]

---

125 *Ibid.*, nos. 1685 and 1694; for Erasmus Bartholin's journey to England see no. 1536.
126 *Ibid.*, no. 1751; see also Schepelern, *Museum*, 176 and 180, and *Museum Wormianum*, 39
127 *Ibid.*, no. 1667; Schepelern, *Museum*, 194 and 289 and *Museum Wormianum*, 319.

The French physician Pierre Bourdelot, who had been part of the French legation travelling through Copenhagen in 1644, returned in the autumn of 1651 on his way to Sweden to become royal physician to Queen Christina. The chaos brought about by the Fronde in France, which had seen Bourdelot's employer, Prince Louis II de Condé, arrested in January 1650, had led him to accept Queen Christina's invitation. He had undoubtedly already visited Worm's museum in 1644 together with his friend La Peyrère and only had to renew the contact in 1651. Worm reminded him in March 1652 that he had promised him a spear made of Amiantus (silicate minerals/serpentine stone) for his museum, while prompting him not to forget his cabinet of curiosity. Worm also forwarded his greetings to 'their mutual friend La Peyrère.[128] By May 1652 Worm had received a cloth and rare asbestos from Pierre Boudelot which he was delighted to give pride of place in his museum with the latter's name attached. The attraction of leading French scholars to the court of Queen Christina of Sweden during these years guaranteed that Worm's cabinet of curiosity saw a steady stream of visitors travelling via Copenhagen to the Swedish court. Among them were Isaak Vossius, who served Queen Christina as royal librarian until her abdication in 1654, and the Calvinist antiquarian and biblical scholar, Samuel Brochart. Ole Worm was particularly impressed by Brochart whom he described as 'a very polite and unusually learned man', and he repeatedly asked Bourdelot to convey his greetings to him. Another casualty of the disturbances of the Fronde was Worm's friend Gabriel Naudé. After having witnessed the forced sale of Cardinal Mazarin's library by the Parlement of Paris he too had accepted an invitation from Queen Christina to join her court in Stockholm. Gabriel Naudé also travelled via Copenhagen and visited Worm and his cabinet of curiosity. Worm was delighted and would have liked him to stay longer so he could enjoy his company.[129]

In his letter from 22 May 1652 Pierre Bourdelot had enclosed some learned observations and interpretations of the recent eclipse of the sun. They were likely to have been the Dutch and French pamphlets which Bourdelot had asked his friend Claude Saumaise to forward to him in Stockholm. Worm asked if he could hang on to these documents while providing Bourdelot with information about what had been observed in Copenhagen. He also informed him that he had read a comprehensive account of the eclipse written by an Englishman from London, William Lilly. A friend of his had provided him with a copy. Worm would have forwarded it to Bourdelot, but his friend wanted it returned. However, its assessment corresponded closely with the French appraisals which Bourdelot had forwarded

128 *Ibid.*, no. 1719; for Bourdelot's visit in 1644, see Popkin, *Isaac La Peyrère*, 10; see also Garstein, *Counter-Reformation in Scandinavia*, 580–83, and A. Guerrini, *The Courtiers' Anatomists: Animals and Humans in Louis XIV's Paris*, Chicago 2015, 44–46.
129 *Ibid.*, 1725 and 1730; see also Schepelern, *Museum*, 191 and Garstein, *Counter-Reformation in Scandinavia*, 569–78.

to him, but, of course, adjusted to English conditions. This exchange clearly wetted Worm's interest and he immediately contacted his son Willum who was then in London with the Danish embassy, and encouraged him to look up the astrologer William Lilly, who had, as Worm put it, made some 'fortunate predictions based on the solar eclipse'. To his father's considerable disappointment Willum never got round to meeting William Lilly while in London.[130]

Most likely it was either Johannes Bureus or Pierre Bourdelot who brought the Swedish royal antiquarian and mystic, Georg Stiernhielm, into contact with Worm. Stiernhielm donated a piece of amber from Mählaren to the cabinet of curiosity in the decade before 1653.[131]

In 1653 Ole Worm published his pamphlet about the Norwegian mouse or lemming which occasionally fell from the sky. Worm did not refute the often repeated claim by Olaus Magnus that the lemmings occurred as a result of cloud formations and then fell to earth. Worm had received a lemming from his son-in-law Jens Pedersen Schelderup, Bishop of Bergen, which he described in detail in his pamphlet, also reporting that rotting lemmings could cause death to cattle by poisoning pastures. Worm sent this lemming with his son Willum as a present to the Duke of Schleswig, pointing out that it was rare and difficult to preserve. In June that year he informed his nephew Erasmus Bartholin in Leiden that he had published his account of the Norwegian lemming which came down with rain. He added that one of his students, Georg Seger, was working on a new catalogue of his museum. This catalogue was published only three months later and Worm was able to send a copy to Joel Langlot on Gottorp.[132]

Worm eventually reproduced his account of the lemming in his museum history, adding a significant observation about the role of the natural philosopher:

> The natural philosopher who is not as preoccupied with the general and distant causes as the immediate and near, cannot be satisfied with this. It is true that God is seen as the cause of all things, but because

---

130 *Ibid.*, nos. 1725, 1726, and 1727. For Bourdelot's letter to Claude Saumaise, see S. Åkerman, 'Queen Christina of Sweden and Messianic Thought', 142 in D. Katz and J. Israel (eds.) *Sceptics, Millenarians and Jews*, Leiden 1990. William Lilly produced an annual almanac from 1647 to 1681 entitled *Merlini Anglici Ephemeris*. It was probably this almanac for 1652 Worm referred to. He may also have seen Lilly pamphlet from 1652 *Annus Tenebrosus, or the Dark Year,* London 1652.

131 Schepelern, *Museum*, 197, and *Museum Wormianum*, 33. For Stiernhielm and Bureus, see S. Åkerman, *Rose Cross over the Baltic. The Spread of Rosecrucianism in Northern Europe*, Leiden 1998.

132 *Breve fra og til Ole Worm*, nos. 1735, 1737, and 1738; see also Schepelern, *Museum*, 289–91 and O. Worm, *Historia Animalis, quod in Norvegia quandoque e nubibus decidit*, Copenhagen 1653.

he does not act directly in order to affect Nature, but through natural causes, it is the task of the natural philosopher to discover these.[133]

8 The importance of donors and objects from Iceland and the Faroe Iles

Ole Worm received a considerable number of objects for his museum from his many friends and acquaintances on Iceland and the Faroe Isles. In June 1637 he was promised a number of items by Gisli Oddsson on Skalholt. A couple of months later Worm received on Icelandic chess set made of whale teeth.[134] In May 1638 Worm sent Thorlak Skulason a short work about the unicorn for his inspection. Here Worm corrected 'the mistakes and fabrications of the multitude' and expressed his opinion about this bone based on what he had been told by his friends. He asked Skulason to tell him if he possessed further information. Worm explained that he had visited Chancellor Christen Friis who had shown him the skull with the tooth and the drawing Skulason had given him, while also mentioning that he had been promised a more detailed drawing. Worm had been told that 'this monster' was not infrequently washed ashore in Iceland, and he would like to receive a complete drawing of it. He did not require the tooth which he knew was extremely valuable, but he would be grateful if Skulason could send him other body parts of this animal, such as the skin, the flippers, and the tail. Worm wanted to have a precise drawing produced. Skulason agreed with Worm that what was perceived to be the horn of the unicorn was, in fact, the tooth of the sea monster. However, as far as he was aware such sea monsters had not been beached on the northern coast of Iceland during the last six to seven years. Skulason forwarded part of a tooth which he had been given 'by an honest man'. He was unable to get hold of the flippers, the hide, and the tail. He had recently forwarded a drawing to the Chancellor, but was happy to send another, if it had been lost.

Worm was extremely grateful for the broken narwhale tooth. He explained that he had once more inspected the cranium of this whale at the Chancellor's residence and noted the common confusion about the tooth. He intended to publish something about it in the near future, if he could receive assistance from those who had greater knowledge about the shape of this animal. Unfortunately, the Chancellor had mislaid the drawing Skulason had sent him so Worm asked him to send another.[135] This duly arrived some months later. Skulason, however, complained about his lack of precise knowledge. The drawing he sent was fairly crude. The animal had no teeth apart from the large prominent and visible one, nor did it have fins but

133 *Museum Wormianum*, 331
134 *Ibid.*, nos. 653 and 664; see also Schepelern, *Museum*, 357, Kat. 239.
135 *Ibid.*, nos. 713, 744, and 785.

some bones covered with flesh and soft skin. The blowhole could be found on top of the lungs behind the head, as Worm could see from the drawing. Skulason estimated its size to be between forty to sixty feet.[136]

Around that time Worm also sought information about whales in general from his antiquarian friend Arngrim Jonsson on Holar. He was informed that it was fairly common for the teeth of a certain type of whales, known as 'Tannfisk', to be covered in some sort of glue. More importantly Jonsson told him that the single tooth, which people assumed was from a unicorn, belonged to 'a sea monster among the whales', rarely referred to in the ancient sources. It was rare and known as 'Naahvalur' after the human corpses it had a preference for eating, and also because it was dangerous to eat and could cause death as opposed to most other whales which could be safely consumed.[137]

Arngrim Jonsson evidently took an interest in Worm's museum too. In August 1640 he sent Worm a stone – which was different from all other stones he had ever seen in shape, colour, weight, and hardness. It had been found on its own at the local beach and Jonsson was not even sure it was a stone. Worm confirmed it was an ironstone (pyrites) which normally contained some ore, but not always. However, the shape, hardness, and beauty of the sample sent to him elevated it above all the common ones, and Worm would display it among his treasures under Arngrim Jonsson's name.[138]

Arngrim Jonsson also received a copy of Ole Worm's first museum catalogue from 1642. He was as always very grateful, and spent a lengthy paragraph in his subsequent letter praising Worm, his talents, and rather oddly in this context, his library. Worm corrected him by pointing out that the catalogue was not concerned with his books, but 'the objects which I have collected because they are recommendable either for their rarity or their exceptional benefit'. He took the opportunity to remind Arngrim that he had previously contributed to his cabinet of curiosity. However, he had sent him a copy in order that Arngrim 'in the common interest', might inform him of objects available in Iceland but not included in his catalogue.[139] As such the catalogue certainly served its purpose encouraging friends, scholars, and students to contribute to his museum.

Arngrim Jonsson sent Worm a couple of items for his museum in August 1643, still calling it a library. He forwarded an arrowhead made of Lapis Lydius, which had been found in the blubber of a big, old walrus. He pointed out that arrowheads made of this material were not found on Iceland and he presumed it came from Greenland. He also included two eagle stones which were presumed to be female and pregnant, because when they were shaken they made a sound proving that there were something within

---

136 *Ibid.*, no. 806.
137 *Ibid.*, no. 738.
138 *Ibid.*, nos. 859 and 955.
139 *Ibid.*, nos. 1065 and 1136.

them. Out of the sea they could not give birth as Worm would be able to confirm through observation. If that was the case 'this secret of Nature would prove highly valuable as an example of matrimonial existence'.[140]

A few months later Worm received another eagle stone among a collection of objects from the Danish minister Christoffer Hansen Nyborg. They included a number of Ombria stones (fossilised sea urchins). Bearing in mind their number Worm wanted a description of the place they had been found to be incorporated into his museum history. He informed Nyborg that the porous and soft bone he had sent him was not whale sperm, but came from the cuttle fish and was well-known among goldsmiths who used it to polish their gold and for making forms and matrixes. In medicine it was used as a toothpowder. Similarly, what Nyborg labelled whale scales were, in fact, oystershells. Whales like dolphins and similar 'fish', Worm explained, were covered with smooth skins without scales.[141]

More objects for Worm's museum arrived in June 1644 from his old friend Arngrim Jonsson. What Arngrim believed was eagle stones Worm identified as West Indian beans. The biggest was known as the heart of St. Thomas because they mainly originated from that island. Worm was grateful for the objects but particularly excited by the rare stone weapon Arngrim had sent him and agreed with him that it was part of a harpoon.[142] The following year Thorlak Skulason sent him a shoe crafted from birch bark which had been found on the beach after having drifted unto land. Worm was very grateful and claimed it would adorn his museum being extremely rare and an example of exceptional craftsmanship. Unfortunately it had arrived too late to be included in his new museum catalogue, but he promised to include it in the next edition where it would be listed among the other gifts Skulason had made.[143]

In April 1647 Ole Worm wrote to the minister in Thorshavn on the Faroe Islands, Hans Rasmussen, acknowledging the receipt of some small birds, while encouraging him to collect rare natural objects for him. Worm wanted him to obtain the skin of a foetus of a whale. Hans Rasmussen thought that it would be impossible to find anyone who could skin and dry a foetus of a whale properly, because the flesh was so thick, but he would try. Meanwhile he forwarded more birds to Worm.[144] Worm also received some swan sloughs from his former student Gisli Magnussen which unfortunately were rotten on arrival.[145] Such disappointments were unavoidable for a seventeenth century collector such as Worm with items regularly being broken or destroyed in transit, or not arriving at all. In June that year

---

140 *Ibid.*, no. 1158; see also Schepelern, *Museum*, 183
141 *Ibid.*, nos. 1167 and 1174.
142 *Ibid.*, no. 1219.
143 *Ibid.*, nos. 1354 and 1425.
144 *Ibid.*, nos. 1493 and 1497.
145 *Ibid.*, no. 1496.

Worm unexpectedly received samples of Icelandic medical soil and petrified water from the Icelandic minister, Torfi Jonsson. He encouraged Torfi to send him other unusual objects which could benefit his museum and add to his fame. Worm explained that the petrified water was not transferred into stone by the spring, but that it had been covered by a crust of stone from the stone forming emanations of the water. Such springs were found in Germany in several places and Worm had recently seen something similar on Sealand.[146]

In September 1648 the exchange about unicorns and narwhales, between Ole Worm and Thorlak Skulason ten years previously, bore fruit. Thorlak informed Worm that 'a monster' of the Cetus family', thirty feet long, had drifted unto the coast with the Greenland ice the previous winter. It was equipped with a single tooth of exceptional length, measuring more than six feet with the point broken off. Thorlak had forwarded the tooth to the King, but kept the cranium for Worm. Worm instructed him to put the cranium, plus the small pieces of skin and blubber of the narwhale he had kept for him in a barrel or box. He was to deliver this to a specific merchant for transport without telling him about the content. Worm had been informed that the new Governor of Iceland was looking for such things and had been ordered, if possible, to ship a complete animal back to Copenhagen. Worm was clearly concerned that the parts of the narwhale he had been promised would not reach him. In that he was proved correct when a few months later Thorlak Skulason was forced to hand the cranium over to the Governor. It was sent to the king, who later donated it to Worm. From the description of the person who found the narwhale it became clear that the drawing made in 1638 was incorrect. The head was small compared to the body and the stomach was so broad that length and width nearly corresponded with each other, while the tail was thin. On the back it had two big bulks. Its skin corresponded to that of a normal whale. Its flesh was not poisonous as rumoured because the fishermen had eaten it without any harm.[147]

Undoubtedly, Ole Worm's renewed enthusiasm for the narwhale resulted in Erasmus Bartholin visiting the Greenland Company in Amsterdam in the autumn of 1649 where a couple of narwhale heads and teeth were kept. As a result he supplied Worm with a drawing of the head of the narwhale depicted from the inside, split diagonally in two following the mouth. The tooth was fixed to the top part, which Erasmus had depicted, so the root of the tooth could be seen. He thought it stuck out like that of a swordfish. He also included another drawing of the other side, but in less detail because it was not as significant. Worm was delighted that the drawings corresponded with what he had already seen.

146 *Ibid.*, no. 1541.
147 *Ibid.*, nos. 1608, 1630, 1644, and 1657; see also Schepelern, *Museum*, 198.

He was particularly excited by having received a number of narwhale bones, especially vertebrae, which were considered rare. Even so Worm remained concerned that he had seen another depiction of the narwhale which differed from Thorlak Skulason's in having two large bulks on the back. He therefore sought further information from the fishermen who had caught it. Eventually, Worm settled for the drawing originally sent to him by Skulason in 1638/39 as the most correct and included it in his museum history.[148]

Many gifts for Worm's cabinet of curiosity arrived from Iceland during these years. Einar Arnfinsson gave him a couple of stones, one of which had been found in a swan's nest. Gisli Magnusson sent him some ancient shields, promising him some swords. Rare stones were donated by Stefan Olafsson, plus a box carved from a whale tooth, and Torfi Jonsson sent him some small crystalline stones and a type of mussel which attached itself to the scales of fish.[149] Worm tried to obtain rare birds for his museum from the Faroe Islands during 1649–50. In particular he wanted the Corvus Variegatus alive or dead. As always the lengthy transportation and preservation proved a problem. The birds and their plumage, which the minister, Hans Rasmussen, had sent him in late 1649, were rotten on arrival. Worm pointed out that new specimens needed to be totally dried out so they could be preserved against worms.[150] Rasmussen fared better in September 1650 when he sent Worm some animal furs and a crow with a mixture of white and black feathers, the much wanted Corvus Variegatus. More birds appear to have arrived in 1651. This time they were well preserved. 1651 was the year Worm made a determined effort to obtain a whale foetus. He wrote to Hans Rasmussen asking him to find him a foetus. Bearing in mind the many whales which were regularly beached on the Faroe Isles Worm was sure he could find a pregnant one. He wanted the foetus without intestines and dried out. By the following spring he had received the much wanted whale foetus cleared of intestines and dried out. By removing the skin and drying it out it had been successfully preserved, but the fat continued to sweat out and had to be dried off regularly.[151] Finally, in 1654 Thorlak Skulason donated the cranium and skin of a walrus which Worm claimed would adorn his museum. Worm also received the slough of the rare Mergus Maximus Farrensis from his former student and amanuensis Stefan Olafsson who among other things had also given him a snuffbox carved from a whale tooth.[152]

---

148 *Ibid.*, nos. 1663, 1667, 1670, and 1713. See also Schepelern, *Museum*, 278, and *Museum Wormianum*, 282–83.
149 *Ibid.*, nos. 1601, 1609, 1611, 1640, 1646, 1649, and 1652.
150 *Ibid.*, nos. 1677, and 1682.
151 *Ibid.*, nos. 1677, 1700, 1710, 1711, and 1720. For Stefan Olofsson see no. 1772 and Schepelern, *Museum*, 184.
152 *Ibid.*, no. 1780.

9 Other donors

The number of noble and royal donors to Worm's cabinet of curiosity grew in the 1640s. The elected-prince donated four items to his museum and later King Frederik III gave nine objects. In the summer of 1647 Worm was given a lance which the nobleman Laurits Ulfeldt thought had belonged to an East-Indian prince and an ancient gold ring or bracelet. Worm was extremely grateful for such valuable, ancient objects. He was particularly fascinated by the ring/bracelet. From its size and shape he deducted that it must have been a ring belonging to a powerful man, possibly a royal, who would have been twice as tall as a normal man. In other words a giant who would have been a third taller than the giant whose corner-tooth Worm exhibited in his museum. The two objects would take pride of position in his museum and he would refer to Ulfeldt by name in his museum history. A few months later Worm reported that the ring's presence in his museum had resulted in him being given another valuable, ancient Indian ring, surrounding a particularly ingenious chrysolithe and several red hyacinth-stones.[153] From the widow of Field Marshal Henrik Holck, who had fought with Gustavus Adolphus at Lützen, Worm received part of the Swedish King's spur which was later completed by a gift from Duke Christian Ranzau.[154]

An ancient shield was donated to Worm's museum in 1650 by Birgitte Thott who declared herself an admirer of his cabinet of curiosity. Worm was informed of the recent find of three daggers/swords made of flint stone in possession of the royal administrator of Dueholm Monastery. Worm was fascinated:

> If you inspect them carefully you cannot help wondering whether they are made by Nature or through craftsmanship. From those I possess clear traces of craftsmanship can be seen. We therefore have to acknowledge that the art of shaping flint like this has been lost.[155]

Some objects obviously had to be paid for before they could be acquired. The German lawyer, Johann Conrad Saur had visited Ole Worm's cabinet of curiosity in April 1646 and had been given a copy of the 1645 catalogue. Worm had shown him a very small horn of the rhinoceros slightly damaged at the top. Saur had given Worm a slightly bigger and undamaged horn of rhinoceros whereupon Worm had given him his, because it was unsuitable for prophylactic treatment. When undamaged the horn could be used against a variety of illnesses such as palpitation, paralysis, and apoplexy when chemically treated. Saur was now offering Worm a much

153 *Ibid.*, nos. 1522, 1524, 1534, 1539, and 1641; see also *Museum Wormianum*, 352, and Schepelern, *Museum*, 166 and 198–99.
154 Schepelern, *Museum*, 166 and Kat. 85.
155 *Breve fra og til Ole Worm*, nos. 1702 and 1706; see also Schepelern, *Museum*, 192.

bigger rhinoceros horn two feet long and weighing seven pounds. He was convinced Worm could get it for sixty Reichsthaler if he responded quickly. Whether for financial or other reasons Worm appears to have refrained from obtaining this horn.[156]

Another German, the student Friedrich Klinger, who had moved to Königsberg gifted Worm a small ball of amber which contained nine or ten pins, two balls, and three small die. He also forwarded a wide variety of objects on behalf of the professor of medicine at the University of Königsberg, Johannes Loesel. They included trumpets, flutes, and other instruments from Lithuania, used at festivities, the beak of a pelican which Worm had long been missing in his collection, pyrites shaped like a nipple, a trunk which looked like a knot, a large tooth from a boar, and the foot of a Eurasian bittern. Klinger mentioned that Loesel also owned other rarities which he would like to give to Worm if he did not already possess them, such as the skin of an 18 feet long Brazilian snake, wasp-nests, Prussian diamonds, not to mention a variety of plants growing along the Prussian coast.[157] Another former student of Worm, Johann Daniel Horstius, who had become town physician in Darmstadt sent him what he thought were some petrified toadstones which had been excavated in the copper mines near Innsbruck. When thanking him Worm told him that they were most likely pyrites. A couple of years later Horstius sent him a rare Hysterolithos stone which Worm had never seen described or depicted before. As promised he included it in his museum history. Never one to miss an opportunity Ole Worm forwarded a copy of his museum catalogue to Johannes Loesel, clearly hoping that more donations might follow.[158]

Not surprisingly Worm was keen to obtain catalogues of other cabinets of curiosity such as that of the Elector of Saxony, even if he realised that his own collection was unlikely to benefit from gifts from such royal collections. In September 1647 his nephew Erasmus Bartholin visited Tradescant's cabinet of curiosity in London. He reported back that he had carefully examined the collection. Erasmus was impressed, even if he politely added that he would have been even more captivated if he had not been convinced that Worm's museum was far superior. Despite not having had Worm's catalogue to hand, nor for that matter seen its most recent edition (1645) he had no doubts. Still, Erasmus had to admit that Tradescant possessed some superb natural objects from India. He also informed his uncle that Tradescant had promised to have a catalogue made.[159] Eventually, Willum Lange

156 *Ibid.* no. 1680; for the objects made from rhinoceros horn in Worm's cabinet of curiosity, see Mordhorst, *Genstandsfortællinger*, 92–96.

157 *Ibid.*, nos. 1699 and 1705; see also Schepelern, *Museum*, 195–96.

158 *Ibid.*, nos. 1701, 1707, and 1733; see also Schepelern, *Museum*, 196 and *Museum Wormianum*, 83.

159 *Ibid.*, nos. 1465, 1521, and 1536. For the catalogue, see John Tradescant, *Museum Tradescantianum, or a collection of Rarities preserved at South Lambert near London*, London 1656.

visited the elector's cabinet of curiosity in Dresden in the autumn of 1650. Having had great expectations he was somewhat disappointed and found Ole Worm's museum and others he had seen better. Even so, he provided Worm with a survey of the rarest items in the six rooms which housed the collection.[160]

While working on the manuscript for his *museum history* queries naturally arose about some of the objects Ole Worm had been given over the years, about their nature, origin, and use. Worm sought to resolve these issues by consulting colleagues and friends. In October he asked his son Willum, who had matriculated at the University of Leiden, to consult a Chinese gentleman who resided with his friend Jacob Golius, the professor in Arabic and mathematics at Leiden University. Worm wanted Willum to show the Chinese gentleman the illustration, in the manuscript of *museum history*, of what he thought was a Chinese compass, hoping that he might provide information which could improve Worm's interpretation. Eventually the issue was resolved not by Willum, but via the Jesuit Willem van Aelst, who resided with the Spanish ambassador in Copenhagen, and who sent a copy of Worm's illustration to his colleague, the sinologist Martino Martinus, who had just returned from China. Martinus identified Worm's Chinese box as an instrument used by the Chinese to find the best burial places which had been in use for thousands of years. Worm received the information just in time to correct his manuscript before it was printed.[161]

Appropriately the last donation to Worm's cabinet of curiosity came from his son Willum who forwarded some rare shells and carnelian stones from Leiden in July 1654 a few weeks before his father's death.[162]

According to the 1642 catalogue Ole Worm's cabinet of curiosity contained 929 objects. Eleven years later when Georg Seger made his catalogue the collection had grown to 1557 objects, a growth of nearly 68%. Evidently, Worm's museum was seeing a rapid expansion during the 1640s and early 1650s. The collection grew at even greater speed in the last year of Worm's life recording an annual growth of 7%.[163]

Throughout his collecting Ole Worm applied a consistent approach. He sought information about the objects he acquired for his museum in the available literature. He then carefully described and compared the object and where necessary undertook experiments. As far as possible Worm sought to determine the natural environment of the object in question, its provenance, which he considered essential for a comprehensive understanding. Finally he often included the name of the donor of the object in order to add further credibility and enhance value.

160 *Ibid.*, no. 1704.
161 *Ibid.*, nos. 1752, 1762, and 1766; see also Schepelern, *Museum*, 197 and *Museum Wormianum*, 372–73.
162 *Ibid.*, no. 1787.
163 See Schepelern, *Museum*, 199–200.

10 The cabinet of curiosity

Over the last decade of his life Worm's cabinet of curiosity and his work on the history and description of it, *Museum Wormianum*, grew in importance until it finally dominated his last couple of years. Having seen the start of the printing of his magnum opus with the Elzevirs Worm still had to decide what was to be done with his collection after his death. Not surprisingly the future of his cabinet of curiosity came to take up a considerable part of his will, dated 7 June 1656. Worm died 10 weeks later, but clearly did not expect to live long after having made his will, stating in the preamble that he considered it very likely 'that God would call him to His eternal Kingdom' soon. Bearing in mind that plague had broken out in Copenhagen by the end of April 1654 and that the epidemic by June was still spreading rapidly, killing a growing number of people, Worm's rather pessimistic outlook for the future seemed justified.[164]

Having made sure that adequate provisions were made for the younger children from his third marriage Worm spent the last third of the will on what he wanted to happen to his cabinet of curiosity.

> Concerning my cabinet of curiosity it is my will and request that it should remain undivided in the hands of my family, in the house where my wife will reside after my death. And that my eldest son, Master Willum Worm, when God returns him home again, shall take care of it, and should he die, then another of my sons who might be suitable shall be in charge. The collection should not be passed on or sold unless my children are in dire need. If so it should be offered to one of my sons who might be interested at a reasonable price. Should he be unable or unwilling to buy it, then it should be offered to his Majesty the King, who undoubtedly will make sure, through the intervention of my beneficent patron, the noble Chancellor Christian Thomesen [Sehested], that my widow and her fatherless children will receive the full value of the collection. Should his Majesty the King not want it then it should be offered to the Duke of Holstein [Christian Rantzau] who is a curious and learned gentleman, and who will probably acquire the collection for an equitable price, as he has done with the collections of Paludanus's and others.[165]

Even if a considerable part of *Museum Wormianum* may well have been printed when Worm died on 31 August 1654, much still remained to be done in editorial terms. This now all fell to Willum who saw the volume

164 For Ole Worm's will, see C. Bruun, 'Ole Worms Testament'. *Danske Samlinger*, I, Series V, 1869–70, 377–378. For the outbreak of plague, see *Breve fra og til Ole Worm*, nos. 1769 and 1774.

165 Bruun, 'Worms Testament', 378.

through to publication in March 1655. In many ways he might well have found it easier on his own. His father's constant changes to the manuscript must have been a burden, not to mention his constant dissatisfaction with the speed and efficiency with which the publication progressed. Willum clearly had found it difficult to keep his father satisfied. Not only did he write the dedication for *Museum Wormianum* to King Frederik III of Denmark, but he also managed to obtain a poem from the famous poet and diplomat Sir Constantijn Huygens to go with the poem already solicited by Worm himself from his nephew Thomas Bartholin, which were both added to Ole Worm's portrait by Karel van Mander.[166]

That Willum did not intend to become the custodian of his father's cabinet of curiosity can be seen from his dedication to King Frederik III. From that it is obvious that Willum hoped that the king would acquire it and incorporate it in the royal cabinet of curiosity which he was busy creating. The fact that the king had already expressed an interest in acquiring Worm's museum before his death served to justify such expectations.[167] Willum returned to Copenhagen from Leiden in the spring of 1655 when his editorial work of *Museum Wormianum* had finished. He remained in Copenhagen over the summer to help with the settlement of his father's estate. As part of the settlement Worm's collection was offered to the king and probably transferred to Copenhagen Castle in connection with the family's vacation of the official professorial residence shortly before 1 August 1655.[168] Around the same time Willum left the city to continue his *peregrinatio academica*, heading for Padua where he obtained his MD in 1657.

Museum Wormianum offers a comprehensive impression of Worm's cabinet of curiosity or collection as it was at the time of his death. It was not just a catalogue of the objects in the collection, but a description and interpretation of the 'rariora' or unusual, natural objects in the first three parts, and the rare man-made objects in the fourth and last part of the book.

Worm's museum would have corresponded closely with most other museums or cabinets of curiosity of the period. The inscription the French physician Pierre Borel had placed over the entrance to his cabinet, 'it is a micro cosmos or compendium of all rare things' would also have been appropriate for Worm's collection. Early modern museums, of course, excluded 99.9

---

166 See *Museum Wormianum*, Amsterdam/Leiden 1655. See also Schepelern, *Museum*, 206, who considers Willum's involvement with the publication as fairly minimal because a fair amount of the manuscript had already been printed by Worm's death. That clearly undervalues the role and significance of Willum in seeing the book published and providing editorial guidance. Simply to blame Willum for the misprints in the volume strikes me as unfair.

167 C. Mordhorst, *Genstandsfortællinger*, Copenhagen 2009, 44–45.

168 Schepelern, *Museum*, 304–05;

percent of the known universe, including all natural and artificial objects, in other words all that was ordinary or common.[169] In other words the ordinary or commonly occurring was of no interest whereas the new, extraordinary, and exceptional, termed rariora, were what early modern collectors focussed on.

Despite the attention given by a number of historians to the role and significance of the early modern museums or cabinets of curiosity the reason why their creators focussed on the exceptional, apart from the scholarly and social prestige attached to it, has yet to be fully understood.[170] Like early modern natural philosophy creating a cabinet of curiosity was, at least for Protestants, ultimately about seeking to understand God through his Creation, Nature.[171] Collecting the new, the rare, and the exceptional was a way of getting a clearer and more complete understanding of the Book of Nature, through the signs God had implanted in his creation, not simply to admire the variety and playfulness of Nature.

Collecting and creating a cabinet of curiosity certainly enhanced its creators' social and intellectual standing. This might be further boosted when collectors published catalogues or histories linked to their collections. Grand examples such as those by Aldrovandi and Calzolari demonstrated this social significance, as did more modest examples such as that of Worm's relation, the physician Henrik Fuiren.[172] Thus, when the French poet and theologian Pierre-Daniel Huet made a stop in Copenhagen in the summer of 1652 on his way to Sweden, he first took time to admire the runic stones which Worm on the King's order had had transported to Copenhagen, while expressing his disappointment by not having been given the opportunity to see Worm's cabinet of curiosity personally, making the following note in his travel description:

> He [Worm] also collected with shrewd care everything rare and unique from nature and art which by accident revealed itself to him in these lands and no appreciator of virtue and learning arrive in Copenhagen without showing his respect for Worm with the ambition to see his collection.[173]

169 See L. Daston and K. Park, *Wonders and the Order of Nature*, New York 1998, 272. The quotation cited by Daston and Park is from Pierre Borel, *Catalogue de choses rares qui sont dans le Cabinet de Maistre Pierre Borel*, 1645.

170 See in particular the works by Daston and Park, and Findlen

171 See P. Harrison, *The Bible, Protestantism, and the Rise of Natural Science*, Cambridge 1998, 64–204.

172 For Aldrovandi and Calceolari, see Daston and Park, *Wonders*, 155; for Henrik Fuiren, see his *Rariora Musaei Henrici Fuiren, M. D., quae Academiae regiae Hafniae legavit*, Copenhagen 1663.

173 Petrus Daniel Huetius, *Commentarius de rebus ad eum pertinentibus*, Amsterdam 1718, 80.

11 Inspirations for Worm's museum history

The typographical model for *Museum Wormianum* was undoubtedly Georg Marcgrave's *Historia Naturalis Brasiliae*, edited by Worm's friend Johannes de Laet and published in Leiden in 1648. It was a richly illustrated book which had impressed Ole Worm. He wanted the illustrations and the typography of *Museum Wormianum* to be as close to de Laet's book as possible.[174] Worm's work differed from the large encyclopaedic works by Conrad Gesner and Ulisse Aldrovandi which sought to describe all known natural objects in detail. As opposed to them Worm was solely concerned with the objects in his own collection. This type of work dedicated to an individual collection would appear to have gained popularity around the middle of the seventeenth century as can be seen from among others the work of Athanasius Kircher.

It has been argued that the matter of fact style of writing used by Ole Worm in *Museum Wormianum*, was adopted from Georg Marcgrave's *Historia Naturalis Brasiliae*, which was considered to be one of the most innovative works of natural history to be published in the seventeenth century, not only in terms of content but also in terms of style and presentation. As we have seen, Worm acquired a copy of this work on publication and was impressed by it, but his own sober and factual style of writing did not result from reading this work. Instead it was a style of writing he had long used when describing natural objects.[175]

Worm drew extensively on the work of Ulisse Aldrovandi, professor of medicine at the University of Bologna, whom he quoted no less than forty-one times in *Museum Wormianum*. Like many others Aldrovandi's cabinet of curiosity was created primarily in order to advance medical knowledge, especially the so-called materia medica. Until the middle of the sixteenth century natural history and materia medica had formed little or no part of the medical curriculum in the universities. By the end of the century this had all changed and it had become a central part of the university curriculum within the leading Italian universities. This interest in natural history inspired not only collecting but also anatomical dissecting, and experimenting, shaping the debates about the preparation and diffusion of medicines. As a result natural history became an important part of early modern medical culture.[176]

By 1642 Worm was trying to acquire some of Adrovandi's works for his library. He wrote to his nephews, Henrik Fuiren and Thomas

---

174 Schepelern, *Museum*, 211 and *Breve fra og til Ole Worm*, no. 1748 [my translation].

175 See W. B. Ashworth, 'Remarkable Humans and Singular Beasts', 133–44 in J. Kenseth (ed.), *The Age of the Marvelous*, Hanover, Hampshire 1991, and Mordhorst, *Genstandsfortællinger*, 159–60

176 Findlen, *Possessing Nature*, 241–87.

Bartholin, who then resided in Padua, asking them to try to obtain these works cheaper than the costly volumes sold by the Amsterdam book-sellers in Copenhagen. Whether he obtained them we do not know, but he clearly had access to these works when finishing his *Museum Wormianum*.[177]

Other works which inspired *Museum Wormianum*, were the natural histories of Ferrante Imperato and Francesco Calzolari. Ferrante Impera-to's work in particular proved important to Worm. It is cited no less than twenty-five times in *Museum Wormianum*. Worm had, of course, seen Im-perato's museum when he visited Naples in 1609 and Imperato had signed his album amicorum. Worm may well have acquired Imperato's work on natural history at the same time. The similarities between the title-page of Imperato's work and that of *Museum Wormianum* are striking, and Worm used Imperato's work as a model for his treatment of soils and stones which he also divided according to their use. In his introduction Imperato men-tioned the scholars and friends who had assisted him in creating his cabinet of curiosity. Among them were scholars who had also inspired Worm's col-lection, such as his supervisor at the University of Basle, Caspar Bauhin and the famous botanist Carolus Clusius in Leiden whom Worm quoted no less than sixty-nine times in *Museum Wormianum*. Unfortunately Worm does not follow Imperato in mentioning the scholars who assisted him in putting his collection together.

The work of Francesco Calzolari, the Verona apothecary, published by his grandson is only referred to nine times by Worm. Ole Worm's work overlaps with Imperato's in terms of those who assisted him in his collec-tion and in the title-page. Worm managed to borrow a copy of Calzolari's work from his friend Otto Sperling in the spring of 1636 which he hung onto for some time.[178]

As a physician Ole Worm was a typical early modern creator of a cabinet of curiosity. The medical use of many of these museums played a promi-nent role and rationale for their creators and Worm was no exception. In fact, the medical raison d'être for his collection was more conspicuous than most. Bearing in mind that Ole Worm added MD to his name on all his publications that should not surprise us. Worm always considered himself first and foremost a physician.

Worm's collecting has been seen as a separate aspect of his interests, de-veloping in parallel with his other concerns such as medicine and antiquar-ianism.[179] Worm's focus and commitment to different fields of research certainly changed over time, but collecting natural objects constituted part

177 Schepelern, *Museum*, 222–23.
178 *Ibid.*, 226–28.
179 *Ibid.*, 229.

of the whole. All his interests formed part of the same drive to observe, describe, and analyse, seeking to understand God's creation through the best knowledge possible about the natural world.

Historians such as Paula Findlen, Krzysztof Pomian, Lorraine Daston, and Katharine Park who have focussed primarily on the museums and collections created by Italian physicians and natural philosophers during the Renaissance have argued that putting together cabinets of curiosity allocated a unique and creative function to Nature, making it possible for Nature to generate all sorts of marvellous objects and creatures.[180] They have emphasised the significance of the rediscovery of the classical concept of lusus naturae, and the significance it gave to the irregular and marvellous as a key to understanding Nature. This resulted not only in the prominence attached to strange and rare natural objects, such as animals, plants, and stones, but also to objects which appeared to represent a hybrid, where art and Nature proved impossible to separate. According to them many natural philosophers and collectors of the sixteenth and seventeenth centuries viewed lusus naturae as the key to 'an efficacious reading of the book of nature'.[181]

The result has been that Ole Worm's rationale for taking an interest in natural philosophy and natural history has been excluded from the story, namely, his Lutheran faith. Consequently Worm's declaration in the introduction to his chapter on rare stones in *Museum Wormianum*: 'Nature has joked uncommonly in all the outward appearances of natural things', has been taken as axiomatic for his research and collecting.[182] This is particularly baffling when borne in mind that a far more significant statement is also to be found in *Museum Wormianum*, namely, that God was the ultimate cause of all natural things, even if He did not act directly in order to affect Nature, but through natural causes. Accordingly it was the task of the natural philosopher to discover those causes.[183]

Worm in other words intended to discover and understand the structure and signs God had placed in his creation by seeking to comprehend exceptional and marvellous creations brought forward by Nature. For Protestants like Worm, the study of the Bible was central to their faith, while the study of Nature was essential for a better understanding of the Book of Nature and God's plan for the world.[184]

180 See in particular Findlen, *Possessing Nature*, K. Pomian, *Collectors and Curiosities. Paris and Venice 1500–1800*, Cambridge 1990, and Daston and Park, *Wonders*.

181 P. Findlen, 'Jokes of Nature and Jokes of Knowledge: The Playfulness of Scientific Discourse in Early Modern Europe', *Renaissance Quarterly*, 43, no. 2, Summer, 1990, 293.

182 For the quote see Worm, *Museum Wormianum*, 81; otherwise see especially Mordhorst, *Genstandsfortællinger*, 146–60.

183 Worm, *Museum Wormianum*, 311 (my translation).

184 Findlen sees a similar approach by the Jesuit Athanasius Kircher, Findlen, 'Jokes', 300–01.

12 The museum history

In his preface to *Museum Wormianum* Ole Worm made his natural philo-sophical views and intentions clear to the reader, stating that since ancient times the learned have complained that the investigations of Nature are like the fox in Aesop's fables which only licked the glass, but failed to touch the porridge. Worm attacked Aristotelianism which he claimed had taken teaching and research in the wrong direction from school to university, focussing on hair-spitting issues such as 'the eternity of the World, the im-penetrability of the celestial spheres and similar sophisms', rather than real insight such as knowledge about the nature, qualities, and character of 'the simplest stone under our feet'. He argued that it had become 'the custom in schools and academies to spurn the most useful books by the philoso-phers on the nature of objects, descriptions of soils, minerals, stones, and plants'. These works are despised as opposed to writings which are best suited to promote disputations and idle bickering. This prevents the young from properly investigating the nature of things. Instead students waste their time and leave their schools and academies more ignorant than when they started their studies. To further prove this point Worm supplied an ex-tensive quote from Pierre Gassendi's anti-Aristotelian book, *Exercitationes Paradoxicæ adversus*, published in Grenoble in 1624, which offered the following conclusion about the student experience when studying natural philosophy:

> They simply have gained no insight into the Nature of the World, be-cause when they start their schooling they step into a different Na-ture which does not at all correspond with the external World. One is accordingly not surprised when experiencing their account of natural objects to find them far removed from our observations outside the Schools. If they encounter real Nature, they become totally befuddled and are made stupid, if they are reminded by people who do not try to understand things through contemplation, but through the teacher of all things: experience and observation.[185]

Worm had been brought into contact with Gassendi by his friend Isaac La Peyrère. Gassendi was then working on his biography of the Danish as-tronomer Tycho Brahe, which was published in 1654. La Peyrère asked his friend Worm to supply Gassendi with information about Brahe.[186] Worm expressed his admiration for Gassendi's *Exercitationes Paradoxicæ* in his response to La Peyrère. He found the book 'ingenious, shrewd and radiat-ing the greatest learning'. He also expressed his disappointment in having only been able to acquire the first of the seven promised books against

185 Cited in Worm, *Museum Wormianum*, Præfatio [my translation].
186 *Breve fra og til Ole Worm*, no. 1545.

the Aristotelians. If on sale in Copenhagen Worm were prepared to pay a considerable sum to acquire them, clearly unaware that they had not been published.[187]

Worm concluded his preface by quoting Galen whom he considered among those natural philosophers who had 'introduced their apprentices into Nature's closet' learning how to use natural objects to preserve and regain bodily health.

> Anyone who wants to own a supply of remedies from all places will have to understand everything about roots, animals, metals, and other objects present in the soil, which we have become used to utilise in medicine.[188]

This was according to Worm the reason why Galen undertook so many journeys to Lemnos and other places, in order that he could personally observe these remedies in their local context.

Ole Worm had been disappointed by the way natural philosophy was taught within the universities with the emphasis on theory and debate. He wanted this approach replaced with investigation, observation and demonstrable proof. To achieve that Worm had begun a collection of the most beautiful natural objects he could find in order that his students could be 'pulled out of the bog of errors and darkness and brought into the clear daylight and the most beautiful observation of God's creation'. He claimed to have started his collection, sparing no effort and expense, when he had been given the Chair in natural philosophy at the University of Copenhagen in April 1621. This would seem to be an exaggeration. As we have seen Worm may have begun to acquire natural objects at this stage, but not in a systematic or organised way with the intent of building a cabinet of curiosity. That began at least a decades later. However, his views of how natural philosophy should be pursued with the emphasis on the study of Nature and sensory observation as the proper means of establishing and authorising knowledge were already present in his inaugural lecture when he took over the professorship of natural philosophy.[189]

Worm very likely made use of his university lectures when writing *Museum Wormianum*, supplementing his text with smaller individually published pamphlets when convenient, such as those on terra sigillata and the Norwegian lemmings. Like most of his contemporaries Worm took his departure in the classical authors, especially Aristotle, Pliny, and Galen and through the natural objects collected and described he aimed at checking and revising their views.

187 *Ibid.*
188 Worm, *Museum Wormianum*, Præfatio [my translation].
189 See Chapter 2 above.

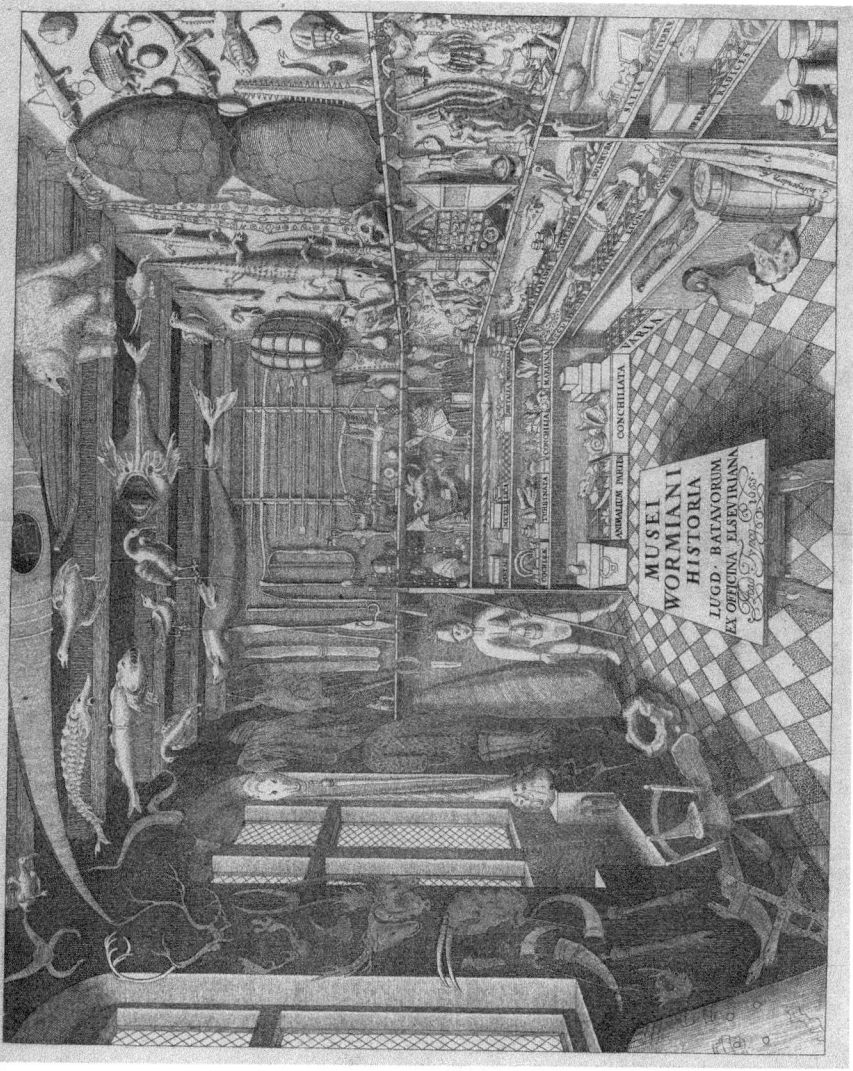

Figure 4.6 View of the interior of Worm's cabinet of curiosity from Ole Worm, *Museum Wormianum*, 1655; courtesy of the Royal Danish Library.

Ole Worm's cabinet of curiosity was not assembled exclusively for pedagogic or didactic purposes, it also served as a research laboratory for natural philosophers who, like Worm himself, could use the collection for study, observation, and experiment.[190]

Worm divided his work into four books each focussed on a particular subject area, generally accepted as a coherent field or unit by contemporary scholars. The first book deals with fossils and is divided into three parts on, soils, stones, and metals. This book repeatedly refers to the works of the physicians Georg Agricola and Anselm Boetius de Boodt.[191] Both authors provided numerous instructions for the medical use of fossils. In his chapter on types of soil and their medical use Worm writes extensively about the uses of terra sigillata. He had no doubt that these soils had the power to fight diseases, because they could generate secretion of sweat. As such he considered them particularly useful against dysentery and diarrhoea.[192] Some, however, were more remarkable for the way they materialised. Thus in November 1642 Worm forwarded some terra sigillata from Scania to his friend Johannes de Laet in Leiden, offering him the following description of what he labelled miraculous soil:

> In the year 1619, at a time when it had become customary among us to colour our clothes on collars and similar adornments with blue, a sumptuousness often criticized in their sermons by the servants of the church, the Almighty God demonstrated in many places in Scania how much he abhorred this vice; He dispatched a rain squall which made this blue soil fall down sullying people's clothes. The lump I possess was given to me by my famous father-in-law, Dr. Thomas Fincke, public professor of medicine at this university, who at the time was attending a noble patient in Scania. With regard to the Icelandic [terra sigillata] which I forward wrapped in a piece of sailcloth the following is the case: In the year 1625, when the Icelandic Hekla known as Mödals Jöckel [volcano], burnt with a terrible roar and destroyed many people and animals, its ash was transported through the air as far as Norway. Here a ship sailing in the sea in the vicinity of Trondheim was covered in ash to such an extent that its thwarts and sails were buried as if they had been filled with snow, and this rain of ash took away their view of sea and air in the middle of the day as if they were sailing in total darkness. However when this ash had water added it turned into soil which could not be washed of the sails; when the sailor told us this on his return and showed us the sails which had been coloured by this soil I received a piece as a memento of the event.[193]

190 A point emphasised by Mordhorst, *Genstandsfortællinger*, 91–92.
191 Schepelern, *Museum*, 231–35.
192 Worm, *Museum Wormianum*, 16.
193 *Breve fra og til Ole Worm*, no. 1089.

Here as with most of the objects Worm collected it was not only the objects themselves that mattered but the context in which they materialised, without which their authenticity and value could not be demonstrated.

In his chapter on magnets it is evident that Worm had consulted Athanasius Kircher's work, *Magnes, sive de arte magnetica*, published in Rome in 1641, even if much of the information appears to have come from his own experiments.[194] Similarly Worm dedicates a couple of chapters to precious stones and jewels, their medical power, and how to use it. He was attracted to the Renaissance teaching on signature, which considered hidden connections to exist between Man and objects such as precious stones. Signatures contained important information often of a medical nature and had been imprinted by God to be identified only by well-trained men such as physicians. This was a view which had been strongly promoted by Paracelsus in particular and it evidently influenced Worm even if he did not accept it uncritically.[195]

The last section of book one is dedicated to metals and here Worm shares the generally held view that metals can be transformed into other metals, and that the fineness of metals depends on mercury. He points out that antimony was Paracelsus's preferred chemical drug while his view of mercury is that it contains all metals except gold. Worm recommends its use for goldsmiths and for physicians as a remedy against the pox. It is evident from this section that Worm had personal hands-on experience of work in a laboratory. In fact, the first book contains substantial artisanal knowledge which can only have been achieved through direct practical involvement in working with metals. Worm like many of his fellow collectors was fascinated by the skill and knowledge which was needed to produce the finest and most unusual works in gold, silver, jewels, stones, and ivory, and considered these artificialia as matching and complementing those of Nature.[196]

The second book is about botany, but only deals with what Worm termed the rarer plants. Worm remained a botanist all his life and as a physician was particularly focussed on the medical use of plants. Not surprisingly most of the references in this book are to Pliny, Carolus Clusius, and the Italian, Padua-educated, physician Pietro Andrea Matthiolo, who had served as royal physician to Emperor Maximilian II. Worm very likely owned a copy of the collected works by Matthiolo published in 1598 by his tutor at the University of Basle, Caspar Bauhin. This was the edition he used when writing *Museum Wormianum*. It is noteworthy that the other great botanist of the sixteenth century Joachim Camerarius, who had inherited Conrad Gesner's manuscripts and his illustrations of plants, is only rarely referred to in *Museum Wormianum*.[197] The second book is to a considerable extent characterised by Worm's own observations and descriptions of plants.

194 Schepelern, *Museum*, 239–40
195 Schepelern, *Museum*, 245 and Mordhorst, *Genstandsfortællinger*, 172–78.
196 Mordhorst, *Genstandsfortællinger*, 165–71; see also Daston and Park, *Wonders*, 277.
197 For this see Worm, *Museum Wormianum*, 250–51.

The third book deals with animals and differ from the previous two not only by having far fewer bibliographical references but also by its near exclusive dependence on the general sources for the whole work, namely, Aristotle, Pliny, Gesner, and Aldrovandi. The animals are split between those containing blood and those without. Worm begins with the insects and follows Aldrovandi's classification of those with and those without wings. He then covers shellfish before moving on to more advanced animals who contained blood, starting with the cold-blooded such as snakes, fish, and whales. The latter offered Worm a chance to return to an issue which had preoccupied him since the mid-1630s, namely, the common mistake of identifying the narwhale tooth as being the horn of the unicorn.[198]

The last five chapters of the third book are dedicated to four-footed mammals and humans. Chapter 23 is unusually long because it incorporates a reprint with a few additions of Worm's tract from 1653 about the lemming, the Norwegian mouse. Towards the end of this book Worm offers some views of the role of the natural philosopher with regard to the sudden appearance and disappearance of animals. Worm considers it the obligation of the natural philosopher to investigate the natural causes for such developments. It is not enough to consider such developments as something supernatural, and as an expression of God's omnipotence.[199]

The fourth and final book of *Museum Wormianum* is concerned with close to 300 man-made objects or 'artificiosa' as Worm labelled them. As opposed to the rest of his collection these items proved more durable, their survival not depending on any treatment or conservation, plus the fact that many of them later found a natural home in the royal collection, the so-called Museum Regium. This part of Worm's cabinet of curiosity did not serve the same clear-cut educational and research purposes as did the rest of his collection, but would undoubtedly have added to its social standing, appealing to the growing, more popular interest, in unusual and surprising objects which characterised the age.

The first three books of *Museum Wormianum*, however, dealing with natural objects, constituted the bulk of the folio edition. They encompassed a total of 345 pages, 89% of the work, leaving only 44 pages for the fourth book on 'artificialia' or around 11% of the book.[200]

Even if *Museum Wormianum* was only one of several works about cabinets of curiosity which was published across Europe around the mid-seventeenth century, aiming in the first instance at the learned republic of letters, it proved one of the more influential. It probably appealed first and foremost to physicians or people with a medical education with its distinct focus on the medical

198 *Ibid.*, 278–80.
199 Worm, *Museum Wormianum*, 331–32
200 Mordhorst, *Genstandsfortællinger*, 43.

utility of many of the objects discussed, but its allure went far beyond this group and proved popular with the broader European republic of letters.

13 The publication of *Museum Wormianum*

By 1648 it would appear that Worm had finished most of his manuscript for *Museum Wormianum*.[201] He was now spending much of his time editing it, claiming he was repeatedly being urged to publish. Even so it took him another five years to finish, because of corrections and amendments, while his collection continued to grow and revisions became necessary.[202] Furthermore Worm was determined to find a leading Dutch publisher to publish his work.

His son Willum who had arrived in Leiden to study medicine in the summer of 1653 was commissioned to start negotiations for the publication of *Museum Wormianum* with Johannes Elzevir, the famous Dutch printing house, who, according to Worm, were able to supply fine quality paper and beautiful types. Worm also wanted the Elzevir Press because of the many relevant illustrations in Elzevir's possession previously used for Johannes de Laet's edition of Marcgrave's *Historia Naturalis Brasiliae*, which he hoped to be able to use. That summer Ole Worm had met with a member of the Elzevir family in Copenhagen and had shown him his manuscript. It had received praise, and Worm had been led to believe that the Elzevirs would be keen to publish it. However, the fact that this member of the Elzevir family left Copenhagen without taking leave of him caused Worm to take a less optimistic view of the prospect.[203]

Meanwhile, Willum served his father well in Leiden and convinced the Elzevirs to publish his book. Worm was delighted when the news reached him in August 1653, and he informed Willum that he would not forward the manuscript until he had found a reliable messenger to deliver what was his only copy to the printers.[204]

Willum was constantly kept informed about his father's plans and did his best to further and execute them. Despite that, Worm proved impatient with his young son whose correspondence he found both too slow and irregular. Worm was totally focussed on the publication of his book in his letters

---

201 *Ibid.*, no. 1712; in this letter dated May 1651 Worm makes it clear in the postscript that more might still be included in his *Museum Wormianum*.

202 *Ibid.*, no. 1576 and 1747.

203 *Ibid.*, nos. 1741–42. Bearing in mind the difficulties his friend Johan Rhode encountered with the Elzevirs in the mid-1640s when seeking to publish his work on Scribonius with them, it is surprising that Worm chose the Elzevirs for his museum history, especially since he had questioned their honesty. For Rhode's difficulties see nos. 1222, 1225, 1293, 1361, and 1405. For Worm's doubt about the honesty of the Elzevirs, see no. 1431. For the influence of the Elzevirs on the Danish book trade and market, see A. Pettegree and A. der Weduwen, *The Bookshop of the World. Making and Trading Books in the Dutch Golden Age*, London 2019, especially 281–93.

204 *Ibid.*, no. 1745.

to Willum and often only inquired about his studies in Leiden as an after-
thought. The letter to Willum of 24 September 1653 was, in many ways,
typical:

> I forward my museum history in order that you can hand it over to
> the Elzevirs for printing on condition that they do not wait, but print
> it immediately. Take care it isn't lost because you know that this is
> my only copy. I hope they will give me some copies for my trouble.
> I shall postpone the dedication until they have forwarded a sample
> of the edition. I would appreciate a learned man with knowledge of
> natural history as my copy-editor. I would prefer if the types which
> were used for the American history [a reference to *Historia Naturalis
> Brasiliae*] could be used for my book. I have indicated in the margins
> where illustrations can be inserted. I would welcome an illustration for
> the title page. ... Write immediately you have received the manuscript
> and inform me what the Elzevirs have decided; do hasten the work as
> much as you can.[205]

Worm was clearly preoccupied with the safe delivery of his manuscript and
the danger of it being lost. Similarly, he was worried that it might not be
printed immediately but shelved until a time when it was convenient for
the printers to send it to press. And then, of course, there was the issue of
quality: Worm wanted the best in both paper and types, not to mention
illustrations. He had always taken great care with his publications, constantly checking on his printers and their copy-editing. Thirty years earlier
he had evidently been deeply disappointed when he first had to abandon
his plans to have his work on Aristotelian natural philosophy, *Liber aureus
philosophum aquilæ Aristotelis de mundi fabrica*, published by the printer
Ferber in Rostock in 1622, because he had proved unreliable, only managing to get the printer and bookseller Johannes Hallerfort in the same city
to print it two years later. Hallerfort's efforts had seriously disappointed
Worm. He complained to Hallerfort about the lack of proper copy-editing
of his work and the lack of inclusion of Aristotle's text De Mundi. He
pointed out that there was hardly a page which had not been disfigured by
mistakes. Neither did he like Hallerfort's title-page with its description of
him as exceptionally learned, which he considered self-praise and in bad
taste. He insisted that the printer added a list of errata at the end. When he
forwarded copies to his friends in October that year he apologised for the
incompetence of the printer, pointing out that there were so many misprints
that he was inclined not to recognise the book as his own. Writing to his
friend Johannes Cabeljau nine years later his anger over the mangling of his

205 *Ibid.*, no. 1748.

work still lingered and he claimed that he was reluctant to trust this printer with any more of his works.[206]

Worm's view of the Copenhagen printers was not much better. As we have seen above Worm faced considerable problems finding a printer for his work on runes and claimed they were not interested in publishing anything but popular pamphlets. But printers were far from Ole Worm's only concern in September 1653. He was worried about Willum's education, telling him to focus on his medical studies in order that he might be well prepared for his trip to Italy to study at Padua the following spring. He was adamant that Willum should not remain in Leiden where he spent far too much money and had fallen in with a crowd of students and drinking companions of whom Worm did not approve.[207] The question remained, however, whether these educational and social concerns would override Worm's need for retaining Willum in Leiden to make sure that the publication of *Museum Wormianum* kept going to plan.

Willum's travels abroad had, of course, proved a constant worry for Ole Worm who feared that his young son might associate with the 'wrong' people and prove profligate. The previous year, in June 1652, when Willum had joined the Danish diplomatic mission to England, Worm had written him a series of letters expressing his concerns. They ranged from distress over the bad exchange rate obtained by Willum, to instructions about not to throw away his old clothes which he could use when in transit on the boat thereby saving his new clothes for important occasions. Worm also warned Willum against imitating the lives of courtiers – presumably the diplomats he travelled with – while simultaneously admonishing him not to associate with the 'common herd' which would prove detrimental to his standing. Willum meanwhile managed to lose or have a substantial amount of money stolen on a journey to Bath and Worm scolded him for his negligence. But the final straw for Worm was what he considered Willum's extravagance on this trip. He found it incomprehensible that Willum had been able to spend 200 Imperial Thalers in two months having had all his daily expenses and travel paid for by others – presumably Willum travelled as part of the diplomatic mission. Worm claimed that he had spent more than others would do in a whole year. Willum was told to return home immediately and make sure that he would not spend on such a lavish scale when he began his study in Leiden, because if so, Worm was convinced that he would squander the inheritance after his mother.[208] The foundations were, in other words, in place for what proved a difficult relationship between a cautious and at times grumpy old parent and his son who found it necessary to spend more freely.

206 *Ibid.*, nos. 109, 158, 163, 167, and 489.
207 *Ibid.*, no. 1749; for this see also nos. 1744 and 1745.
208 For the London trip see *ibid.*, nos. 1726–29.

Finally, in the second week of October 1653 Ole Worm managed to dispatch his manuscript to the Netherlands. It had evidently been difficult to find a reliable messenger. But a lady from Amsterdam had been recruited in Copenhagen who would deliver it to the Amsterdam merchant, Niclas Relinkhuysen, who was closely associated with the Elzevirs. Four days later, however, Worm had to inform Willum that this arrangement had fallen through, and that the manuscript had instead been dispatched through another two Amsterdam merchants, Gerrit Jansson and Abraham van Cossart. Worm, however, was still concerned that the Elzevirs might not be the right publishers for his work. Could they be trusted to take good care of it and would he receive the same number of copies as they had given to De Laet? He advised Willum to consult the Leiden professor of Arabic and mathematics, Jacob Golius, and some of his other Leiden friends such as the professor of medicine, Otto Heurnius. Golius, had been brought into contact with Worm by Thomas Bartholin in 1640 and was still active within the university in 1653, whereas Worm's friend Heurnius had died over a year earlier. Worm also used the opportunity to include a separate sheet of paper with additions to his manuscript which Willum was asked to insert at the right places. Worm had in other words hardly dispatched his manuscript before he started to change it and make additions.[209]

Meanwhile, Ole Worm was impatiently awaiting confirmation that the manuscript had arrived safely. Only seventeen days after having dispatched it he complained to Willum that he had yet to confirm its arrival, claiming that he had been waiting for news for more than a month. A fortnight later Worm received no less than two letters from Willum written a week apart. But they did not contain the hoped for news that the manuscript had safely arrived. Consequently Worm instructed Willum to visit the Amsterdam merchant Abraham Cossart and enquire about it. He added that daily he found things to add to the manuscript which he would forward to Willum for insertion. Worm, however, remained concerned about Willum's expenditure, pointing out that Willum had spent 350 Imperial Thalers in five months in Leiden. 'For what my Willum? Either you are providing loans for others or abandoned yourself to considerable extravagance. What am I to say?' Worm pointed out that if Willum continued to spend that much he would not have enough for another two years study abroad.[210] Money clearly continued to be a major issue between father and son. Willum undoubtedly had a more relaxed attitude to spending than his father. Worm, of course, drew on his experience as a student in Leiden forty years earlier and appeared at times out of touch. Furthermore, Worm was now an elderly man and his health was failing.

209 *Ibid.*, nos. 1752 and 1753.
210 *Ibid.*, no. 1757.

Fifteen months later Worm received the long awaited good news from the Netherlands. In two letters dated 21 and 28 November 1553 Willum informed his father that his manuscript had arrived safely and had been handed over to the Elzevirs. Worm was delighted and he immediately sent off a letter instructing Willum about necessary additions and illustrations. He certainly knew how to keep his son busy. Worm wanted his illustrations – presumably drawings – turned into woodcuts by a competent artist so that they would match those he planned to use from the volumes by Johannes de Laet and Anselm Boetius de Boodt, court physician to Rudolph II (*Gemmarum et Lapidum Historia*, 1609), and inserted according to his indications in the margins. Worm also wanted only a single illustration per page. Willum had included a sample page from the Elzevirs for how *Museum Wormianum* would look and Worm expressed his satisfaction. Worm elaborated his preference for woodcuts, which he found clearer and cheaper than engravings. They could be used together with the illustrations from Le Maire's edition of de Boodt and Elzevir's of de Laet which he was convinced could be obtained cheaply. He suggested that the new illustrations should be done, if possible, by the same artist who had supplied the illustrations for these two works in order that consistency could be achieved.[211]

Worm's constant changes and additions to his text, not surprisingly, caused problems. At times he was not sure whether Willum had received all his letters, and was therefore in doubt whether all his additions had been inserted. He therefore suggested that in future they both listed the letters they had received from each other with the dates they were written on top of their responses. Willum had included a sample of the work of the woodcutter he proposed to hire for his father's work in his latest letter, dated 1 January 1654. Worm expressed his satisfaction as long as the woodcutter showed similar care with the work for *Museum Wormianum*. Towards the end of his response Worm repeated his worry about the high costs of Willum's study in Leiden. A fortnight later he conveyed his satisfaction with the agreement Willum had reached with the Elzevirs. It would appear, that the printers had promised him more copies than expected. Worm also addressed the queries which Willum had raised about his manuscript. The enterprise clearly kept Willum busy, and the constant and repeated changes and additions from his father cannot but have been challenging to deal with. Worm was rightly concerned that everything appeared in the right place and only once. That only two sections were eventually repeated – the one about the eider and the one about the statue of the Norwegian king – plus some to be expected misprints, is a rather remarkable outcome bearing in mind the many changes and additions.[212]

211 *Ibid.*, nos. 1759 and 1760.
212 Schepelern, *Museum*, 211.

By February Worm had become seriously impatient. He inquired why the Elzevirs were delaying the publication and asked Willum to make urgent inquiries.[213] Worm added that friends in Copenhagen had informed him that the Elzevirs had a reputation for letting manuscripts remain unpublished for more than a year. Willum was told to make sure that 'our hopes are not disappointed' and to inform his father the moment printing had begun.[214]

Instructions for Willum continued to be sent through March, mainly about illustrations and corrections with little or no recognition of all the work he was doing apart from a short sentence praising him for keeping the Elzevirs up to the mark.[215] However, by mid-April Worm had begun to despair and began to blame Willum for the delays. He sternly inquired whether Willum had forgotten the Fourth Commandment: honour they father and mother. He accused him of having totally forgotten his 'old and decrepit father' and for having failed to keep him informed about what was happening to his manuscript. Worm even pointed out that he now regretted having sent Willum abroad.[216] Worm's health was in decline again and may well explain the excessive anger and disappointment he expressed, but undoubtedly it was also generated by the fact, that he had received no response to his three most recent letters. Rather than the fairly regular problems with the postal connections between Leiden and Copenhagen Worm was convinced that this time it was all Willum's fault. Accordingly, by the end of April Worm decided to leave Willum 'to his own dreams' and deal directly with the Elzevirs himself. He wrote two letters to find out what was happening to his manuscript and enclosed a drawing of his cabinet of curiosity. This was clearly the illustration which was eventually used as a frontispiece for *Museum Wormianum*.

While writing this angry letter to his son Ole Worm received a response from Willum dated 5 April. This served to alleviate the distress of his 'troubled mind,' as he put it, even if he still felt that Willum had not sufficiently explained his tardiness in writing. Meanwhile plague had broken out in Copenhagen and Worm was concerned, especially because of his dual role of physician and vice chancellor of the university. In his next letter Worm made a vague apology for his angry outburst, pointing out that his parental concern for the welfare of his son was natural and had been unduly strained by Willum's lack of communication. By then Willum had acknowledged that his letter-writing had been amiss and promised to write more often. More importantly Willum was able to inform his father that the Elzevir Press was now engaged in printing his book. Worm's attempt to communicate directly with the printers had evidently failed in generating any response. He was delighted and expressed the hope that the Elzevirs would continue to show their zeal while Willum would remain in Leiden to sort

213 *Breve fra og til Ole Worm*, nos. 1761 and 1762.
214 *Ibid.*, no. 1763.
215 *Ibid.*, nos. 1765 and 1766.
216 *Ibid.*, no. 1767.

out any queries. Worm also hoped that the Elzevirs would make sure that his book was included in the catalogue for the next Frankfurt Book Fair.[217] He remained in other words totally dependent on Willum to further the printing of his book with the Elzevirs.

Even so, Worm was keen for Willum to leave Leiden for Padua in the summer of 1654, primarily for financial reasons. Not only did he find his expenditure far too high, but he remained concerned that Willum had fallen in with the wrong sort. Willum had forwarded the first couple of the printed pages of *Museum Wormianum* to his father in June and Worm informed him that he found them 'quite neatly' printed. Rather modest praise especially since Worm proved far more effusive about the sample he had received when writing to one of his students in Schleswig, describing the pages from the Elzevirs as printed 'on rather fine paper and with elegant types'.[218]

Still Worm remained dissatisfied with Willum's correspondence – he didn't write often enough nor did he provide the information required. Worm had hired the royal court painter Karel van Mander to draw his portrait, which he intended to send directly to the Elzevir Press with instructions to employ a better artist for making the engraving than the one who had recently supplied the engraving for Thomas Bartholin's portrait. His nephew Thomas Bartholin had written him a verse which was to be added below the portrait. He instructed Willum to return the drawing to him when work was finished because it had proved a rather expensive undertaking, while also telling him to order an extra hundred copies of the printed portrait at his own expense which Worm planned to give to his friends.[219]

Worm was not easy to satisfy and he constantly found reasons to be worried and concerned, if not about the lack of information reaching him, then about issues relating to the printing of his book. By mid-July Willum must have informed him that the Elzevirs were not inclined to use the drawing of his museum. Worm was annoyed and baffled, because he had no doubt that it would make it possible for the Elzevirs to charge more for the book if it was included. Consequently, he became concerned that the Elzevirs might not use his expensively obtained portrait by Karel van Mander either.[220] As it turned out his worries proved unnecessary.

In his last letter to Willum written only a fortnight before his death on 31 August 1654 Worm remained concerned about the difficulties of staying in regular communication by letter. It would appear that Willum had not received his last three letters and Worm complained about the lack of reliable and dependable carriers. Overall Worm appears to have had greater faith in merchants than students to deliver letters expeditiously. He had sent his portrait with a Dutchman who should deliver it to an Amsterdam merchant,

217 *Ibid.*, nos. 1769 and 1770.
218 *Ibid.*, nos. 1777 and 1779.
219 *Ibid.*, nos. 1783, 1785 and 1786.
220 *Ibid.*, no. 1787

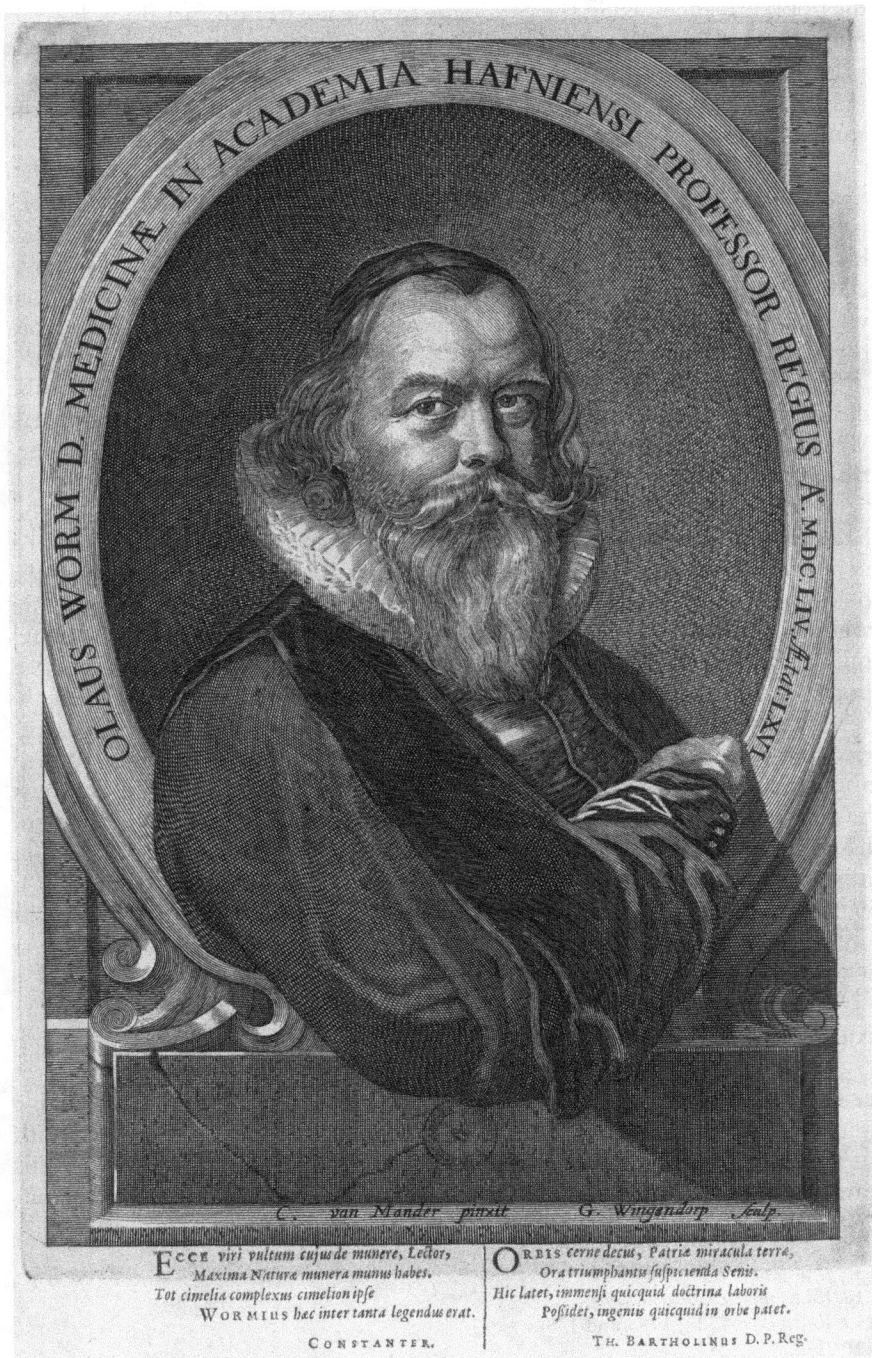

Figure 4.7 Ole Worm (1588–1654) age 66, by Karel van Mander; courtesy of the Royal Danish Library.

Johan Fige. However, he was worried it had been lost. Willum had heard nothing about it during a visit to Johan Fige, nor had Fige mentioned it in his recent letter. Furthermore, Worm was clearly irritated that the Elzevirs had complained about the cost of having plates made of his portrait. According to him they would more than cover their expenses by being able to sell his book for a higher price. Willum was firmly instructed to have *Museum Wormianum* included in the catalogue for the forthcoming Frankfurt Fair. Even at this late stage Willum was asked to make further additions to the manuscript and make sure they were inserted in the right places. Worm was clearly a publisher's nightmare constantly revising his manuscript even while it was being printed, and asking his young son to make sure that all his changes and additions were done correctly.[221]

The book was close to publication when Ole Worm died on 31 August 1654. It appeared the following year, and had he lived Worm would undoubtedly have been pleased with the result. He may even have been appreciative of the efforts and patience of both the Elzevirs and his son Willum, who stayed on in Leiden to steer the book through to publication.[222]

14 Conclusion

Ole Worm clearly collected the odd object or souvenir during his educational journey prior to taking up his professorship in Copenhagen in 1613. From then on during the next decade he was predominantly focussed on botany and creating a garden for which he collected plants. Gradually his interests in gardening declined until in 1630 he took over the house which had belonged to his brother-in-law Caspar Bartholin, and which had a much bigger garden. This inspired Worm to renew his interest in botany and gardening until in 1638–39 these interests once more declined reaching a low point by 1644.

Parallel to these interests Worm slowly started to collect rare natural objects. By 1623 Worm began to bring a more systematised approach to his collecting, and by the end of the 1620s he started to include man-made objects, the so-called artificia in his collection. Gradually his cabinet of curiosity came into existence and by the end of the 1620s visitors started to arrive. However, the 1640s proved the age of real expansion for Worm's museum. His friendship with the wealthy natural historian and director of the Dutch West India Company, Johannes de Laet, proved crucial. Through de Laet Worm obtained and received information about objects, plants, and animals which would otherwise have been virtually impossible for him to collect. Between 1642 and 1648 the two men corresponded regularly, exchanged objects and described and discussed issues of natural historical importance. In 1642 Worm had the first of two catalogues printed – the second appeared in 1645 – listing the objects present in his cabinet of curiosity. It was distributed widely among friends and colleagues not only with the

---

221 *Ibid.*, no. 1793.
222 See Hovesen, *Ole Worm*, 275–76.

intent of showing the content and importance of his collection but also as an aid and guide to what was still needed. The collection grew rapidly during the 1640s and 1650s until Worm's death in 1654. Worm's nephews from the Fuiren and Bartholin families proved particularly important for new acquisitions and gifts for his museum during their study trips abroad from the mid-1640s, and for the many international contacts they organised for him, as did his old friend Johan Rhode who resided in Padua. They brought him into contact directly and indirectly with some of the leading lights of the age such as the Jesuit polymath, Athanasius Kircher, and Cassiano dal Pozzo. The 1640s also witnessed a growing number of donations from Worm's many Icelandic friends not to mention from his contacts on the Faroe Isles, many of which such as the narwhale tooth proved particularly significant for the growing international reputation of Worm and his cabinet of curiosity. To those should be added a growing number of gifts from princes and nobles during the decade leading up to his death in 1654.

The growing fame of Worm's museum guaranteed that most prominent men travelling to or through Copenhagen at this time paid him a visit. Visits by members of the French diplomatic mission on its way to peace negotiations in Sweden established friendships with leading French libertines of the age such as Isaac La Peyrére, the royal physician Pierre Bourdelot, and Gabriel Naudé.

By 1648 Ole Worm had his first draft of his *Museum Wormianum* ready. He spent the next six years editing and expanding it. This was evidently his magnum opus for which he had found inspiration from a number of similar publications. Worm was determined that his work should be published by one of the leading publishing houses of the day, the Elzevirs in Amsterdam. His previous experience and low opinion of printers meant that Worm took a keen interest in the publishing process, making sure that only the best paper, types, and illustrations were used, constantly seeking to make sure that no unnecessary delays took place, no mistakes made, and that all his amendments and corrections were included in the right places.

The book was close to publication when Ole Worm died on 31 August 1654. It appeared the following year and had he lived Worm would undoubtedly have been pleased with the result. He may even have been appreciative of the efforts made by both the Elzevirs and Willum to see the book through to publication.

The *Museum Wormianum* was the crowning glory of a life-time preoccupation with natural philosophy and history by a Lutheran scholar who through study, observation, description, and experiment, sought to understand God's creation as revealed in the Book of Nature. Through describing, analysing, and observing rare and unusual natural objects Worm hoped ultimately to be able to find the key to, or reach a better if not definitive understanding of the created world.

Index

For Product Safety Concerns and Information please contact our EU
representative GPSR@taylorandfrancis.com
Taylor & Francis Verlag GmbH, Kaufingerstraße 24, 80331 München, Germany